Treatment Resource Manual

for Speech-Language Pathology

Seventh Edition

Treatment Resource Manual

for Speech-Language Pathology

Seventh Edition

Froma P. Roth, PhD
Colleen K. Worthington, MS

PLURAL
PUBLISHING
INC.

9177 Aero Drive, Suite B
San Diego, CA 92123

email: information@pluralpublishing.com
website: https://www.pluralpublishing.com

Typeset in 11.5/14 Adobe Caslon by Flanagan's Publishing Services, Inc.
Printed in China by Regent Publishing Services Ltd.

Library of Congress Cataloging-in-Publication Data:

INames: Roth, Froma P., author. | Worthington, Colleen K., author.
Title: Treatment resource manual for speech-language pathology / Froma P.
    Roth, Colleen K. Worthington.
Description: Seventh edition. | San Diego, CA : Plural, [2025] | Includes
    bibliographical references and index.
Identifiers: LCCN 2023037129 (print) | LCCN 2023037130 (ebook) | ISBN
    9781635506532 (paperback) | ISBN 1635506530 (paperback) | ISBN
    9781635504514 (ebook)
Subjects: MESH: Speech Therapy--methods | Language Therapy--methods |
    Communication Disorders--therapy
Classification: LCC RC423 (print) | LCC RC423 (ebook) | NLM WL 340.3 |
    DDC 616.85/5--dc23/eng/20230824
LC record available at https://lccn.loc.gov/2023037129
LC ebook record available at https://lccn.loc.gov/2023037130

Dedication

*For **Eli**, in memorium, and **Ilana**, my inspirational guides;*
and to my brightest lights:
***Graydn Robert**, **Harper Rose**, **Evelyn Brady**, and **Chloe Indigo**.*
FPR

•

*For **Leigh-Anne**, the small miracle*
who will always be the heart of my heart.
CKW

Contents

PART ONE   Preparing for Effective Intervention

CHAPTER 1

CHAPTER 2

Information Reporting Systems and Techniques 45

PART TWO   Providing Treatment for Communication Disorders

CHAPTER 3

INTRODUCTION TO CHAPTERS 4 AND 5

CHAPTER 4

CHAPTER 5

CHAPTER 6

Intervention for Autism Spectrum Disorder (ASD) 197

CHAPTER 7

Intervention for Adult Aphasia With Introduction to 223
Traumatic Brain Injury

CHAPTER 8

Intervention for Motor-Speech Disorders: The Dysarthrias, Apraxia of Speech, and Dysphagia

CHAPTER 9

Intervention for Stuttering

CHAPTER 10

CHAPTER 11

CHAPTER 12

Multicultural Issues in Intervention/Diversity, Equity, Inclusion, and Accessibility (DEIA)

CHAPTER 13

Contemporary Issues

Whole-Book Appendices located on the PluralPlus companion website (not included in print version)

    APPENDIX A: ASHA Code of Ethics

    APPENDIX B: International Phonetic Alphabet Symbols

    APPENDIX C: Glossary of Selected Medical Terms

    APPENDIX D: Schematic of the Vocal Tract

    APPENDIX E: Cultural Competency Check-Ins

Case Examples by Disorder

List of Tables

List of Forms and Figures

List of Forms located on the PluralPlus companion website (not included in the print version of the book)

List of Forms located in the printed chapters and on the PluralPlus companion website

List of Figures

Preface

The original purpose of this manual was to provide beginning speech-language pathology graduate students with a practical introductory guide to intervention. It also provided practicing clinicians with a single resource for specific therapy techniques and materials for a wide variety of communication disorders. This new edition continues to fulfill these aims and also reflects the changing information and recent advances in the field of speech-language pathology that are essential to address in a text of this kind. The revisions made in this seventh edition provided important changes in content compared to previous editions. Selected examples include (a) a new focus on a social model of disability (diversity-affirming approach to intervention); (b) expanded and reorganized information on treatment approaches for autism; (c) expanded information on intervention with traumatic brain injury (TBI); and (d) updated discussion of multicultural issues relevant to clinical work. We carefully updated each chapter in the areas of treatment efficacy and evidence-based practice to ensure that the book reflects the most current thinking in the research and clinical spheres. Two main factors created the need for a resource of this kind for students. First, speech-language pathology programs across the country are rapidly adopting a preprofessional model of education that minimizes clinical practicum experience at the undergraduate level. Thus, even students with undergraduate degrees in communication disorders are entering graduate school with very little direct knowledge of basic therapy approaches, techniques, and materials. Second, master's programs in speech-language pathology are attracting an increasing number of students with bachelor's degrees in areas other than the hearing and speech sciences. These students enter clinical training without any supporting background. As a result, a genuine need exists for a user-friendly and comprehensive source of effective, practical suggestions to guide beginning clinicians through their first therapy experiences.

Another primary use of this book is as a text for undergraduate and graduate-level courses in clinical methods. Traditional textbooks for such courses tend to be largely theoretical in nature and lack useful information on how to do therapy. Thus, instructors are often faced with the task of assembling their own clinical materials to complement the text. One of the aims of this text is to provide such supplementary information in a single source. In response to requests from readers, this new edition is accompanied by a premium website that provides substantial new content to enhance classroom instruction and strengthen student learning. It also includes the forms and appendices in the book for easy download and use.

This manual also was written with the practicing clinician in mind. Speech-language pathologists are handling caseloads/workloads with a broader spectrum of communication disorders than ever before. This trend is occurring in all clinical settings, from hospitals to public schools to early childhood centers. Moreover, there has been a dramatic increase in private practice as a service-delivery model in the field of speech-language pathology. Many practitioners work independently, particularly since the pandemic, and may not be able to consult readily with colleagues about the management of communication disorders that are outside of their main areas of expertise. This manual can serve as an accessible and reliable source of basic treatment information and techniques for a wide range of speech and language disorders.

The information in this book is based on existing knowledge about communication disorders and available research data, as well as the combined clinical experiences of the authors. It is not intended as a cookbook approach to intervention. The complexities of communication disorders preclude such a parochial approach. The therapy targets and activities we included are meant to serve as illustrations of basic intervention practice, and only as starting points in the therapeutic process. By their very nature, therapy programs for communication disorders should be designed to accommodate each client's unique strengths and weaknesses as well as individual learning styles.

Text Organization

The manual is organized into two main sections. The first section (Chapters 1 and 2) covers basic principles of speech-language intervention and information reporting systems. The second section includes eight chapters (Chapters 3 to 10) devoted to therapy strategies for specific communication disorders. Each of these chapters includes a brief description of the disorder, example case profiles, specific suggestions for the selection of therapy targets, and sample therapy activities. These have been designed to illustrate the most common characteristics of a given disorder, as well as typical approaches to treatment. Each chapter concludes with a set of helpful hints on intervention and a selected list of commercially available therapy materials

The second section also includes Chapter 11, which offers practical suggestions for beginning clinicians regarding effective client and family counseling skills. Chapter 12 offers discussion and guidelines regarding multicultural issues in speech-language interventions. And, this seventh edition of the book concludes with Chapter 13 that incorporates a discussion in profession-wide areas of interest to educators, students, and clinicians. Reference tables, charts, and reproducible forms are included throughout the manual.

The focus of this text is on the most common characteristics and treatment approaches for a given disorder. Unusual or atypical populations are beyond the scope of this book. This book is written from the perspective of Standard American English. The information, procedures, and activities contained in each chapter should be adapted in a culturally appropriate manner.

New to the Seventh Edition

This new edition includes updated citations and references throughout as well as current information on treatment efficacy in all disorder chapters to reflect recent developments in the field. In addition, we added the following:

- New focus on a social model of disability (diversity-affirming approach to intervention)

- Substantial update on treatment efficacy of intervention approaches for autism

- Expanded discussion of the use of telepractice to remotely conduct intervention

- Expanded information on cultural/linguistic diversity and cultural responsiveness/competence within the context of therapeutic intervention.

- Updated information on incidence/prevalence of aphasia and expanded discussion of treatment efficacy in TBI, spasmodic dysphonia, and goals for treatment of motor speech disorders

- Additional Helpful Hints in each disorder chapter

- Updated lists of Additional Resources and Recommended Readings for each chapter

- QR codes in the margins lead to websites of the key resources discussed

- Enhancements to the online ancillary materials as mentioned below

PluralPlus Companion Website

This edition comes with access to a PluralPlus companion website containing updated PowerPoint lecture slides, self-study quizzes, and essay questions for each chapter. In addition, it incorporates the book's reference section along with a list of clickable URL citations organized by chapter. All book appendices can be found on this ancillary website. A new feature of this edition is a collection of video clips and suggested student learning activities as well as all of the book's forms in digital format for easy duplication and customization to specific experiences. **See the inside front cover of the book for the website URL and access instructions.**

Acknowledgments

We are very grateful to the many people who have contributed their time, efforts, and talents to the preparation of this revised edition. As in previous editions, we wish to acknowledge the invaluable technical support of our colleague, Emily (Mineweaser) DeAngelis, MA, CCC-SLP. In this seventh edition, we also express our deep gratitude and respect for her continued contribution as author of the substantive section on traumatic brain injury. Emily's content knowledge, her enthusiasm for clinical practice, her superlative copy-editing skills, and her ability to consistently produce excellent work under tight timelines continue to serve as a genuine source of inspiration to both of us.

For Leigh-Anne and Joe, your thoughtfulness delivered in the form of emergency tech support and endless pots of perfectly-brewed coffee made all the difference.

We also want to express our appreciation for all the people at Plural Publishing who make this book possible. The efforts of Valerie Johns, Lori Asbury, Jessica Bristow, Megan Carter, and as always, Angie Singh, have carried this book over the finish line once again.

About the Authors

Froma P. Roth, PhD

is a Professor Emeritus at the University of Maryland, College Park, Maryland, in the Department of Hearing and Speech Sciences. Professor Roth received her bachelor's degree from Hunter College, her master's degree from Queens College, and her doctoral degree from the Graduate Center of the City University of New York. Dr. Roth's current research and clinical interests focus on language/literacy and learning disabilities. In 2020, Dr. Roth was awarded the Honors of the Association from the American Speech-Language-Hearing Association.

Colleen K. Worthington, MS

is a Clinical Professor Emeritus and served for 30 years as the Director of Clinical Education in Speech-Language Pathology within the Department of Hearing and Speech Sciences at the University of Maryland, College Park. She received her bachelor's degree from the University of Maryland and her master's degree from Loyola College, Baltimore. Worthington's primary professional interests include diagnostic principles/methods, articulation/phonology, and the supervisory process.

Part One

Preparing for Effective Intervention

Chapter 1

The Essential Ingredients of Good Therapy: Basic Skills

Philosophy

In the field of communication disorders, the domains of research and clinical practice are frequently regarded as distinctly separate entities. It is true that the aims of the two activities are very different. The main purpose of research is to add to the existing knowledge base in a given area, whereas the ultimate goal of clinical work is to change behavior. However, the two activities also share many common characteristics, and these similarities outweigh the differences. The most fundamental similarity is that both research and clinical practice are scientific processes based on the highest quality of evidence available (often referred to as evidence-based practice). Therefore, it is our view that intervention, like research, should be based on the principles of the scientific method. Both research and intervention involve the following:

- identification of a problem

- review of existing knowledge regarding the problem area

- formulation of hypotheses about how to solve the problem

- manipulation of the independent variable(s)

- collection and analysis of data

- formulation of conclusions about the validity of the original hypotheses

Based on the authors' experiences, an essential ingredient to successful intervention is critical thinking. Critical thinking is the objective analysis and evaluation of an issue to form a judgment, which goes beyond memorization/recall of information and is free from feelings or personal biases. Teaching beginning clinicians critical-thinking skills supports their ability to manage complex issues inherent in clinical work. This important topic is discussed more extensively in Chapter 13.

Speech and language intervention is a dynamic process that follows a systematic progression. It begins with the diagnosis of a communication disorder and is followed by the selection of appropriate therapy targets. Training procedures are then implemented to facilitate the acquisition of the target behaviors. The intervention process is complete when mastery of these behaviors is achieved. Periodic follow-up is performed to monitor retention and stability of the newly acquired behaviors. Throughout all stages of therapy, advocacy is an important role for the speech-language pathologist (SLP). All clinicians should be aware of the Americans with Disabilities Act (1990). This federal legislation (Public Law 101-336) and its amendments (Public Law 110-325) prohibit discrimination and ensure equal opportunity in public accommodations, employment, transportation, government services, and telecommunications (see https://www.ada.gov for more specific information). Speech-language pathology is a dynamic profession that is continually evolving. The **scope of practice** in speech-language pathology is delineated by the American Speech-Language-Hearing Association, or ASHA (ASHA, 2007b). SLPs are responsible for fully understanding the areas of communication and swallowing that they are qualified to address (e.g., voice, language, fluency) as well as the range of services that they are eligible to deliver (e.g., screening, consultation, treatment). A related document of major importance to all SLPs is the 2023 **ASHA Code of Ethics** (see Appendix A on the companion website). This document outlines standards for professional behavior with regard to several areas (e.g., client welfare, SLP competence level, public understanding of the profession).

Universal Design Principles for Learning: An Overarching Framework

In 2000, Rose and Meyer put forth a framework based on the premise that every individual—regardless of physical, cognitive, sensory, learning, or other type of disability—is entitled to universal access to information and to learning. Their model is characterized by three universal design for learning (UDL) principles: multiple means of representation, multiple means of expression, and multiple means of engagement. As applied to educational and clinical settings, it is meant to be a theoretical framework for providing the most appropriate supports for children and adults and includes the following:

- *Multiple means of representation:* There must be multiple methods available by which individuals can access and learn important information and skills (e.g., traditional textbook augmented by supplemental internet resources, speech-to-text media).

- *Multiple means of expression:* Various methods and modalities must be available for individuals to demonstrate their mastery of information and skills.

- *Multiple means of engagement:* Individuals must be provided with enough successful learning opportunities and meaningful interactions to maintain adequate motivation for learning.

The crux of UDLs is instructional flexibility to provide the most suitable options for different learners. For individuals with disabilities, UDLs include accommodations, modifications, and assistive technology. **Accommodations** are changes that help clients overcome or compensate for their disability, such as preferential seating or allowing written rather than spoken communication. **Modifications** are changes in informational content or expectations of an individual's performance. Examples include a decreased amount of classwork/homework or reduced goals for productivity or learning.

Also inherent in UDLs is the use of **assistive technology (AT)** as support for students and adults with disabilities (Dalton et al., 2002; Hall et al., 2012; Ralabate, 2011; Strangman, 2003). AT may include speech-to-text software that converts speech into text documents, translation software for English-language learners, and internet access as a means of information gathering. In all cases, adequate training must be provided so that individuals can use the AT successfully and reliably. We must emphasize that these technologies are supportive and do not replace direct instruction.

General Principles of Intervention

The basic principles of effective intervention are consistent with a UDL framework and apply to clients of all ages and disorders. These include the following:

- Intervention is a dynamic rather than static process in which the clinician continuously assesses a client's progress toward established goals and modifies them as necessary.

- Intervention programs should be designed with careful consideration of a client's verbal and nonverbal cognitive abilities. Knowledge of a client's level of cognitive functioning is critical to making decisions about eligibility for treatment and selecting appropriate therapy objectives.

- The ultimate goal of intervention is to teach strategies for facilitating the communication process rather than teaching isolated skills or behaviors (to the extent possible). Whereas skills are required to achieve specific outcomes in given situations, strategies enable the individual to know when and how to use these skills in new and varied learning contexts.

- Speech and language abilities are acquired and used primarily for the purpose of communication and therefore should be taught in a communicative context. To the extent possible, therapy should occur in realistic situations and provide a client with opportunities to engage in meaningful communicative interactions.

- Intervention should be individually oriented, based on the nature of a client's specific deficits and individual learning style.

- Intervention should be designed to ensure that a client experiences consistent success throughout all stages of the therapy program.

- Intervention is most effective when therapy goals are tailored to promote a client's knowledge one step beyond the current level.

- Intervention should be terminated once goals are achieved or the client is no longer making demonstrable progress.

- Intervention practices must be based on the best scientific evidence available.

- Intervention should be sensitive to a client's values and beliefs as well as cultural and linguistic background.

To provide effective intervention for any type of communication disorder, SLPs must acquire certain essential clinical skills. These skills are based on fundamental principles of human behavior and learning theory. The following categories of clinical skills are the building blocks of therapy and serve as the foundation for all disorder-specific treatment approaches:

- *Programming:* Selection, sequencing, and generalization of therapy targets

- *Behavior modification:* Systematic use of specific stimulus-response-consequence procedures

- *Key teaching strategies:* Use of basic training techniques to facilitate learning

- *Session design:* Organization and implementation of therapy sessions, including interpersonal dynamics

- *Data collection:* Systematic measurement of client performance and treatment efficacy

Successful intervention requires the ability to effectively integrate these five parameters into a treatment program. Appendix 1–A, listed on the companion website, provides a checklist of clinician behaviors that correspond to each of the parameters. This checklist can be used by students as a guide for observing therapy sessions or by supervisors for evaluating student clinician performance. The remainder of this chapter is devoted to a detailed discussion of each basic skill area.

Programming

Programming involves the selection and sequencing of specific communicative behaviors. New behaviors are introduced and taught in highly structured situations with multiple prompts and maximal support provided by the clinician. Subsequent activities progress through a hierarchy of difficulty and complexity, with decreasing support from the clinician. The client demonstrates generalization of each newly learned behavior by using it in novel situations or contexts. The programming process culminates with a client's habitual and spontaneous use of a behavior in everyday speaking and listening situations.

In recent literature (e.g., DeThorne & Gerlach-Houck, 2023), there is a growing call for intervention that is based on a **social model of intervention**. This approach does not focus on how to bring the client up to typical societal expectations. Instead, it identifies ways to modify the attitudes and structures of society to accommodate the client's communication profile. Rather than targeting specific skill deficits demonstrated by the client, a social model focuses on reducing barriers to successful communication found within the individual's environment or interpersonal relationships. This framework focuses on enhancing communicative daily function in society by providing supports, accommodations, and modifications that address physical, environmental, and sensory barriers experienced by the client.

Selection of Therapy Targets

The first step in programming is identification of the communication behaviors to be acquired over the course of the treatment program. These therapy targets are often referred to as **long-term goals**. Initial information about potential therapy targets should be obtained by reviewing the results of previous diagnostic findings. Frequently, assessment data are based, in part, on the administration of standardized tests. These tests typically are designed to sample only one or two exemplars of a given communication behavior. However, a single incorrect response does not constitute a sufficient basis for the inclusion of a behavior as a target in a treatment program. It indicates only a potential area of weakness, which then must be sampled more extensively to determine whether a genuine deficit exists. In addition, it is essential that a clinician consider the client's cultural and linguistic background when identifying potential therapy targets. Speech and language differences arising from dialect usage or a non-English native language do not constitute a communicative disorder. Refer to Chapter 12 for common characteristics of African American English, Spanish-influenced English, and Asian-influenced English.

This sampling is accomplished through the administration of **pretreatment baselines**. Baselines are clinician-designed measures that provide multiple opportunities for a client to demonstrate a given communicative behavior. A good rule of thumb is to include a minimum of 20 stimuli on each pretreatment baseline. The ratio of correct versus incorrect responses is calculated; the resulting percentage is used to determine whether the behavior should be selected as a therapy target. Many clinicians view a performance level of 75% accuracy or higher as an indication that the communication skill in question is not in need of remediation. Baseline measures that fall below the 75% accuracy level represent potential intervention targets. Ultimately, however, the selection of appropriate therapy targets relies heavily on clinical judgment. Some clinicians believe that behaviors that occur with at least 50% accuracy represent targets with the best potential for improvement. Other clinicians argue strongly that behaviors with much lower baseline rates of accuracy may be the most appropriate choices based on individual client characteristics (e.g., intelligibility level, age).

Often, clients present with several behaviors that qualify as candidates for remediation. For individuals who demonstrate a large number of errors, clinicians may choose a *broad* programming strategy that attacks as many targets as possible in a given time frame. Alternatively, clinicians may select a *deep* programming strategy for clients who demonstrate either relatively few or highly atypical errors. In addition, clinicians typically employ one of two basic approaches for choosing among potential targets: developmental/normative or client specific.

The Developmental/Normative Strategy

This strategy is based on known normative sequences of communicative behaviors in typically achieving individuals. Therapy targets are taught in the same general order as they emerge developmentally. When two or more potential targets are identified from baseline procedures, the earliest emerging behaviors are selected as the first therapy objectives. Following are two examples that illustrate use of the **developmental** strategy.

 A 5-year-old child with an articulation disorder produces the following speech sound errors on baseline procedures:

- /p/ for /f/ as in *p*inger for *f*inger
- /t/ for /ʃ/ as in *t*ip for *sh*ip
- /d/ for /dʒ/ as in *d*uice for *j*uice
- /d/ for /b/ as in *d*oat for *b*oat

Use of the developmental strategy guides the clinician to select /b/ as the initial therapy target, because typically developing children demonstrate mastery of this sound earlier than the others. According to a developmental progression, /f/ is the next logical target, followed by /ʃ/ and /dʒ/.

 A 4-year-old child with a language disorder exhibits the following grammatical errors on baseline procedures:

- Omission of present progressive tense, as in "The boy *play*" for "The boy is play*ing*"
- Omission of the plural marker on regular nouns, as in "I see two *bike*" for "I see two *bikes*"
- Overgeneralization of regular past tense, as in "He *runned* down the street" for "He *ran* down the street"

Use of the developmental strategy dictates that the first target for therapy is the present progressive form (**is + verb + -ing**), because it is the earliest of the three structures to emerge. The plural marker is the next behavior to be targeted, followed by the regular past-tense form.

Note: With clients from different cultural/linguistic backgrounds, these grammatical forms may reflect a language difference rather than a language disorder. Therefore, intervention may not be warranted.

The developmental strategy tends to be most effective for articulation and language intervention with children. This strategy has less application for adults and disorders of voice and fluency.

A developmental strategy for target selection should be implemented with careful consideration of at least two factors. The sample population from which the norms were derived may have been too small to permit valid generalization of the findings to other populations. Moreover, the characteristics of the standardization sample (e.g., ethnicity, gender, socioeconomic status) may differ significantly from those of an individual client. Consequently, it may be difficult to draw direct comparisons between the client's performance and the group norms.

For clinicians who choose to approach therapy from a social model of intervention, potential goals might include training peers to initiate communication with an autistic child, encouraging teachers to provide written as well oral instructions in the classroom, or educating coworkers on best practices for conversational interactions with a colleague who stutters.

The Client-Specific Strategy

Using the **client-specific** strategy, therapy targets are chosen based on an individual's specific needs rather than according to developmental norms. Relevant factors in the selection of treatment objectives include (a) the frequency with which a specific communicative behavior occurs in a client's daily activities; (b) the relative importance of a specific communicative behavior to the client, regardless of how often it occurs; and (c) the client's potential for mastery of a given communication skill. This last factor addresses the notion of *stimulability*, which is typically defined as the degree to which a client can approximate the correct production of an error pattern on imitation. Following are two examples that illustrate the use of the client-specific strategy.

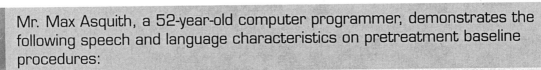
Mr. Max Asquith, a 52-year-old computer programmer, demonstrates the following speech and language characteristics on pretreatment baseline procedures:

- Omission of final consonants such as /s/, /k/, and /θ/

- Distortion of vowels in all word positions

- Misarticulation of consonant blends, such as /br/, /pl/, /fl/, /ks/, and /skw/

- Omission of the copula forms (*is* and *are*) as in "He sad" for "He is sad"

- Difficulty with the accurate use of spatial, temporal, and numerical vocabulary

- Difficulty with subject-verb agreement, especially third-person singular constructions, as in "He *drink* milk" for "He *drinks* milk"

From the client-specific perspective, initial speech intervention targets could consist of /ks/ and /skw/, because these blends occur in the client's name and therefore constitute a high priority for him. An appropriate initial language target for this client would be vocabulary words that convey number concepts, because his position as a computer programmer relies heavily on the use of this terminology.

A 6-year-old child with an articulation disorder exhibits the following speech sound errors on baseline procedures:

- /θ/ for /s/ as in *th*un for *s*un
- /g/ for /d/ as in *g*uck for *d*uck
- /w/ for /l/ as in *w*ight for *l*ight
- /ʃ/ for /ʧ/ as in *sh*ew for *ch*ew

Using the client-specific strategy, the initial therapy target would be /s/, regardless of developmental considerations. The results of stimulability testing conducted during the diagnostic test indicated that this child's ability to imitate /s/ was superior to performance on the other error sounds. In addition, /s/ occurs far more frequently in English than /l/, /w/, and /ʧ/.

Unlike the developmental approach, a client-specific strategy can be implemented across a wide range of communication disorders with both pediatric and adult populations. In addition, a combination of the two strategies is often an effective way to approach therapy target selection for children with speech and language impairments.

Sequencing of Therapy Targets

Following therapy target selection and prioritization, programming involves the development of a logical sequence of steps that will be implemented to accomplish each objective. Three major factors determine the progression of the therapy sequence: *stimulus type*, *task mode*, and *response level*. The following outline presents a hierarchy of complexity for each of these factors.

Stimulus Type (Nature of Input Used to Elicit Target Responses)

- Direct physical manipulation
- Concrete symbols
  - Objects
  - Photographs/color pictures
  - Black-and-white line drawings
- Abstract symbols
  - Oral language
  - Written language

Task Mode (Type of Clinician Support/Scaffolding Provided to Obtain Desired Responses)

- Imitation
- Cue/prompt
- Spontaneous

Response Level (Degree of Difficulty of Target Responses)[1]

- Increase length and complexity of desired response
  - Isolation
  - Syllable
  - Word
  - Carrier phrase (e.g., "I see a _____.")
  - Phrase
  - Sentence
  - Text (conversation, narration)
- Decrease latency (actual time) between stimulus presentation and client response

The sequencing process starts with a decision regarding the most appropriate level to begin training on each target behavior. Pretreatment baseline data for a given target are analyzed to determine the entry training level. Rules of thumb that can be used are as follows:

- If a client obtained a baseline score lower than 50% accuracy, training on that behavior should begin just below the level of difficulty of the baseline stimulus items.

- If the score was between 50% and 75% accuracy, training can begin at the same difficulty level as the baseline stimuli.

For example, a 5-year-old client scored the following on baseline measures for initial /s/: word level = 65%; carrier phrase level = 40%; and sentence level = 30%. In this example, therapy would begin at the word level of difficulty.

Adherence to these procedures generally will result in a progression of targets at the appropriate levels of difficulty. However, there may be occasions when a client does not perform as predicted; a chosen task turns out to be too difficult or too easy for the individual at this time. The clinician must recognize this situation when it occurs and immediately modify the task rather than persist with the original plan. This modification is known as **branching** and is achieved by increasing or decreasing the difficulty level by one step according to the therapy sequence hierarchies listed previously.

As the client's performance improves and initial training objectives are mastered, the stimulus type, task mode, and response level should be manipulated systematically to gradually increase the difficulty of therapy tasks until the final criterion is met for a given target. This criterion level is generally set at 90% accuracy or higher in everyday conversational interactions.

The following sample behavioral objectives illustrate the manipulation of each of the three factors:

Behavioral objective: The client will imitatively produce /s/ in the initial position of single words with 90% accuracy while naming 20 photographs.

Modified stimulus type: The client will imitatively produce /s/ in the initial position of single words with 90% accuracy while naming 20 *written* words.

---

[1]This response-level hierarchy pertains to oral responses only. Other response types—such as gesture, sign, and writing—may require alternative hierarchies of difficulty.

Modified task mode: The client will *spontaneously* produce /s/ in the initial position of single words with 90% accuracy while naming 20 photographs.

Modified response level: The client will imitatively produce /s/ in the initial position of words in carrier phrases with 90% accuracy in response to 20 photographs.

Generalization/Carryover

A crucial consideration in programming involves a client's ability to transfer newly mastered communicative behaviors from the clinical setting to the everyday environment. Generalization is enhanced when intervention is provided in the most authentic, realistic contexts possible. Generalization should not be viewed as a distinct event that occurs only in the final phase of the therapy process. Rather, it is an integral part of programming that requires attention from the very beginning. Three main factors can influence the degree to which successful generalization occurs. A variety of **stimuli** (objects, pictures, questions) should be used during therapy activities to avoid tying learning to only a small set of specific stimulus items. Similarly, the clinician should vary the **physical environment** (location in room, location in building, real-world locations) in which therapy occurs as soon as a new target behavior has been established. This will minimize a client's natural tendency to associate target behaviors with a particular setting. Finally, clinicians should bear in mind that target behaviors frequently become attached to the individual who consistently reinforces them (i.e., the clinician). Therefore, it is important to vary the **audience** (familiar adult, sibling, unfamiliar adult) with whom therapy targets are practiced, to maximize the likelihood of successful generalization.

Termination of Therapy

It is difficult to definitively state the point at which intervention services are no longer warranted. At the current time, there are no valid empirical data that can be used to determine appropriate dismissal criteria for any particular communicative disorder. Therefore, it is beyond the scope of this book to indicate realistic time frames for the duration of intervention. General discharge guidelines used by many clinicians include (a) attainment of communication skills that are commensurate with a client's chronological/developmental age or premorbid status, (b) attainment of functional communication skills that permit a client to operate in the daily environment without significant handicap, and (c) lack of discernible progress persisting beyond a predetermined time period. The authors strongly believe that the establishment of reliable treatment outcome measures is critical in the current climate of professional accountability in both the public and private sectors. Within the past few years, the availability of efficacy data has increased significantly for a variety of communication disorders. This information is presented throughout the book in pertinent chapters.

Formulation of Behavioral Objectives

Once long-term goals and initial treatment levels have been identified, the clinician develops short-term objectives designed to culminate in the achievement of the selected long-term goals. (In education settings, student progress is measured through *benchmarks*, which are sets of skills required to achieve specific learning standards.) These objectives must be clearly delineated to ensure appropriate and effective intervention programming. A widely used approach to task design is the formulation of **behavioral objectives**. A behavioral objective is a statement that describes a specific target behavior in observable and measurable terms. There are three main components of a behavioral objective:

1. "Do" (action) statement

2. Condition

3. Criterion

The **"do" statement** identifies the specific action the client is expected to perform. Thus, behavioral objectives should contain verbs that denote observable activity; nonaction verbs should be avoided. List 1 contains examples of verbs that are appropriate for inclusion in behavioral objectives; list 2 is made up of verbs that are unacceptable because they refer to behaviors that cannot be observed.

List 1		List 2	
point	say	understand	know
label	write	think	appreciate
repeat	count	learn	remember
match	vocalize	believe	apply
name	ask	improve	comprehend
tell	elevate	discover	feel

An easy way to check the appropriateness of a verb is to ask yourself, "Will I be able to count (tally) how many times this behavior occurs?" (Mowrer, 1988). For example, consider the following pair of statements: (a) "to repeat single-syllable words" and (b) "to learn single-syllable words." Only the first is an appropriate "do" statement. Number of repetitions can be easily counted, whereas "learning" is a behavior that cannot be directly observed.

The **condition** portion of a behavioral objective identifies the situation in which the target behavior is to be performed. It specifies one or more of the following: when the behavior will occur, where it will be performed, in whose presence, or what materials and cues will be used to elicit the target. Following are common examples of condition statements:

- Given the clinician's model

- In response to a question from the teacher

- In the presence of three classmates

- During book report presentation

- Given a list of written words

- In the home environment

- During a job interview

- Using pictures

- During free play

- In the presence of other group therapy members

- During storybook reading time

Condition statements are critical parts of behavioral objectives, because clients may demonstrate adequate mastery of a communicative behavior in one situation and yet be completely unable to perform the same behavior under different conditions. For example, a client's ability to perform a "do" statement, such as "Produce 1 min of connected speech without disfluency," is likely to be quite different if the condition statement specifies "while talking to a familiar clinician" versus "while talking to a potential date."

The **criterion** specifies how well the target behavior must be performed for the objective to be achieved. It can be expressed in several ways, including percent correct, within a given time period, minimum number of correct responses, or maximum number of error responses. Criterion measures typically used in speech-language therapy are as follows:

- 90% accuracy

- Eight correct out of 10 trials

- Less than four errors over three consecutive sessions

- 80% accuracy over two consecutive sessions

- 90% agreement between clinician and client judgments

- Continuously over a 2-min period

A well-formulated behavioral objective allows the client, as well as the clinician, to know exactly what the therapy target is, how it is to be accomplished, and what constitutes successful performance. It also is helpful to consider that unexpected changes can occur in caseloads. Clear behavioral objectives help ease the transition of care by clearly defining the focus of therapy for the next clinician. The following examples illustrate how to formulate behavioral objectives.

Example A

1. "Do" statement: Verbally segment words into syllables

2. Condition: Given a written list of 100 multisyllabic words

3. Criterion: With no more than four errors

Behavioral objective: The client will verbally segment 100 written multisyllabic words into their component syllables with no more than four errors.

Example B

1. "Do" statement: Use a slow rate of speech (four syllables per second)

2. Condition: Read single sentences

3. Criterion: With 85% accuracy or better over two consecutive sessions

Behavioral objective: The client will use a slow rate of speech (four syllables per second) with 85% accuracy or higher while reading single sentences over two consecutive sessions.

Example C

1. "Do" statement: Say /s/ in the initial position of single words

2. Conditions: Given the clinician's model
   Name pictures of animals

3. Criterion: With 90% accuracy

Behavioral objective: Given the clinician's model, the client will say /s/-initial single words with 90% accuracy while naming animal pictures.

In the authors' opinions, beginning clinicians tend to put too much focus on the "condition" aspect of behavioral objectives. While this aspect is important, the "do statement" should be the primary focus. In other words, the hierarchy of objectives should be built to move the client to higher levels of skill mastery rather than focusing on the incremental differences in teaching input strategies used by the clinician. A brief comparative example is listed in Table 1–1. A slightly modified version of behavioral design is known as SMART (Marsland & Bowman, 2010). In this paradigm, the following characteristics are the essential components of therapy objectives:

Specific—establish a clear goal behavior.

Measurable—ensure progress can be assessed on each established goal.

Achievable—ensure that the goal is a behavior within the skill set of a client.

Relevant/realistic—ensure that the goal is directly related to the desired outcomes.

Time based—establish a projected timeline for achievement.

Table 1–1
Comparison of Behavioral Objective Hierarchies

Objective Hierarchy Focused on Clinician Input ("condition" aspect)	Objective Hierarchy Focused on Client Skill Level ("do statement" aspect)
Given a model, Jeremiah will produce the regular past tense forms of single verbs with 80% accuracy.	Given a model, Jeremiah will produce the regular past tense forms of single verbs with 80% accuracy.
Given maximal verbal and visual cues, Jeremiah will produce the regular past tense forms of single verbs with 80% accuracy.	Jeremiah will produce the regular past tense forms of single verbs with 80% accuracy.
Given visual cues, Jeremiah will produce the regular past tense forms of single verbs with 80% accuracy.	Given visual or verbal cues, Jeremiah will produce the regular past tense forms of verbs in simple sentences with 80% accuracy.
Given brief verbal cues, Jeremiah will produce the regular past tense forms of single verbs with 80% accuracy.	Jeremiah will produce regular past tense forms of verbs in spontaneous speech.

Additional examples of behavioral objectives and worksheets are provided in Appendix 1–B and Appendix 1–C on the companion website for this book. Appendix 1–D on the companion website contains a sample Daily Therapy Plan that illustrates the following components of a single session: behavioral objectives, client data, and clinician comments. (A reproducible copy of the Daily Therapy Plan form is provided in Appendix 1–E and on the companion website, along with a sample form for documenting observation hours in Appendix 1–F.)

Theories of Learning

Different philosophies regarding the nature of human learning have led to the development of a variety of theories of how we learn information and skills. Different theories result in different intervention approaches and strategies. No single theory is applicable to all clients. To evaluate how well a model fits a specific client, clinicians may find it helpful to ask themselves the following questions:

- Has this approach been evaluated experimentally?

- Have the results been favorable?

- Has the approach been replicated across settings, clinicians, and clients?

- Is the model appropriate for my client (e.g., cognitive issues, cultural issues)?

- Can the environment be manipulated to implement procedures that are required for this approach (e.g., hospital versus school versus clinic)?

- Is my client improving?

Three of the major theoretical approaches to learning are the innateness/biological model, the behavioral model, and the constructivism model. An overview of each model is presented in the following sections. The behavioral model is discussed at length in this chapter, and the other models are incorporated into later chapters as they relate to specific communication disorders.

Innateness Theory/Biological Model
(Chomsky, 1965; Fodor, 1975; Piaget, 1973)

The hypothesis is that human beings have an innate predisposition to acquire knowledge. Children use these innate capacities to develop concepts, ideas, and linguistic rules. Exposure to the environment serves as an "on–off" switch that activates the linguistic system.

When applied to clinical intervention,

- clinical programming follows patterns of typical developmental sequences in areas such as cognition, language, and motor skills; and

- variations of the biological approach stress different facets of development.

For example, a cognitive model emphasizes the experiences necessary to activate cognitive capacities, whereas a linguistic model stresses teaching semantic-syntactic relationships.

Behavioral Model (Skinner, 1957)

The hypothesis is that children learn because their behaviors are selectively rewarded by significant others in their environment. This is the "tabula rasa" view and claims that human minds begin as blank slates and that the environment is the major determinant of learning. In this manner, children's responses to their environmental experiences are gradually shaped through feedback; desirable behaviors are reinforced and unwanted behaviors are faded.

When applied to clinical intervention,

- clinical programming emphasizes development of functional behaviors without the assumption of a stage-wise progression or prerequisite behaviors; and

- there is a heavy reliance on systematic application of behavior-modification techniques such as reinforcement, punishment, and extinction.

Constructivism/Interactionist/Integrative Model
(Bruner, 1960; Piaget, 1973; Vygotsky, 1978)

The main hypothesis is that children are biologically predisposed to learn, and their experiences help them to construct knowledge (an integration of the two previous models). Learning is an active process in which children construct ideas and concepts through experience. Learners continuously test and refine knowledge through interactions with others as well as their environment. This allows the learner to extract unique meaning from information and experiences.

When applied to clinical intervention,

- this model fosters client-centered learning in which learners play an active role;

- clinical programming is designed as a reciprocal process between clients and clinicians and emphasizes intervention tailored to an individual's specific needs and abilities; and

- because learning is a combination of inborn capacity and extrinsic environmental factors, it can be affected by certain constraints (e.g., attention/memory deficits, severe disabilities). Some individuals with severe disabilities may learn primarily through behavioral principles that emphasize repetition and practice.

Another way of capturing the variation among theoretical approaches is through the lens of a "continuum of naturalness." According to Fey (1985), the continuum represents the degree to which intervention contexts reflect everyday communication situations and interactions (Figure 1–1). According to this view, intervention approaches fall along a continuum into one of three groups: *clinician directed, hybrid,* and *client-centered.* In directive strategies, the clinician takes charge of all aspects of therapy, including the selection of goals, therapy materials, procedures, and the order of tasks and target responses to be elicited. Imitation and indirect modeling (response is not expected from the client) are two examples of clinician-directed techniques. Directive approaches are not considered naturalistic because of the degree of clinician control and the absence of natural reciprocal communication.

Client-centered approaches emphasize the use of authentic communication in natural communication situations. In contrast to directive strategies, these approaches involve following the client's

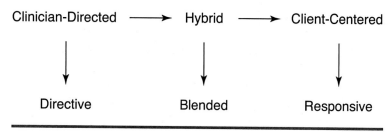

Figure 1–1
Continuum of naturalness. *Sources:* Adapted from Fey
(1985) and the American Speech-Language-Hearing
Association (2015).

lead (waiting for the client to initiate a behavior), treating the client's verbal and nonverbal initiations as intentional communications, and providing natural responses. These approaches are based on the premise that individuals will attain therapy goals more quickly and transfer newly learned behaviors more spontaneously when they are taught in natural contexts using familiar activities. Examples of responsive strategies used with children are expansions, extensions, and recasts (see the section "Key Teaching/Scaffolding Strategies" later in this chapter for definitions). For adult clients, two examples of client-centered techniques are functional communication (practicing communication activities of daily living, such as making a doctor's appointment) and conversational group therapy with other clients and the clinician. Both of these strategies permit clients to receive natural feedback on the relevance, intelligibility, and appropriateness of their turns from others in the group and the clinician.

Hybrid approaches represent a blending of clinician-directed and client-centered approaches. Hybrid approaches promote generalization by teaching new behaviors in natural environments using behavioral strategies. An example of a hybrid approach that is used with both children and adults is focused stimulation (concentrated exposure to a target form in a natural context, such as reading a book or restaurant menu).

The continuum of naturalness also applies to clients who use assistive technology (AT) to augment their speech production capabilities and those who rely completely on alternative modes of communication (AC), because speech is not a realistic communication mode. These accommodations are known collectively as AAC (augmentative and alternative communication).

Behavior Modification

The fundamental purpose of intervention is to either increase desired behavior or decrease unwanted behavior. (The term *behavior* refers to communication targets as well as a patient's degree of cooperation and attentiveness.) This is accomplished through application of the principles of behavior modification. **Behavior modification** is based on the theory of operant conditioning and involves the relationship among a stimulus, a response, and a consequent event (Skinner, 1957). A **stimulus** (or antecedent event) is an event that precedes and elicits a response. A **response** is the behavior exhibited by an individual on presentation of the stimulus. A **consequence** is an event that is contingent on and immediately follows the response. There are different types of consequent events. Consequences that increase the probability that a particular behavior will recur are known as **reinforcement**. Those that are designed to decrease the frequency of a behavior are termed **punishment**.

Types of Reinforcement

There are two basic types of reinforcement: **positive reinforcement** and **negative reinforcement**. Both types are used to increase the frequency of a target response.

Positive Reinforcement

Positive reinforcement is a rewarding event or condition that is presented contingent on the performance of a desired behavior.

Primary. These are contingent events to which a client reacts favorably due to the biological makeup or physiologic predisposition of the individual. Food is the most common example of a primary reinforcer. This type of reinforcer is very powerful and is used most effectively to establish new communicative behaviors (i.e., behaviors not previously present in the client's repertoire). Low-functioning clients often respond well to the basic nature of primary reinforcers. There are known disadvantages of primary reinforcement. First, it can be difficult to present the reinforcement immediately after every occurrence of the target behavior. In addition, this type of reinforcement is susceptible to **satiation**; that is, it loses its appeal as a reward if presented too often. Finally, skills that are taught using these contingent events are often difficult to generalize outside the therapy setting, because primary reinforcers do not occur naturally in the real world.

Secondary. These are contingent events that a client must be taught to perceive as rewarding. This category includes the following subtypes of reinforcers:

- **Social:** This group of reinforcers consists of events such as smiling, eye contact, and verbal praise. It is the most commonly used type of reinforcement in speech-language remediation programs. Social reinforcers are extremely easy to administer after each target response and generally do not disrupt the flow of a therapy session. In addition, this type of contingent response is not very susceptible to satiation (although it is not totally immune) and does occur in a client's natural daily environment.

- **Token:** This group of reinforcers consists of symbols or objects that are not perceived as valuable in and of themselves. However, the accrual of a specified number of these tokens will permit a client to obtain a previously agreed-on reward. Examples include stickers, check marks, chips, and point scores. These reinforcers are generally regarded as very powerful, because they are easy to administer contingent on each occurrence of a target behavior and are relatively resistant to satiation.

- **Performance feedback:** This category of reinforcers involves information that is given to a client regarding therapy performance and progress. Many individuals find it rewarding to receive information about the quality of their performance. It is not intended to function as praise and need not be presented verbally. Feedback regarding client performance can be delivered in various formats, including percentage data, frequency of occurrence graphs, numerical ratings, and biofeedback devices. Provision of this type of contingent event decreases a client's reliance on external sources of reinforcement by encouraging the development of intrinsic rewards (i.e., internal satisfaction and motivation) for mastering and maintaining a target behavior.

Negative Reinforcement

An unpleasant event/condition is removed contingent on the performance of a desired behavior.

Escape. This type of reinforcer requires the presence of a condition that the client perceives as aversive. Each performance of the target behavior relieves or terminates this aversive condition, thus increasing the probability that the specified behavior will recur. For example, a clinician might place her hands firmly over a child's hands and remove them only when the child exhibits the target behavior of imitatively producing /s/.

Avoidance. With this type of negative reinforcer, each performance of a target behavior prevents the occurrence of an *anticipated* aversive condition. This contingent event results in increased rates of performance of the desired response on subsequent occasions. For example, a clinician might inform a child that each imitative production of the target /s/ will prevent the imposition of hand restraint.

Use of negative reinforcement is relatively uncommon in the treatment of communication disorders because it repeatedly exposes clients to unpleasant or aversive situations. Use of positive reinforcement is the preferred method for increasing the frequency of desired responses. Positive reinforcement also can improve a client's motivational level and foster an effective interpersonal relationship between clinician and client.

Punishment

An event is presented contingent on the performance of an undesired behavior, to decrease the likelihood that the behavior will recur.

Type I. This involves the prompt presentation of an aversive consequence after each demonstration of an unwanted behavior. Examples of this consequence type that might be used in speech-language remediation programming include verbal utterances such as "No!" frowning, or the presentation of bursts of white noise.

Type II. This type of punishment requires withdrawal of a pleasant condition contingent on the demonstration of an unwanted behavior. Time-out and response cost are the two most common forms used in speech-language intervention. **Time-out** procedures involve the temporary isolation or removal of a client to an environment with limited or no opportunity to receive positive reinforcement. A modified version can be accomplished by turning the client's chair toward a blank wall in the therapy room or simply withholding direct eye contact from the client for short periods of time. **Response-cost** contingencies occur when previously earned positive reinforcers are deducted or taken back each time the undesirable behavior is demonstrated. This type of punishment can take various forms, including removal of stickers earned for previous correct responses or the partial subtraction of points already accrued by the client earlier in a therapy session. Sometimes, the clinician may choose to give a client several unearned tokens at the beginning of a session or task to institute response-cost procedures.

Several factors influence the effectiveness of punishment procedures (adapted from Hegde & Davis, 2010):

- Punishment should be delivered after *every* instance of the unwanted behavior.

- Punishment should be presented *immediately* following the undesirable behavior.

- Punishment should occur at the *earliest* signs of the unwanted behavior rather than waiting until the behavior is full blown.

- Punishment should not be programmed in graduated levels of intensity; this creates the potential for client habituation to the punishing stimulus, thus reducing its effectiveness.

- Punishment duration should be as brief as possible; lengthy periods of punishment call into question the strength of the chosen punishing stimulus.

Punishment procedures should be employed with caution in the therapy setting because there are undesirable effects associated with their use. These may include client anger, aggression, a reluctance to engage in any communicative behavior with the therapist, and the avoidance or actual termination of treatment.

If no contingent consequences occur following a targeted behavior, the frequency of that behavior will gradually decrease and ultimately disappear from a client's repertoire. This phenomenon is known as **extinction** and is used in therapy to eliminate behaviors that interfere with effective communication. Extinction does not occur immediately. In fact, a temporary increase in emission rate may be observed when the behavior is initially ignored. Behaviors that receive reinforcement on a continuous basis are most vulnerable to extinction, whereas those that are only periodically reinforced over a long period of time are least susceptible to this procedure. It is recommended that extinction procedures that are implemented for an undesired behavior (e.g., ignoring crying behavior) be combined with positive reinforcement for the converse behavior (e.g., rewarding noncrying behavior).

Positive Behavioral Interventions and Supports

Application of all the principles just discussed does not guarantee that a therapy session will run smoothly. The clinician should anticipate the possibility that a patient may not pay attention or cooperate with the session plan. This may occur due to a patient's developmental level of attention, boredom, frustration, lack of self-motivation, or a neurological behavior disorder. The clinician must now focus on **behavior management** in addition to behavior modification.

Currently, a system of positive behavioral interventions and supports (PBIS) is recommended for dealing with challenging behaviors. PBIS is a proactive approach that uses interpersonal and environmental strategies to minimize opportunities for problematic behavior and encourages more socially useful behaviors. Thus, PBIS shifts the emphasis of behavior management from a reactive, aversive approach to one that is more preventative, positive in nature, and prioritizes patient's success. Helpful information on this topic can be found at several websites, including the Center for Effec- tive Collaboration and Practice and the Center on Positive Behavioral Interventions and Supports. A PBIS plan can be developed for individuals, classrooms, school districts, or statewide systems. These plans utilize a continuum of behavioral and instructional strategies to promote complementary improvements in academic and social learning.

A positive behavior support plan (see Appendix 1–H on the companion website) generally identifies the following information:

- A description of the problematic behavior(s), an explanation of why it impedes learning, and an estimate of its severity (frequency, intensity, duration)

- Antecedent events that appear to trigger the behavior(s)

- The desired or alternative behavior(s)

- The intervention and supports (teaching strategies or environmental modifications) that will help the client achieve the desired behavior(s)

From the SLP's perspective, most behavior problems can be prevented if the therapy materials are creative, the activities are interesting, and the session is well paced.

Schedules of Reinforcement

Once the appropriate type of reinforcer has been selected for a given client, the clinician must decide how often the reinforcer will be delivered. The two main schedules of reinforcement are *continuous and intermittent*.

Continuous Reinforcement

A reinforcer is presented after *every* correct performance of a target behavior. This schedule, sometimes characterized as "dense," tends to generate a very high rate of response. It is most commonly used to shape and establish new communication behaviors. It also can be used when transitioning an already established skill from one level of difficulty to the next (e.g., from word to sentence level). Use of a **continuous** schedule reduces the risk that a client's production of a target behavior will "drift" from the intended response. The primary disadvantage of this schedule is that behaviors reinforced at such a high density level are very susceptible to extinction. It also may interfere with a client's production of a steady flow of responses.

Intermittent Reinforcement

With this schedule, only some occurrences of a correct response are followed by a reinforcer. **Intermittent** reinforcement, often termed *lower density*, is most effective in strengthening responses that have been previously established. This reinforcement schedule reduces the probability of satiation during treatment and results in behaviors that are extremely resistant to extinction. The four types of intermittent schedules are as follows.

Fixed Ratio. A specific number of correct responses must be exhibited before a reinforcer is delivered (e.g., every two responses, every 10 responses, every 35 responses). The required number is determined by the clinician and remains unchanged throughout a therapy task. This reinforcement schedule generally elicits a high rate of response.

Fixed Interval. Reinforcement is delivered for the first correct response made after a predetermined time period has elapsed (e.g., every 3 min, every 50 s). The main disadvantage of this schedule is that response rate tends to decline dramatically immediately following presentation of the reinforcer; therefore, a fixed interval schedule may be an inefficient use of therapy time.

Variable Ratio. The number of correct responses required for the delivery of a reinforcer varies from trial to trial according to a predetermined pattern set by the clinician. For example, the pattern might be as follows: after the third response, then after the tenth response, then after the fourth response, then after the seventh response. This ratio—represented as variable ratio (VR): 3, 10, 4,

7—would be repeated throughout a therapy task. This schedule tends to be more effective than a fixed ratio schedule, because the client cannot predict the seemingly random pattern of delivery and anticipates that every response has an equal chance of being reinforced.

Variable Interval. This schedule is similar to a VR except that the clinician varies the time period required for reinforcement delivery rather than the number of responses. For example, one variable interval (VI) pattern might be as follows: after 3 min, then after 10 min, then after 1 min, then after 4 min. This pattern—represented as VI: 3, 10, 1, 4—would be repeated throughout a therapy task.

In general practice, continuous reinforcement is used to establish a new target behavior. Intermittent schedules are introduced in subsequent stages of therapy to promote maintenance and generalization. One rule of thumb is to switch to lower density intermittent schedules when the target response rate increases 30% to 50% over the original baseline measures.

Key Teaching/Scaffolding Strategies

Several basic training techniques are commonly used in intervention programs to facilitate the acquisition of communication behaviors. The following strategies are used for a variety of purposes and are implemented at different points throughout the remediation process:

- *Direct modeling:* Clinician demonstrates a specific behavior to provide an exemplar for the client to imitate.

- *Indirect modeling:* Clinician demonstrates a specific behavior frequently to expose a client to numerous well-formed examples of the target behavior.

- *Shaping by successive approximation:* A target behavior is broken down into small components and taught in an ascending sequence of difficulty.

- *Prompts:* Clinician provides additional verbal or nonverbal cues to facilitate a client's production of a correct response.

- *Fading:* Stimulus or consequence manipulations (e.g., modeling, prompting, reinforcement) are reduced in gradual steps while maintaining the target response.

- *Expansion:* Clinician reformulates a client's utterance into a more mature or complete version.

- *Recast:* Clinician reformulates a client's utterance into a different sentence type.

- *Negative practice:* The client is required to intentionally produce a target behavior using a habitual error pattern. This procedure is generally employed to facilitate learning by highlighting the contrast between the error pattern and the desired response.

- *Target-specific feedback:* The clinician provides information regarding the accuracy or inaccuracy of a client's response relative to the specific target behavior. This type of feedback contrasts with generalized feedback or consequences.

Direct modeling is the teaching technique most frequently used in the early stages of therapy. It is also employed whenever a target behavior is shifted to a higher level of response difficulty, because this type of modeling provides the maximum amount of clinician support. Typically, clinicians augment direct models with a variety of visual and verbal cues to establish correct responses at the level of imitation. Direct modeling also minimizes the likelihood that a client will produce his or her customary error response. Initially, a direct model is provided before each client response.

Once a target behavior is established, continuous modeling should be eliminated, because it does not facilitate strengthening or maintaining a target response. Direct modeling can be terminated abruptly or faded gradually. Gradual **fading** can be accomplished in at least two ways. One requires a client to produce multiple imitations for each model demonstrated by the clinician (e.g., three imitative responses are required after each direct model). The second method involves the progressive reduction of the length of the behavior modeled by the clinician. For example, the direct model of "The boy is running" is shortened first to "The boy is . . ." and then to "The boy . . . ," while the client's imitative response in all three cases is the production of the complete target sentence, "The boy is running." In general, fading procedures can be initiated once a client is able to produce at least five consecutive correct imitative responses.

In some cases, the stimulus alone is not sufficient to elicit the desired response. **Prompts** are extra verbal and nonverbal cues designed to help a client produce the target behavior. Prompts can be categorized as attentional or instructional. **Attentional** cues improve performance by focusing a client's concentration on the task at hand. Examples include "Look at me," "Watch my mouth," "Remember to pay attention," and "Are you ready?" Clinicians also can draw attention to a target by modeling the behavior with exaggerated loudness and duration. **Instructional** cues provide information that is directly related to the specific target behavior being attempted. This may include verbal prompts such as "Remember to elevate your tongue tip at the beginning of each word," "Don't forget to segment your words into syllables if you get stuck," or "Be sure that your answer has at least three words in it." Instructional cues also can be nonverbal, such as an index card with the name of the targeted fluency technique written on it, a gesture to indicate that voice loudness should be increased, or drawings that represent the grammatical categories of subject, verb, and object.

Some target behaviors are too complex for a client to perform successfully, and even the provision of a direct model accompanied by prompts may not elicit a correct imitative response. In such instances, procedures for **shaping by successive approximation** are usually instituted. The simplification of a difficult target into a series of more manageable tasks fosters client success at each step. Each successive step moves progressively closer to the final form of the desired response.

Target-specific feedback is a technique that is useful throughout all phases of the therapy process. It serves three main functions. First, clients benefit from feedback that consists of more than simple accuracy judgments regarding their responses. Target-specific feedback provides precise information about why responses are correct or incorrect (e.g., "Good, I didn't see your tongue peeking out when you said, 'Soup'," rather than simply "Good job!"). Second, use of this strategy tends to maintain a client's awareness of the exact response being targeted without the need for continuous reinstruction during a therapy activity. Finally, this type of feedback assists clinicians in maintaining client focus on the communication behavior being targeted by a given therapy activity. It is a particularly helpful strategy for beginning clinicians who may get too involved in the details or rules of an activity and lose sight of the true purpose of the therapy task.

Negative practice is a strategy intended to enhance a client's awareness of the salient characteristics of his or her error pattern. It is used primarily to illustrate the differences between an "old" response and the intended target. This procedure generally is implemented only after a client demonstrates the ability to produce a given target consistently at the level of imitation. Negative practice is a powerful technique that is best used on a short-term basis. Devoting a significant amount of therapy to client practice on incorrect responses is of questionable value.

In addition to the specific training techniques just discussed, clinicians frequently use the general stimulation procedures of **indirect modeling, expansion, and recasting**. These strategies can be employed at any stage in the therapy process. They provide a client with increased exposure to instances of desirable speech, language, or communication behaviors but are not intended to elicit immediate specific responses. For example, a clinician working with a client on the production of /s/ may implement indirect modeling by including a significant number of /s/-initial words in her off-task comments throughout a session. Expansions are used almost exclusively in language therapy programs and may involve the clinician's interpretation of the client's intended meaning (e.g., Client: "Daddy cookie"; Clinician: "Yes, Daddy is eating the cookie."). An example of recasting is changing the client's declarative statement to an interrogative form (e.g., Client: "Doggie is barking"; Clinician: "Is the doggie barking?").

Homework

Once a target communication behavior has been established in therapy using the teaching strategies specified in the previous section, **homework assignments** can be given to strengthen the response and facilitate its generalization outside the clinical setting. Certain guidelines for the design and implementation of homework can increase its effectiveness as an intervention strategy:

- The purpose of homework is to provide the client with practice on an *existing* skill rather than teaching something new. Therefore, it should focus only on targets that have been solidly established in therapy.

- Homework should be instituted only after a client has demonstrated a basic ability to accurately evaluate his or her performance on a given target.

- To increase the likelihood that homework will be completed, it should be assigned in amounts that are perceived as manageable by a client or family. For example, activities that involve a daily commitment of 5 to 10 min may be more effective than those that require 30 to 45 min once a week.

- Homework should be assigned on a regular basis throughout the course of therapy.

- Homework assignments should always be accompanied by simple written instructions that specify exactly what the client is expected to do.

- Review and check homework during the initial portion of the next therapy session.

- Homework activities can be supervised by a variety of individuals (e.g., teacher, spouse, babysitter).

Session Design

Once therapy targets have been appropriately programmed, the clinician must determine the organizational flow of each therapy session. The first decision to be made is whether treatment will be delivered in an individual or group setting. **Session design** for both of these formats requires consideration of the basic factors discussed in the sections that follow. Elements that are specific to design for a group session are addressed later in this chapter.

Basic Training Protocol

Regardless of disorder type or severity level, speech, language, and communication therapy is carried out using the same basic training protocol. This protocol is the distillation of the therapy process and consists of the following five steps (Table 1–2 provides guidelines on giving instructions):

1. Clinician presents stimulus.

2. Clinician waits for the client to respond.

3. Clinician presents appropriate consequent event.

4. Clinician records response.

5. Clinician removes stimulus (as appropriate).

This sequence represents a single trial for a given target and is repeated continuously throughout a therapy session. The acceptable latency period between stimulus presentation and client response may vary according to disorder type as well as individual client characteristics. It is critical that the consequent event (reinforcement/punishment) follow the response immediately, so that the contingent relationship between the two is obvious to the client. For this reason, data recording should not delay the delivery of the consequence.

Table 1–2
Guidelines for Effective Instructions

- Instructions should be worded as clearly and concisely as possible. Long, complicated explanations can be counterproductive to a client's understanding of the intended task. (Beginning clinicians may benefit from writing an actual script of instructions prior to a session.)

- State instructions in the declarative form. Directions that are presented indirectly in the form of requests (e.g., "Would you say /s/ for me?") are pragmatically confusing and understandably may elicit negative replies (e.g., "No" or "I don't want to.").

- Be sure to allow clients sufficient time to respond before repeating the instructions. Resist the temptation to repeat instructions or stimuli too quickly, because individuals with communication impairments often require increased processing time. Waiting is a strategy that may facilitate correct responses more consistently than repetition of instructions.

- If it becomes necessary to readminister instructions, try to avoid significant reformulation of the original wording. This is particularly important with clients who have language disorders, because rewording tends to become a source of confusion rather than clarification.

- The main emphasis of instructions should always be on the targeted behavior rather than on the details of the activity or game being used to elicit the behavior. (This aspect poses particular difficulty for beginning clinicians, who must learn to create the appropriate balance between the amount of time spent explaining elaborate therapy activities versus working on target behaviors.)

Task Order

Another important component of session design is the order in which tasks are conducted. Appropriate task order enhances the overall effectiveness of treatment. An ideal progression follows an "easy–hard–easy" pattern. A session should begin with therapy tasks with which a client can be relatively successful without excessive expenditure of effort. This could entail a review of completed homework assignments or nearly mastered targets from a previous session. The central portion of the session should consist of behavioral objectives that are most challenging to the client. The final segment should return to tasks that elicit fairly accurate performance with minimal effort. This task order increases the likelihood that a given therapy session will begin and end on a positive note. This success-oriented session design promotes high levels of client motivation even during difficult stages of the therapy process.

Dynamics of Therapy

Thus far, this chapter has focused on the technical aspects of intervention. However, the therapy process involves another critical dimension: the dynamics of therapy. Therapy dynamics contribute significantly to session design and include factors such as the clinician–client relationship, work efficiency/pace, materials, and proxemics.

The Clinician–Client Relationship

The nature of the clinician–client relationship influences the success of a therapy program as powerfully as the technical design. One of the most important aspects of the therapeutic relationship is the professional personality of the clinician. Clearly, personal attributes among clinicians vary tremendously. In general, a calm, positive, and firm demeanor is most effective in enhancing clinician–client interaction.

Some therapists consistently generate better client outcomes than other clinicians regardless of the intervention approach used. The literature on treatment efficacy tends to focus on differences between specific intervention methods/techniques. One frequently overlooked factor in these outcome studies is "therapist effects." In other words, what is the contribution of therapist skill in establishing therapeutic relationship to differences in treatment outcomes? Wampold (2015) identifies the *therapeutic alliance between clinician and client* as an important concept in understanding the degree to which a client experiences success in treatment. It is the clinician's responsibility to establish this relationship, which consists of three main elements: (a) creating the interpersonal bond between clinician and client, (b) ensuring alignment between clinician and client/family regarding the long-term goals of treatment, and (c) ensuring alignment between clinician and client/family regarding the nature of tasks necessary to achieve these goals. This therapeutic alliance enhances the likelihood of a more positive treatment outcome.

In practice, clinicians need to maintain a conscious awareness of their body language, intonation patterns, and social speaking style to prevent client confusion. Body language and voice intonation patterns must be monitored to ensure that they do not conflict with accompanying verbal messages. For example, the message, "You're doing a great job!" may not be perceived by a client as a positive remark if it is delivered without eye contact and in an apathetic tone of voice. Further, the use of overly diplomatic forms of speech should be minimized because they may contradict the message that a clinician intends to convey. For example, beginning clinicians who are reluctant to risk hurting a client's feelings may react to an incorrect response with a big smile while saying, "Good! Let's try that again!" rather than clearly stating that the attempt was inaccurate.

In any interpersonal interaction, there may be a mismatch between an intended message and the perceived message. A persistent mismatch can have a negative influence on the therapeutic alliance. It is the responsibility of clinicians to adapt their interactive styles (comprising energy level, humor, talkativeness, and vocabulary) to accommodate the comfort level of each client rather than the other way around. It is also important to remember that clients can be easily overwhelmed and intimidated by the excessive use of unfamiliar technical jargon. To maintain a professional yet warm atmosphere, clinicians need to determine on a case-by-case basis the appropriate balance between their use of technical versus more colloquial language forms.

Moreover, clinicians must establish the parameters of the therapeutic relationship from the very first session. This entails an explicit definition of the roles and responsibilities of each partner. This will clearly differentiate the nature of a professional relationship from a personal one. At the beginning of a therapeutic relationship, clients do not always feel comfortable volunteering information about their goals for therapy. Clinicians should make a point of asking clients about their expectations. Whenever possible, clients (and their families) should be active participants in the target selection phase of therapy, by identifying the communication behaviors that are the highest priorities in their daily lives. Clinicians can minimize client anxiety and confusion by providing a clear rationale regarding the purpose of each activity implemented in a therapy session. Intervention tends to be less effective if clients do not understand why they are being asked to perform particular tasks. Further, difficult client questions should be addressed in a manner that allows the clinician to maintain credibility. For instance, instead of responding with "I haven't had that course yet," it is more effective to simply say, "I don't know. I'll do some research on the topic and give you the information at our next session."

Clinicians need to create a balance between responding to and ignoring off-task comments made by clients. Sometimes clients genuinely need to talk about topics that are not part of the clinician's original lesson plan but are important to address (e.g., questions regarding lack of progress, comments concerning family reactions to new communicative behaviors). At other times, off-task comments are meant simply to distract the clinician from a therapy task that a client perceives as difficult or boring.

Ultimately, the success of any therapeutic relationship will be influenced by the clinician's recognition that it is the client, and not merely the disorder, that is the main focus of treatment.

Work Efficiency/Pace

This aspect of session dynamics entails consideration of two main issues. First, every session should be efficiently designed to provide a client with the maximum number of opportunities to practice target behaviors. Second, the pace of each session must be geared to the learning rates and styles of individual clients. A pace that is either too fast or too slow may cause frustration for a client and interfere with successful performance.

Materials

The materials selected for therapy must be appropriate for a client's age, developmental status, language level, gender, cultural background, and linguistic needs. In addition to these criteria, it is important to consider the interest value of therapy materials based on individual client preferences. For example, when selecting materials for a 12-year-old boy with a learning disability who reads at a second-grade level, the clinician must ensure that any stories used in therapy are sufficiently interesting for a preteen, yet written at a manageable difficulty level. Finally, clinicians should avoid the use of time-consuming and complicated materials or activities. Materials that require lengthy physical manipulation (e.g., cutting, gluing, intricate board games) may negatively affect the efficiency of a session by reducing the amount of time available for client responses.

Proxemics

For the purposes of the present discussion, **proxemics** involves the spatial arrangement or relationships between the clinician and client(s) within the therapy setting. Proxemics should take into account the spatial factors that affect any social interaction. One of the most important considerations for SLPs is to determine a socially acceptable (and, in some cases, culturally acceptable) physical proximity between the clinician and the client. Seating arrangements that are extremely far apart may be perceived by the client as an indication of aloofness or lack of interest on the part of the clinician. In contrast, clients may be very uncomfortable with clinicians who sit too close and invade their personal space. Clinicians may deliberately use proxemics as a strategy to influence client behavior (e.g., reducing impulsive or distractible behavior by sitting very close to a child).

In addition to having social implications, proxemics also influence the effective implementation of certain therapy procedures. For example, monitoring the degree of tongue protrusion for an interdental lisp (i.e., /θ/ for /s/) will be difficult if the clinician cannot see the client's face. Alternatively, a face-to-face seating arrangement may interfere with an activity that requires the clinician and client to read from the same stimulus sheet. Seating arrangements should always be selected based on the goal of a given therapy objective. The three most common sitting arrangements (chair or floor) for conducting individualized therapy are face to face, side by side, and side by side in front of a mirror.

Group Therapy

The use of a group therapy model requires attention to several unique aspects of session design that are not pertinent to individual treatment. Unfortunately, there is a paucity of information on group intervention and even less empirical study of this process in the field of speech-language pathology. However, group therapy is critical to any discussion of session design, because it is a frequently used service delivery mode—in fact, it is becoming the dominant model in many therapeutic settings (such as the public schools). Therefore, group therapy is treated as a separate topic in this chapter to provide clinicians with fundamental information on the effective design and execution of these programs.

Clinicians implement a group intervention model for a variety of purposes. Some groups are intended to teach new communication skills at introductory levels. Others are designed primarily to provide clients with practice on skills previously established in individual sessions. Still others have socialization, self-help, or counseling as their main purpose.

The stage of therapy at which group intervention is initiated also varies. Some clinicians employ a group model from the very beginning of the therapy process; others use it mainly in the final stages to facilitate carryover. In many cases, a combination of individual and group formats is used throughout all stages of the therapy process.

Group Size

The size of a group will vary depending on its purpose, the setting, and client age. Groups whose primary purpose is to teach new skills tend to be smaller than those geared for the generalization of previously mastered skills. Group size is also determined by the availability of clients in different service delivery settings. Institutions such as metropolitan hospitals and public schools lend themselves more readily to the formation of larger therapy groups than do private practices or small clinics.

Based on the available literature, the recommended group size for children is approximately two to six members (Blosser & Neidecker, 2002; Gordon-Brannon & Weiss, 2007). Guidelines for adults differ. For example, Cooper and Cooper (2003) recommend 7 to 12 members for adult stuttering groups. They also caution that groups of fewer than five clients are undesirable for several reasons: (a) personality characteristics of individual group members are more prominent, (b) the absence of a single member can interfere with the group's ability to function, and (c) small groups are more susceptible to domination by a single member.

Group Composition

The primary client characteristics to be considered in the formation of a group are age, gender, disorder type, and disorder severity. Other factors that may be relevant to some groups include cognitive level, socioeconomic status, education level, and personality type. As a general rule, the two most important factors are client age and disorder type. Effective groups tend to be relatively homogeneous with respect to one or both of these variables. Clinicians may choose to organize groups in either a closed or open format. *Closed groups* frequently operate for predetermined time periods and maintain the same membership throughout. In contrast, *open groups* have revolving membership and accept new individuals whenever space becomes available. One rule of thumb for pediatric groups is that the age or developmental level of the members should be within 2 or 3 years of one another, because cognitive abilities and social maturity can significantly influence group interaction. See Farquharson et al. (2020) for an interesting discussion of group versus individual therapy formats for pediatric speech sound production.

Clinician's Role

The role of the clinician is to function as group leader. Leadership style can be directive or nondirective. A *directive* style is typically used with groups composed of young children. In addition, it is more common in the early stages of therapy when a group model is being used to teach new communication behaviors. In this role, the clinician sets the agenda, chooses the materials and activities, provides specific instruction, and gives corrective feedback. A *nondirective* approach is more commonly used in the carryover stages of therapy and with self-help groups. In this style, the clinician does not perform a primary teaching function. Instead, group members take charge of session activities, while the clinician serves as a facilitator who oversees rather than directs group interactions. Regardless of style, a group leader is responsible for establishing and maintaining group cohesion, mediating conflicts between members, and ensuring that each member of the group is progressing adequately toward established therapy goals.

Procedures

Several procedures can be used in group settings to maintain the active participation of all members throughout the entire session. In one method, the clinician presents a stimulus and pauses before choosing a particular group member to respond. This strategy increases the likelihood that all members will pay attention and prepare answers to every stimulus in anticipation of being called on. In another strategy, clients can take turns modeling target behaviors for other group members to repeat in unison. Finally, clients can be required to listen, watch, and evaluate the performance of a target behavior by fellow group members.

Clinicians can use a variety of techniques to facilitate group interaction. The following examples are applicable to any type of communicative disorder:

- Reinforce client behaviors and comments that are consistent with treatment goals.

- Model the target behaviors or techniques group members are attempting to develop.

- Focus attention and group time on members who are making progress toward established goals.

- Encourage interaction within the group by asking one member to demonstrate a target behavior for the other members.

- Ask open-ended questions that require longer than one- or two-word responses.

- Cue a group member to focus on a particular therapy target before she or he begins speaking.

- Restructure comments or topics so they have appeal for all members of the group.

- Use behaviors of individual members to form generalizations that are applicable to the group as a whole.

Advantages and Disadvantages

The delivery of therapy services through a group model has both advantages and disadvantages. The main advantages are as follows:

- Carryover is facilitated.

- Clients stimulate and motivate each other.

- More opportunities exist for natural-speaking situations.

- Clients recognize that others have problems similar to their own.

- More occasions exist for clients to engage in critical listening.

- A broader variety of activities and materials can be used.

- The setting provides for socialization and peer interaction.

- Increased opportunities exist to learn by observing others.

- Self-monitoring is encouraged by reducing the client's dependence on the clinician as the sole evaluator of communication behavior.

The primary disadvantages of group intervention include the following:

- Each group member receives less direct attention from the clinician than is given in individual sessions.

- Fewer opportunities exist to address the specific weaknesses of each client, especially when the group is not homogeneous with respect to disorder.

- Clients who are shy, reticent, or of different cultural backgrounds may be reluctant to participate.

- One or two members may become dominant and monopolize the group.

- The group's rate of progress may be too fast for the slowest members and too slow for the most advanced members.

Perhaps the heart of successful group therapy is a clinician's ability to establish and maintain a true group dynamic; otherwise, the sessions merely consist of multiple clients receiving individualized treatment in a group room.

Data Collection

SLPs are accountable for the efficiency as well as the effectiveness of the intervention services they provide. Clients and their families invest valuable time, resources, and effort in the therapy process. The primary mechanism for ensuring clinician accountability is data collection. Information obtained from the data collection process serves two important functions. It allows the clinician to monitor a client's progress from one session to the next. Data collection systems also can be designed to permit documentation of the efficacy of a given treatment strategy. Clinicians need to recognize that best practices in service delivery are data driven.

Recording Session Data

Data recording is greatly facilitated by behavioral objectives that are written properly (i.e., in specific and measurable terms). In most cases, data collection difficulties occur because objectives are written in a vague and unclear manner. Following are guidelines for a comprehensive approach to data collection:

1. Appropriate data-recording sheets should be designed or selected prior to the onset of a therapy session. (Samples of reproducible data forms and instructions for their use are included in Appendix 1–G on the companion website.)

2. The notation system should provide the type of information that is most relevant to a specific client or disorder. A binary system of "correct" versus "incorrect" is not the only option. Interval scales can be developed to rate responses on a continuum (e.g., degree of correctness or latency of response).

3. The data collection system must allow the clinician to clearly distinguish among imitative, cued/prompted, self-corrected, and spontaneous responses.

4. Once therapy tasks reach the conversational level of complexity, it is often more efficient to use a data-recording system that is based on time rather than on total number of responses. For example, it may be easier to document the number of errors per minute rather than to identify all occurrences of a target behavior to calculate the percentage correct.

5. Reinforcement tokens or stimulus items can be used as an alternative to paper and pencil or online recording of client responses. One useful approach is to organize the items or tokens in groups of 10 or 20. The number and percentage of correct responses can be calculated easily by (a) counting the number of unearned reinforcement tokens remaining at the end of an activity or (b) checking the number of stimulus items (e.g., picture cards) that the clinician has placed in a "correct response" pile.

6. Record *every* stimulus-response event. Even the absence of a response to a particular stimulus should be recorded. However, good clinicians should recognize when powerful teaching moments arise during therapy sessions. To take maximum advantage of these moments, the clinician may choose to engage in a brief period of teaching using a variety of strategies and reinforcers without adhering to strict data-recording procedures.

Data collection systems are used to maximize a clinician's effectiveness. It is important to recognize that data yield information regarding a client's status on a particular objective. However, data alone do not identify specific programming changes that may need to be made or how to implement them. These clinical decisions can be made only through a clinician's careful analysis and interpretation of the recorded data.

Probes

Probes are instruments administered periodically throughout treatment to measure a client's progress. They are designed to assess generalization of a trained target behavior (Hegde, 1998). Probes consist of a set of novel stimuli that are equivalent to, but different from, those used for treatment. For example, after teaching the production of initial /s/ with a set of picture cards, the clinician may probe a client's generalization by presenting a new set of unfamiliar pictures to elicit this phoneme (a good rule of thumb: 20 stimulus items for each probe).

Probes are similar to baselines in that client responses are elicited without target-specific instruction and do not receive any reinforcement. However, lengthy periods of nonreinforcement may be undesirable for some clients, particularly in the early stages of therapy. Therefore, a **mixed probe** may be instituted, whereby both trained and untrained stimulus items are presented in an alternating sequence. In this procedure, the client continues to receive reinforcement for responses to the trained stimuli.

The findings obtained from probe procedures are used by the clinician to determine the next step in the therapy program. If the predetermined criterion from the behavioral objective has not been achieved, training should continue at the current level. If the criterion has been met, the clinician may choose to shift to a higher level of response complexity in the same target area or move on to a new communicative behavior. Periodic administration of probes is especially important, because it minimizes the risk of continuing therapy that is no longer effective or necessary.

Collaborative Service Delivery Models

The traditional approach to providing speech-language intervention has been the individual model, where clients receive therapy in a one-to-one setting. There is a growing trend toward the provision of therapy in a variety of different service-delivery models. The hallmark characteristic of this trend is collaborative partnership.

Collaboration is critical to promoting better communication among different professionals, all of whom possess specialized knowledge and skills. For example, SLPs have a deep understanding of the linguistic underpinnings of literacy in both typically developing children and children with learning problems. Teachers and special educators have expertise in strategies, materials, and standards for teaching literacy. In medical and educational settings, health professionals from different disciplines regularly team with one another to problem solve and provide interprofessional patient care (Golom & Schreck, 2018).

Often, professionals do not have an appreciation for the knowledge and skills possessed by one another. Partnerships offer an opportunity for professionals to engage in focused and frequent exchanges about effective intervention and instruction. They are able to leverage their combined knowledge and skills to implement best practices and improve outcomes for diverse groups of clients (Roth & Troia, 2006). Further, collaboration with parents/family members is an important aspect of effective treatment in all settings (Klatte et al., 2020; Smart et al., 2022).

Collaboration is highly valued by SLPs and other professionals, and although research findings suggest that it is a service-delivery model of choice, collaboration often does not occur, because it requires a substantial degree of coordination and planning (Pfeiffer et al., 2019; Wallace et al., 2022). One means of making collaboration more manageable is to strategically select a client(s) for whom the potential benefits of cotreatment are most evident. Once success is experienced in this initial venture, collaborative efforts can be extended more broadly across a clinician's workload.

Eight guiding principles for effective collaborations (Paul et al., 2006) that promote effective communication and build good relationships among professionals and families are as follows:

1. Engage in mutual problem solving and shared responsibility for positive client outcomes.
2. Establish communication goals and priorities for clients on the basis of their strengths and needs.
3. Form partnerships that are nonhierarchical and based on coequal participation.
4. Recognize that collaboration is a dynamic process: the size, composition, goals, and function of teams change as client needs change.
5. Respect different professional perspectives.
6. Make partnerships a priority.
7. Establish realistic expectations for the partnership.
8. Celebrate success.

Effective implementation of these principles across a wide variety of service delivery settings can be maximized with the following strategies:

- Maintain ongoing communication with collaborative partners to promote clear understanding of roles and responsibilities of different partners.
- Use technology to maintain communication and exchange of information.
- Involve people who have significant relationships with the student (e.g., teachers, families, spouses, and peers).
- Engage in preprofessional training and professional development opportunities to learn and implement partnership models.

Many collaborative partnership models are easily adapted to the educational setting and can be used instead of or in combination with the traditional pull-out model, in which a student leaves the classroom and receives therapy in either individual or group sessions. Some of the most commonly used collaborative models are as follows:

Consultative: The clinician acts as a resource for professionals who work directly with a child and parents to help solve problems related to the child's communicative deficit. In this model, the agent of intervention is someone other than the SLP.

Team teaching: The clinician and the teacher share the responsibility for classroom instruction on a regular basis. In this model, a comprehensive program with strong language and academic components can be provided within the context of the classroom.

Self-contained: The clinician alone serves as the classroom teacher and is responsible for developing and implementing all aspects of the curriculum. Classroom activities in all topic areas are specifically designed to promote the development of language skills.

Many states and localities now use an inclusion model of education in which students with disabilities receive all needed services and supports in the general education classroom. In addition, there has been a growing trend toward the provision of therapy in a wider variety of service-delivery models.

An increasingly well-regarded collaborative model is interprofessional practice (IPP), more recently referred to as interprofessional collaborative practice (ICP), in which multiple service providers with different areas of professional expertise work together to provide high-quality, comprehensive educational or health care services to improve patient/client outcomes. SLPs have key roles on ICP teams. They educate others about their unique knowledge and skills and share this expertise with other team members. SLPs also acquire increased understanding about the expertise of colleagues from other professions. ICPs have some elements, or core competencies (ICP Core Competencies, 2016), that differentiate them from other types of interdisciplinary teams and that create a "collaborative culture." The following are examples of ICP team characteristics:

- Open, deliberate, continuous communication

- Shared goals and/objectives

- Clearly defined roles and responsibilities

- Equal status/value of each team member

- Shared values and ethics

- Mutual trust, respect, and support

- Collaborative decision-making at each stage of the process

- Highly coordinated services with quality monitored on a consistent basis

- Reflective practice (decisions about what is working and what needs to be changed)

- Conflict resolution (agreed-upon procedures for handling disagreements as they arise)

Notably, all ICP core competencies aim to enhance communication among SLPs and other practitioners.

Along with the IPP model, current health care and education reforms are prompting some rethinking about the academic and clinical preparation of future professionals in health-related professions (including speech-language pathology and audiology). One iteration of this rethinking is **interprofessional education** (IPE). The core feature of IPE is interactive student learning, in which students from different disciplines (e.g., speech-language pathology, physical therapy, occupational therapy, nursing, social work, and nutrition) learn and work side by side, both academically and clinically.

The goals of IPE are to (a) develop students' knowledge, skills, and attitudes that result in ICP team competencies; (b) learn how to function successfully on ICP teams; and (c) prepare students to integrate interprofessional collaborative services into future clinical practice.

Multitiered Systems of Support/Response to Intervention

The term multitiered systems of support (MTSS) is an umbrella term for response to intervention (RTI) and PBIS (see discussion on PBIS earlier in this chapter). MTSS models most often focus on educational and behavior issues at the same time, because these concerns usually "go hand in hand" in the same student.

In the reauthorization of the **Individuals with Disabilities Education Act** (2011), **response to intervention (RTI)** was sanctioned as an approach for identifying students with learning disabilities and determining their eligibility for services. It was developed as an alternative to the traditional discrepancy criterion approach. With the *discrepancy criterion*, students need to demonstrate a significant gap (usually defined as 1.5 standard deviations) between cognitive ability and academic achievement. Researchers and educators have long viewed this approach as a "wait-to-fail" model, because most children do not demonstrate the needed discrepancy until the third or fourth grade. RTI focuses on earlier identification and intervention when students first experience academic difficulties. Its goal is to improve the achievement of all students, including those with language-learning disabilities. RTI models involve a collaborative, problem-solving process with the following components (Fuchs & Fuchs, 2006; Roth & Troia, 2009):

- Universal screening/assessment

- High-quality classroom-wide instruction

- Progress monitoring

- Multitiered instruction/intervention

- Family engagement

The most widely used RTI model includes the three tiers described in Table 1–3 along with suggested roles for SLPs within each tier. The intensity and duration of services (i.e., progression through the tiers) are determined by a student's responsiveness to intervention.

In RTI, the identification of a learning disability (LD) is based on a "dual discrepancy" (Fuchs, 2003). That is, despite *high-quality instruction* and *remedial instruction*, a student does not progress at the expected rate. Although originally conceived as a model for primary grades, there is growing support for applying developmentally appropriate RTI approaches in preschool settings as a means of prevention, earlier identification, and early intervention for children at risk for educational failure (Coleman et al., 2009; Justice, 2006).

The existing body of evidence shows that tier-based early intervention approaches can improve the academic performance of at-risk students (e.g., Murray et al., 2010; Orosco & Klingnen, 2010). Results of a statewide survey of RTI implementation (Hoover et al., 2008) indicated that tier-based models are currently in use or are in development in almost every state. Survey findings also revealed that (a) statewide RTI professional development training efforts are under way in 90% of the states

Table 1–3
Response to Intervention Tiers

Tier	Description	Suggested Roles of Speech-Language Pathologists
1	All students receive high-quality, scientifically based core classroom curriculum in the general education setting. Teachers monitor student learning on an ongoing basis (compared to age, grade, classmates' performance) to track child progress and guide differentiated instruction for children according to their needs.	• SLPs can use their extensive knowledge of the structures and functions of language (e.g., phonological awareness, vocabulary, morphology/syntax) to educate school staff about the fundamental relationships between oral language, literacy, and academic learning. • Help teachers make appropriate adaptations in academic language (e.g., reducing linguistic complexity, marking important information, providing concrete and relevant examples for abstract concepts). • Contribute to the creation of literacy-rich classroom learning environments. • Help teachers systematically implement screening and progress monitoring measures and interpret the results. • Provide in-class modeling or coteaching of language-based emergent literacy activities (e.g., phonological awareness, shared book reading).
2	Students whose performance and rate of progress lag behind that of peers receive more specialized instruction within the general education curriculum.	• Adapt their training in "diagnostic" observation and analysis to assist in the delivery of targeted interventions for struggling learners (e.g., provide specifically tailored instruction retrieval strategies for students who read slowly). • Continue professional education efforts to help school staff with progress monitoring and identification of students with learning disabilities. • Consult with school staff to ensure consistency and continuity among the multiple individuals who provide instruction to the same struggling learners (e.g., reading specialists, English as a second language/bilingual education teachers, paraeducators, community volunteers).
3	Students who show continued need for support are considered for more intensive, individualized instruction and/or are referred for comprehensive evaluation to determine eligibility for special education services.	• Implement direct treatment for students with language or learning deficits who have not benefited from Tier 1 or Tier 2 services. • Confer with special educators to focus resources on students who need the greatest amount of support to succeed in the classroom. • Provide services in the quickest possible time frame to minimize the gap between struggling students and their classroom peers.

Source: Adapted from "Applications of Responsiveness to Intervention and the Speech-Language Pathologist in Elementary School Settings," by F. P. Roth and G. A. Troia, 2009, *Seminars in Speech & Language, 30,* p. 75–89.

and that (b) most states are using or plan to use a combined problem-solving assessment and treatment model for making tier-based educational decisions (Hoover & Patton, 2009). A systematic review of 16 well-designed studies indicated that five factors were constant across effective programs. Of these five, at least three involved collaborative efforts (i.e., involvement of all school personnel, administrative support at the building and system levels, adequate meeting time for teaming, and coordination; Hughes & Dexter, 2011). Few treatment efficacy and effectiveness studies have been conducted in the last several years. For a more recent comprehensive discussion of RTI issues, see Fuchs and Fuchs (2017) and Swaminathan and Farquharson, (2018).

Current Challenges of RTI

Information about the effectiveness of RTI models is still evolving. Clinicians should be aware of several issues that require further study:

- RTI models have focused on early identification and intervention. No studies are available that report the long-term effects of Tier 1 and Tier 2 services on later academic achievement and learning outcomes. RTI may miss identifying and addressing the needs of students with late-emerging reading or writing disabilities (Badian, 1999; Catts et al., 2005; Leach et al., 2003; Nation, 2005).

- Application of RTI has largely been limited to the domain of reading and writing; consequently, its applicability to other domains (e.g., oral language, writing) is unknown.

- It is unclear how long a student should remain in a particular tier of service and what specific criteria should be met to judge responsiveness as adequate or inadequate (e.g., Duhon et al., 2009; Speece & Hines, 2008).

- RTI models evaluate risk and disability status in the classroom setting (Fuchs, 2002, 2003).

- This context is relative, because demands vary not only across grades but also across teachers, schools, districts, and states. When discrepancy is based on comparisons between performance of the struggling student and his or her peers at the local level, identification of LDs becomes much more relative (Kavale et al., 2003).

Treatment Efficacy/Evidence-Based Practice

Treatment efficacy is a general term that encompasses three basic factors: effectiveness (Does treatment work?), efficiency (Does one treatment work better or faster than another?), and effects (In what ways does treatment alter behavior?). For certain communicative disorders, such as those involving voice and fluency, the definition of successful treatment should account for subjective variables (e.g., client feelings, willingness to communicate) as well as objective variables (e.g., number of stuttered words, maintenance of specified optimal pitch).

In the context of clinical intervention, the most typical approach to data collection is the following single-subject design: pretreatment baseline of a target → treatment → posttreatment baseline of the same behavior (in which the baseline measures are identical to one another and different from the treatment items). The information obtained from this data collection method is useful in documenting the amount of change or progress for a specific client. However, it does not address treatment efficacy in that this design does not permit the clinician to determine whether the intervention itself was responsible for the observed change.

To more adequately document the efficacy of treatment, a **multiple-baseline** design can be implemented. A simple multiple-baseline procedure involves the selection of at least three target behaviors of similar complexity that are in need of remediation. It is important to choose a set of targets for which direct transfer of learning is not expected to occur from one behavior to the others. For example, it is inappropriate to include phonemes that differ from each other by only one feature (e.g., voicing). Baseline measures are used to ascertain pretreatment status of the targets, and treatment procedures are then implemented for one of them. After the criterion has been reached on the trained behavior, the clinician repeats the baseline measures on the untrained targets. If the results show no significant change from the original baseline scores, the clinician can be confident that the treatment, and no other factor, was responsible for the client's improvement on the trained target. One of the remaining targets is then selected for training, and the treatment/post-treatment baseline sequence is repeated. This procedure is continued until all therapy targets have been trained.

An **evidence-based practice (EBP)** approach to intervention is best conceptualized as the integration of three main components: (a) current best scientific evidence; (b) clinician expertise; and (c) client values, beliefs, and preferences, including cultural/linguistic factors. Information in the professional literature can be categorized according to levels of scientific design and quality. TEKA (Total Evidence and Knowledge Approach) is a version of EBP that incorporates a stronger focus on knowledge as an important aspect of clinical decision-making (McCurtin et al., 2019). Table 1–4 provides an evidence rating hierarchy that ranges from most to least scientifically robust. ASHA provides a valuable compendium of systematic literature reviews that clinicians can consult to guide their "best practices." Another resource, the National Center for Evidence-Based Practice in Communication Disorders (N-CEP), can be accessed online and facilitates clinicians' ability to incorporate evidence into their clinical decision-making in a variety of disorder areas.

From a practical perspective, clinicians should realize that "gold-standard" evidence (Levels I and II) is frequently unavailable in the research literature for our profession. Clinicians should evaluate existing information from the other levels of the hierarchy to guide their decision-making, to the extent possible. Implementation of an EBP approach may take many forms. Key steps in the process generally include the following:

Table 1–4
Evidence Rating Hierarchy

IA	Well-designed meta-analysis of more than one randomized, controlled study
IB	One well-designed, randomized, controlled study
IIA	One well-designed, controlled study without randomization
IIB	One well-designed, quasi-experimental study
III	Well-designed, nonexperimental studies (i.e., correlational and case studies, including multiple-baseline designs)
VI	Expert committee report, consensus conference, clinical experience of respected authorities

Source: Adapted from Robey, R. R. (2004). Levels of evidence. *The ASHA Leader, 9*(7), 5.

1. Ask an answerable and intelligent clinical question.

2. Search for the best available evidence.

3. Critically evaluate the evidence.

4. Consider individual client characteristics and needs.

5. Make a clinical decision with client input.

6. Implement treatment plan and document progress/outcome(s).

Treatment Intensity and Dosage

In 2007, Warren et al. presented a formal definition of treatment intensity: "the product of rate [teaching episodes] per minute or hour, the number of hours of intervention per specified time period (e.g., a day or a week), and the full length of the interventions in weeks, months, or years ..." (p. 71). This definition has been interpreted many different ways by both researchers and clinicians, resulting in considerable variability in treatment intensity (McManus et al., 2019). From the clinical practice perspective, the heart of the issue is, "How much therapy, of what frequency and overall duration, and in which forms is necessary to attain treatment goals?" Because little scientific evidence exists, clinicians must base their decisions on the individual characteristics and circumstances of each client.

Following is a list of the most common terminology used to describe treatment intensity: dose, dose form, dose frequency, total intervention duration, and cumulative intervention intensity (adapted from Breit-Smith et al., 2009; Warren et al., 2007). An explanation of each of these terms follows:

- *Dose:* The number of times a strategy or technique is presented within a session
  - Example: 10 wh- questions produced in one session

- *Dose form:* The delivery form for presenting the stimuli
  - Example: Semantic maps

- *Dose frequency:* How often the intervention is provided
  - Example: Three times per week

- *Total intervention duration:* The entire length of time the intervention is provided
  - Example: 14 weeks

- *Cumulative intervention intensity:* The numerical result of multiplying the values from dose, dose frequency, and total duration time
  - Example: 100 treatment sessions

The assumption that learning is facilitated by more exposure to the important elements of an intervention may be erroneous (i.e., more therapy is better therapy). Rohrer and Pashler (2010) provide evidence regarding the "spacing effect," which stipulates that distributing learning opportunities over time results in improved long-term outcomes in comparison to massed learning opportunities, for both basic/rote skills and more complex goals. Clinicians can manipulate this effect within sessions (e.g., the time between presentations of stimuli during a specific task) and also across sessions (e.g., scheduling sessions weekly versus daily). Dispersing learning opportunities within or between sessions also may be referred to as *distributed practice*. Cepeda et al. (2006) argue that distributed practice allows for periods of skill consolidation and increased client engagement. It is important to consider the elements of treatment intensity described in the previous bulleted list collectively rather than in isolation. The literature on treatment intensity in the field of speech-language pathology is far from settled. However, a number of studies (Baker, 2012; Fey et al., 2013; Schmitt et al., 2017) indicate that there may be a point of diminishing return when all elements of intensity (i.e., session dose, session frequency, and overall duration) are increased simultaneously. In fact, these studies suggest that therapeutic intervention that is delivered in a regimen of *low-frequency/ high treatment dose over longer periods of time* is associated with the best learning outcomes. Given the caseload management responsibilities of most clinicians, efficient manipulation of these treatment intensity factors to optimize client learning warrants serious consideration.

Setting-Specific Professional Terminology

In the field of speech-language pathology, clinicians work in a variety of settings. Much of the information in the profession is considered "core" and applicable across settings. However, some jargon or terminology is specific to certain populations or work environments. Clinicians need to adapt the information contained in this book to their settings. To illustrate this point, Table 1–5 provides key examples of terminology used in two different settings: medical/hospital and educational/school.

Troubleshooting Tips for Therapy Sessions

If your client is not making adequate progress or seems bored and inattentive, ask yourself the following questions:

1. Are the reinforcers that I am using during therapy activities really motivating for this client?

2. Am I delivering the reinforcers fast enough for the client to connect them with the target behavior?

3. Did I shift from a continuous reinforcement schedule to an intermittent schedule too soon?

4. Am I teaching the target behavior in small enough steps?

5. Am I presenting the stimuli when the client is not paying attention or not making eye contact?

6. Is the patient bored because the same therapy materials are being used too often?

7. Is the client confused because I tend to phrase instructions in the form of requests rather than directions?

8. Am I programming a sufficient variety of target behaviors during each session to maintain the client's interest and motivation level?

9. Am I providing enough prompts/scaffolding during difficult therapy tasks to ensure that the client is relatively successful?

10. Am I allowing the client to make too many errors in a row without modifying the task?

11. Am I telling the patient what he or she does well or giving feedback only about incorrect responses?

Table 1–5
Examples of Terminology

Medical/Hospital Setting	Educational/School Setting
Modified barium swallow study: X-ray images are analyzed by a radiologist and speech-language pathologist (SLP) to evaluate the structure and function of the swallowing mechanism. This is also known as VFSS (videofluoroscopic swallow study).	**Decodable texts:** A type of text used in beginning reading instruction in which words are restricted to spelling patterns that students can already decode given their existing knowledge of letter-sound correspondence.
Fiber-optic endoscopic evaluation of swallowing (FEES): SLP uses a flexible tube with a light attached to evaluate an individual's ability to swallow food/liquid safely and comfortably.	**Differentiated instruction:** Adapting teaching strategies to the needs of individual students or groups of children within a classroom to ensure that all students can learn effectively regardless of ability differences.
Skilled nursing facility (SNF): A facility that primarily provides inpatient care and rehabilitative services but does not provide the level of care or treatment available in a hospital.	**Embedded phonics:** An approach to classroom reading instruction in which letter-sound correspondence training is woven into authentic reading experiences.
Tracheostomy tube: A small plastic tube placed in a surgically created airway opening in the trachea to facilitate breathing.	**Guided reading:** Small-group reading instruction strategy in which teachers use a variety of prompts/scaffolds (e.g., context cues, definitions, word pronunciations) to improve the reading ability of students.
Ventilator: A machine designed to mechanically move breathable air in and out of the lungs.	
Passy-Muir speaking valve (PMSV): A one-way valve that attaches to the outside opening of a tracheostomy tube. It allows air to pass into the tracheostomy but not out through it. The valve opens when the client breathes in, but stays closed during exhalation. This directs airflow around the tube and up through the vocal folds, permitting speech production.	**Language experience approach:** A reading instruction strategy that utilizes the personal experiences of students or a shared class experience to increase young readers' abilities to decode and understand written text.
NG (nasogastric) tube: A long, flexible tube is placed through the nose into the stomach to allow liquid nutrition to be provided to individuals unable to eat by mouth.	**Leveled texts:** A system for organizing texts/books at different difficulty levels. Books are generally categorized by grade level using alphabetic lettering (A to Z) or by stages of difficulty (e.g., Stage 1, Stage 2, etc.).
G (gastrostomy) tube: A tube is placed in a surgically created opening to the stomach to allow nutrition to be provided to individuals unable to eat by mouth.	**Locus of control:** Refers to a person's beliefs about the causes of good and bad predicaments in one's life. There are two main forces: external (fate, luck) and internal (one's own decisions and efforts). Belief in internal forces is associated with high levels of motivation.
Acute rehab: Rehabilitation services provided in a medical setting for patients whose health status requires continued hospitalization.	
Subacute rehab: Programs/facilities that provide comprehensive inpatient rehabilitation services to clients after their discharge from the hospital.	

continues

Table 1–5
continued

Medical/Hospital Setting	Educational/School Setting
NPO: An abbreviation for a Latin term meaning "nothing by mouth."	**Readability:** An estimate of the relative difficulty or ease of a reading passage, based on counting the number of syllables, words, or sentences in a passage. There are three levels:
Arteriovenous malformation (AVM): An abnormal collection of blood vessels that block the flow of blood to brain tissue.	• *Independent:* Level at which student can read without adult support
RUE/LUE: An acronym for right and left upper extremity (i.e., arms).	• *Instructional:* Level at which student can read with adult guidance
Functional independence measure (FIM): A seven-level scale sensitive to client changes over the course of a comprehensive inpatient rehabilitation program.	• *Frustration:* Level at which student cannot read even with adult assistance
Functional assessment measure (FAM): An adjunct set of items to the FIM that specifically address cognitive, behavioral, and communicative skill areas.	**Structural analysis:** A teaching strategy to help students understand the meaning of new words. It involves dividing words into their parts (i.e., roots, prefixes, suffixes) and figuring out the meaning of the word parts.
Cerebrovascular accident (CVA): Damage to brain cells due to the lack of oxygen that occurs when blood flow is impaired by blockage or rupture of an artery. This is also referred to as a *stroke*.	**Think-alouds:** An instructional strategy in which students are asked to say out loud what they are thinking about before, during, and after reading, solving math problems, or responding to questions posed by the teacher or other students. The think-aloud process is first modeled by the teacher to demonstrate practical ways of approaching difficult/new tasks or materials.
ICD codes: Alphanumeric codes that are used to uniformly describe every medical diagnosis, description of symptoms, and cause of death.	**Thinking map:** A type of visual graphic organizer that shows the structure of different text genres (e.g., description, cause–effect, compare–contrast).
CPT codes: Numbers assigned to every task and service a practitioner may provide to a client, including medical, surgical, and rehabilitation diagnostic services.	

12. Am I giving the client enough time to respond before repeating or rephrasing the stimuli?

13. Did I anticipate the unexpected and prepare 50% more material than I thought I needed?

Conclusion

This chapter has presented basic information, protocols, and procedures for intervention for communicative disorders at an *introductory* level. This information is intended only as a starting point in the reader's clinical education and training. For in-depth coverage of this area, the following readings are recommended:

Edwards, M., Stedler-Brown, A., & Houston, K. T. (2012). Expanding use of telepractice in speech-language pathology and audiology. *The Volta Review, 112*(3), 227–242.

Efficacy information on the Internet in speech-language pathology and audiology. (n.d.). http://www .mnsu.edu/comdis/efficacy/efficacy.html

Evidence-based practice. (n.d.). http://www.asha.org/members/ebp/

Hegde, M. N., & Kuyumjian, K. (2019*). Clinical methods and practicum in speech-language pathology* (6th ed.). Plural Publishing.

Paul, R., & Schoen Simmons, E. (2020). *Introduction to clinical methods in communication disorders* (4th ed.). Brookes Publishing.

Speech and Language Forum: Evidence-Based Practice (EBP) Briefs. (n.d.). http://www.speechand language.com/ebp-briefs

Additional Resources

TheraSimplicity
Website: http://www.therasimplicity.com

TheraSimplicity
A series of "books" that allow clinicians to access and print therapy materials such as cards, sequences, photographs, and pictures for a wide range of communication disorders. Also includes a medical encyclopedia and graphics for creating cards, templates, and certificates. Provides information on products in 23 areas (e.g., feeding, motor development).

Tactus Therapy
Website: https://tactustherapy.com

Professional Apps for Speech Therapy
A series of apps designed to target the adult rehabilitation population. A variety of strategies and programs are provided to target skills such as language comprehension, naming, conversation skills, and memory/recall. Programs can be altered to allow clients to receive varying amounts of prompting and supports throughout the treatment process. The programs also enable clients to continue working on therapy targets at home.

Chapter 2

Information Reporting Systems and Techniques

Philosophy

The main purpose of clinical reports is to summarize and interpret information regarding a client's performance or status. In this chapter, the term *report* is used to refer to written records that may vary in length from multiple-page documents to brief notations in client charts. (Note: Many facilities use electronic records; thus, the format of reports may be dictated by the electronic platform that is being used.) A well-written document does more than report test scores and performance data. It provides an explanation of each data point and specifies its relation to a client's overall communication profile and needs. Numbers alone do not yield this interpretive information. Inferential statements always must be substantiated by supporting data. Adherence to this philosophy of clinical writing promotes clinician accountability by providing justification for the judgments and decisions that occur throughout the treatment process.

Accountability also requires that reports be written with ethical considerations in mind. Prognosis and recommendation statements, in particular, must be written carefully to ensure that they are not misleading or unrealistic. For example, consider the following prognostic statement for a 60-year-old male with moderate aphasia who suffered a stroke 10 years ago:

> Based on Mr. Hanks's high level of enthusiasm, the prognosis for improvement in therapy is good.

This statement is inappropriate for two important reasons. First, a client's degree of enthusiasm is not a reliable indicator of future success. Moreover, the amount of time that has elapsed since Mr. Hanks's stroke (a more meaningful indicator) may warrant a more guarded statement of prognosis. Ethical considerations also significantly influence the development of treatment recommendations. These statements must be based on client needs and preferences rather than on the type and frequency of service that a particular therapist or facility can provide.

Technical Writing Style

Clinical reports are formal documents that must be written in an appropriate technical style (Hegde & Davis, 2010). In many cases, written reports may be the first or the only avenue of contact between a speech-language pathologist (SLP) and other professionals. Poorly written reports can severely compromise a clinician's professional credibility. Imagine the reaction of a physician when reading the following section of an SLP's progress report:

> Shirley was initially nervous in the therapy room, particularly when her mother, she thought was going to leave her, she cried. Difficult to illicit spontaneous utterances from her, though she was willing to imitate.

For this reason, the ability to communicate effectively in writing is as important as a clinician's knowledge of communication disorders and their treatment. The following guidelines can assist in the development of professional reports that are clear, concise, and well organized:

- Avoid writing clinical reports in a conversational style (e.g., "He just didn't get the point" versus "He did not appear to understand the task").

- Use correct spelling, grammar, and punctuation, and write in complete sentences.

- Write in the third person (e.g., "The Peabody Picture Vocabulary Test-IV was administered") rather than first person ("I administered the Peabody Picture Vocabulary Test-IV").

- Avoid use of contracted verb forms (e.g., isn't, can't, I've).

- Give the full names of tests on first mention, then use acronyms and other abbreviations in the remainder of the report.

- Express information in behavioral terms (e.g., "followed two-step commands" versus "is able to follow two-step commands").

- Present information (particularly case history) in chronological sequence.

- Differentiate clearly between information reported by others and information obtained directly through clinician observation.

- List all data such as test scores, baseline measures, or progress-monitoring measures before providing any interpretative statements. This approach facilitates interpretation of a client's overall profile rather than presenting unrelated descriptions of isolated communication skills.

- Include information about a client's strengths as well as weaknesses in the body of the report.

- In any report, avoid presenting information in the summary section that was not introduced previously in the body of the report.

- Write reports to communicate with colleagues using professional terminology, but include simple explanations and clear examples to make reports meaningful to family members and other nonprofessionals.

- Use language that is specific and unambiguous (e.g., "He demonstrated language skills characteristic of 4-year-old children" rather than "He demonstrated poor language skills").

- Avoid exaggeration and overstatement (e.g., "*completely* uncooperative," "*absolutely* intelligible," "never produces /s/," "*extremely* motivated").

Report Formats

In the context of intervention, clinical reports serve three main purposes: (a) to outline the intended intervention plan at the beginning of therapy, (b) to document client performance on a session-to-session basis throughout the course of treatment, and (c) to summarize client status periodically and at the end of the treatment program. Report formats for each of these functions can vary greatly among clinicians and service-delivery settings. Regardless of the particular format, however, a basic core of information is important in each of the three types of reports. Following is a framework for each report type.

Initial Therapy Plan

An **initial therapy plan (ITP)** is developed at the beginning of treatment for each client. It specifies long-term goals and short-term objectives based on diagnostic findings and pretreatment baseline results. Following are the basic content and organization of an ITP.

Identifying Information

List identifying information at the top of the report. This section may include a client's name, age, address, type of disorder, date of report, and so on.

Example	
Name: José Rodríguez	Date of Birth: July 15, 2016
Parents: Carlos and María Rodríguez	Age: 7 years, 2 months
Address: 1800 Knox Street	Category: Language/Articulation
College Park, MD 20740	Graduate Clinician: Gary Frost
Phone: (301) 555-2379	Clinical Supervisor: Melanie Barr, MA,
Date of Report: 09/25/23	CCC-SLP

Background Information/Pertinent History

In paragraph form, state the full name and age of the client, note the location and date of the initial evaluation, and summarize highlights of relevant diagnostic information in a few sentences. If the client was referred from another source, give the date, referral source, and reason for referral. For clients who have received previous therapy, this section should specify the provider, identify the dates of most recent service, and briefly summarize goals and progress.

> **Example**
>
> José is a 7-year-old boy who was first seen at the University of Maryland Speech and Hearing Clinic for a diagnostic evaluation in March 2023. At the time of this testing, José demonstrated a number of language and articulation difficulties, including weaknesses in oral expression. José's parents are bilingual, and Spanish is sometimes spoken in the home. However, they identify José's primary language as English. José is currently in the second grade at Maple Elementary School. He is reportedly doing well in school.
>
> Past therapy began on January 15, 2023, in his elementary school and focused on the production of fricatives (v, z, th), consonant blends, regular plurals, and irregular past tense. These are no longer notable areas of difficulty for José. He did not demonstrate mastery on goals that focused on vowel + /r/ production and irregular plurals.

Goals and Objectives

In outline form, record pertinent speech-language goals and objectives in a hierarchy of complexity ranging from least to most difficult. (Recall that goals are general statements of desired outcomes over the course of the treatment program, whereas objectives specify measurable behaviors that lead to mastery of the long-term goals.) Under each long-term goal, specify relevant test results/baseline data that have been collected and used as the basis for development of the short-term objectives. Baseline data are generally obtained over the initial therapy sessions. Make note of any unusual or clinically significant behavior patterns. Materials and procedures generally are not included as part of this section.

Example

Articulation

Goal I: To improve production of /ɚ/ in spontaneous speech

Initial Status/Baseline 9/23/23

0% accuracy for spontaneous speech

45% of /ɚ/ productions were at a rating of 2 on a 3-point scale, when produced imitatively in isolation

Note: Productions were scored on a 3-point scale, where 1 = "uh" and 3 = accurate production.

Objectives

A. Given visual and verbal prompts for correct tongue positioning, José will pronounce /ɚ/ imitatively in isolation at a rating of 3 in 9 out of 10 trials over two consecutive sessions.

B. Given pictures or printed stimuli, José will spontaneously produce /ɚ/ in the initial and final position of words, with a rating of 3 in 9 out of 10 trials over two consecutive sessions.

C. Given pictures or printed stimuli, José will produce /ɚ/ in the initial and final position of words in carrier phrases, with a rating of 3 in 9 out of 10 trials over two consecutive sessions.

D. Given pictures, printed stimuli, or objects, José will produce /ɚ/ in the initial and final positions of words in spontaneous sentences during structured activities, with a rating of 3 in 9 out of 10 trials over two consecutive sessions.

E. Given a variety of stimulus prompts (e.g., pictures, objects), José will produce /ɚ/ in the initial and final position of words in structured discourse with a rating of 3 in 9 out of 10 trials over two consecutive sessions.

Language

Goal I: To use irregular plurals in spontaneous speech

(Target set: *sheep, fish, deer, feet, teeth, children, women, men, geese, mice, knives, loaves, wives, wolves, calves, thieves, halves, shelves, leaves*)

Initial Status/Baseline 9/23/23

15% correct plural form at the single-word level, given picture prompts

Objectives

A. José will provide the correct irregular plural, given a singular word from the target set, with 90% accuracy over two consecutive sessions.

B. José will use irregular plurals in carrier phrases, when given a singular word from the target set, with 90% accuracy over two consecutive sessions.

C. José will use irregular plurals in spontaneous sentences, when given a singular word from the target set, with 90% accuracy over two consecutive sessions.

D. José will use irregular plurals in structured discourse, given a set of singular words from the target set, with 90% accuracy over two consecutive sessions.

Reinforcement

In paragraph form, indicate the type and schedule of reinforcers to be used for shaping target productions and attending behaviors.

Example

A continuous schedule of verbal reinforcement, coupled with token reinforcers, will be used to shape target behaviors. This will be faded to an intermittent schedule as José demonstrates progress. A separate response-cost system will be used to reduce José's tendency to initiate responses prematurely.

Family Engagement

In paragraph form, discuss how family members will be involved in observation of therapy sessions, conferences/counseling, and homework.

Example

Parent(s) will observe José's therapy sessions at least once every 2 weeks. Brief, informal discussions of José's progress will take place following every session; formal conferences will be held every 3 months. Periodic training will be provided to help parents participate in homework assignments.

Generalization Plan

In paragraph form, specify strategies for transfer of target objectives to home, school, or work settings.

> **Example**
>
> José will be given weekly homework assignments to facilitate the generalization of target behaviors. The parent will be provided with written instructions for these assignments. The clinician will also contact José's teacher bimonthly to discuss his status and to give suggestions for how therapy objectives can be incorporated into the classroom.
>
> The initial therapy plan can be viewed as the clinician's best prediction of what a client can accomplish in a given amount of time. The client's progress in therapy should be monitored on a periodic basis through the administration of probes to determine whether the plan's original objectives remain appropriate or require modification. (A complete sample ITP is included in Appendix 2–A on the companion website.)

Session Notes

Once therapy has begun, client performance is documented on an ongoing basis. Session notes are short and are written during or after each session. They may be filed in a client's medical chart or a client's folder or written on the therapy plan itself. Daily notes serve at least three important functions: (a) they enable the clinician to monitor the treatment program on a continual basis and implement any necessary changes immediately, (b) they provide information on a daily basis to other professionals who also may be working with the client (e.g., occupational therapist, social worker), and (c) they facilitate the continuity of treatment by allowing another clinician to provide services in the event of unexpected clinician absence.

One common format of daily session notes, particularly in medical settings, is known as SOAP notes. **SOAP** is an acronym that refers to the terms *subjective, objective, assessment,* and *plan.*

Subjective: Write your opinion regarding relevant client behavior or status in a brief statement.

Objective: Record data collected for each task during the therapy session.

Assessment: Interpret data for the current session and compare to client's previous levels of performance.

Plan: Identify proposed therapy targets for the next session.

> **Example**
>
> S: José appeared tired and reluctant to cooperate with the tasks presented.
>
> O: Final /ɚ/ in single words = 85% (17/20); irregular plurals in spontaneous phrases = 50% (20/40).
>
> A: Fading of clinician model to a 5:1 ratio on irregular plural task may have been premature. Today's score of 50% constitutes a decrease in accuracy compared to José's performance of the same task over the two previous sessions (70% and 75%).

> P: Continue work on both tasks at the same levels, but increase clinician modeling for the irregular plural task to a 2:1 ratio..

Progress and Final Reports

A report is written for each patient at specific intervals throughout treatment and when intervention services are terminated. These reports also may be referred to as interim summaries, annual reviews, discharge reports, or final summaries, depending on the clinical setting. Progress and final reports document a client's mastery of the goals and objectives outlined in the ITP and implemented over the course of treatment. Following are the basic content and organization of these reports.

Identifying Information

List identifying information at the top of the report. This section may include a client's name, age, address, type of disorder, dates of service, date of report, and so on.

Example

Name: José Rodríguez
Parents: Carlos and María Rodríguez
Address: 1800 Knox Street
College Park, MD 20740
Service Dates: October 13, 2023 to
               November 21, 2024

Date of Birth: July 15, 2016
Age: 8 years, 4 months
Date of Report: November 25, 2024
Disorder: Articulation and Language
Graduate Clinician: Gary Frost
Clinical Supervisor: Melanie Barr, MA,
                     CCC-SLP

Background Information/Statement of Problem

In paragraph form, state the full name and age of the client and include the following information: (a) date of first therapy session, (b) client's speech and language status at that time, and (c) session frequency and duration. In some cases, it may be useful to include a brief description of previous therapy goals.

Example

José is an 8-year-old boy who was first seen at the University of Maryland Hearing and Speech Clinic for a diagnostic evaluation in March 2023. At the time of the initial diagnosis, José demonstrated language and articulation difficulties. He began therapy during the fall semester of 2023 and has continued through the present. He has been seen twice weekly for 50-min sessions. Past therapy has included the production of fricatives (v, z, th) and consonant blends, regular plurals, and irregular past tense. These are no longer areas of notable difficulty for José. José began therapy for the fall 2023 semester on October 13. Producing vowel + /r/ (e.g., mother) continues to be a target for therapy. Work on irregular plurals was added as a target this semester.

Therapy Objectives and Progress

In outline form, restate all the short-term objectives listed for each goal in the ITP, indicate the client's level of mastery for each objective, and cite supporting data for mastery for each objective. Compare the client's current performance levels to the pretreatment baseline data for that target area. Comment on the degree of improvement represented by this comparison (e.g., significant, moderate, minimal). Note any special procedures, strategies, tasks, or cues that facilitated the client's performance.

Example

Articulation

Note: Productions were scored on a 3-point scale, where 1 = "uh" and 3 = accurate production.

Objectives

A. Given visual and verbal prompts for correct tongue positioning, José will pronounce /ɚ/ imitatively in isolation, with a rating of 3 in 9 out of 10 trials over two consecutive sessions (in progress: 89% on 11/18, 86% on 11/24).

B. Given pictures or printed stimuli, José will spontaneously produce /ɚ/ in the initial and final positions of words, with a rating of 3 in 9 out of 10 trials over two consecutive sessions. [Not yet addressed]

C. Given pictures or printed stimuli, José will produce /ɚ/ in the initial and final positions of words in carrier phrases, with a rating of 3 in 9 out of 10 trials over two consecutive sessions. [Not yet addressed]

D. Given pictures, printed stimuli, or objects, José will produce /ɚ/ in the initial and final positions of words in spontaneous sentences during structured activities, with a rating of 3 in 9 out of 10 trials over two consecutive sessions. [Not yet addressed]

E. Given a variety of stimulus prompts (e.g., pictures, objects), José will produce /ɚ/ in the initial and final positions of words in structured discourse with a rating of 3 in 9 out of 10 trials over two consecutive sessions. [Not yet addressed]

Comments

José demonstrates the ability to describe where his tongue should be in order to say /ɚ/ correctly. He has made moderate progress in improving his /ɚ/ sounds in isolation, although he continues to need occasional prompting to achieve a rating of 3. On occasion, he can produce the sound accurately at the word level, particularly when /ɚ/ occurs in the final position. José lifts his tongue up at the back of his palate while not holding the sides of his tongue to the hard palate near his teeth. The method José seemed to find most successful in facilitating correct productions was moving from an /i/ sound into an /ɚ/ sound by sliding his tongue back along the palate.

Language

Objectives

 A. José will provide the correct irregular plural, given a singular word from the target set, with 90% accuracy over two consecutive sessions (criterion met at 100% accuracy on 10/23 for first half of the set and 11/18 for the second half of the set).

 B. José will use irregular plurals in carrier phrases, when given a singular word from the target set, with 90% accuracy over two consecutive sessions (criterion met at 100% accuracy on 10/28 for first half of the set and 11/24 for the second half of the set).

 C. José will use irregular plurals in spontaneous sentences, when given a singular word from the target set, with 90% accuracy over two consecutive sessions (criterion met at 100% accuracy on 11/12 for first half of the set and 12/5 for the second half of the set).

 D. José will use irregular plurals in structured discourse, given a set of singular words from the target set, with 90% accuracy over two consecutive sessions (criterion met at 100% for all 20 words on 12/7).

Comments

José was familiar with the concept of plurals from previous therapy; however, he was not familiar with plural formation that did not follow the usual rules. Requiring José to write down the plural forms of regular plurals and target words from the set helped him differentiate these forms. Once he was familiar with the new words, they were practiced using a variety of game formats. For example, for the carrier-phrase level, José played Go Fish and asked questions such as, "Do you have any *geese*?" When working at the structured-discourse level, José formulated short stories using the target words; this was a particularly functional activity for him, because he enjoys telling stories.

Summary and Additional Information

Summarize all of the preceding "criterion met" statements. This summary should provide an overall profile of the client's progress over time rather than a simple reiteration of previously stated information. In separate paragraphs, include information about the following:

- Reinforcement (for both targets and attending behaviors)

- Completion of homework assignments

- Family participation/observation

- Parent/client conferences

- Other pertinent issues, such as results of additional testing, significant medical information (e.g., changes in medication), change in educational placement, and so on

> ### Example
>
> Overall, José has made moderate progress in improving his pronunciation of /ɚ/ this semester. His knowledge and use of irregular plurals has improved considerably; he learned the set of target words very quickly and was able to generalize to other contexts. From a functional perspective, José's parents report that his general intelligibility seems to have improved based on the increasing number of verbal messages he conveys without adult and peer requests for clarification or repetition.
>
> A continuous verbal reinforcement schedule was used to establish target behaviors. As accuracy improved, an intermittent schedule was introduced. A behavior-management system was implemented, in which José was given 10 tokens at the beginning of each session. He was told that these could be traded in at the end of the session for a small prize. However, one token would be subtracted from his pile for each instance of noncompliant behavior (e.g., off-task talking) during therapy activities.
>
> Homework practice was assigned weekly. Mrs. Rodríguez reported working with José on homework assignments on a daily basis. Mrs. Rodríguez observed a therapy session at least once every 2 weeks. José's progress was discussed with her informally after each session and formally during parent conferences held every 3 months.

Recommendations

State whether continued speech-language intervention is warranted. If so, give suggestions for specific goals and objectives. Make any other pertinent recommendations (e.g., psychological testing).

> ### Example
>
> It is recommended that José continue to participate in speech and language therapy primarily to improve his vowel + /r/ pronunciation. José learns rules and patterns quickly; therefore, it is felt that specific syntax and word-usage problems that may arise in his spontaneous speech can be addressed successfully in the school setting.

A complete sample progress report is included in Appendix 2–B on the companion website.

Tips for Proofreading Clinical Reports

Students, beginning clinicians, and supervisors can use the following set of proofreading questions to edit and monitor the quality of clinical reports:

- Are spelling, grammar, and punctuation correct?
- Are professional terms used accurately?
- Is there redundancy of word usage or sentence type?

- Are any sentences too lengthy, rambling, or unfocused?

- Is all the important client information included in the report?

- Is information presented only in the germane sections of the report (e.g., no recommendation statements in the background information section)?

- Does the report follow a logical sequence from one section to the next (i.e., from background, to data and interpretation, to summary and recommendations)?

- Are raw data interpreted and not merely reported?

- Are all conclusions and assumptions supported by sufficient data?

- Are speculative statements explicitly identified as such?

- Does the report contain seemingly contradictory statements without adequate explanation?

- Is the wording clear, or are some statements vague and ambiguous?

- Is content presented with appropriate emphasis? Has any critical information been overlooked? Has any minor point been overemphasized?

- Is the report written with ethical/legal considerations in mind?

Individualized Education Program

The Education of All Handicapped Children Act (PL 94-142) was passed in 1975 to ensure that all children ages 3 to 21 years with special needs receive a free, appropriate public education (FAPE). Speech-language pathology is a designated special education service under this law. This legislation was most recently reauthorized in 2011 through PL 108-446 and is known as the Individuals with Disabilities Education Improvement Act (IDEA). Final regulations for Part B of this legislation were released in 2006. These regulations pertain to services in school settings.

Each eligible child must have an annual written **Individualized Education Program (IEP)**, which documents the need for the provision of special education services. The purpose of this program is to identify specific areas for remediation. Unlike other clinical reports, the IEP generally does not include a description of the actual intervention procedures that will be used to accomplish the specified annual goals.

The IEP is generated as part of a process that begins with a referral. A comprehensive assessment is then conducted by an appointed team, and the findings are reviewed at a meeting of all involved parties (including therapists, teachers, and parents). The participants develop and approve a written IEP, which is implemented over the subsequent school year and reviewed periodically. When speech-language therapy is the sole or primary special education service to be provided, the SLP may assume principal responsibility for writing the IEP. (For an overview, summary, and questions and answers about IDEA and the IEP process, see the American Speech-Language-Hearing Association's website).

To ensure a measure of uniformity and accountability nationwide, federal law requires that all IEPs contain the following basic information:

- *Present levels of academic achievement and functional performance:* This section of the document describes how the disability affects the child's involvement and progress in the general education curriculum. For preschool children, this section describes how the disability affects the child's participation in appropriate activities. For speech-language pathology, test scores and clinical analysis of observed performance are presented.

- *Measurable annual goals:* These goals must be linked to academic and functional performance within the general education curriculum. There is no mandate concerning the number of goals that must be included in an IEP.

- *Progress monitoring:* This section of the IEP describes how the child's progress toward the annual goals will be measured. It also specifies when periodic progress reports will be provided.

- *Special education and related services:* This section identifies the special services needed by the child to achieve the annual goals. Statements about needed supplementary aids, services, and program modifications must be included.

- *Placement recommendation and justification:* This section indicates the specific educational setting into which preschool or school-age children will be placed. By law, this setting must be the **least restrictive environment (LRE)** that provides an appropriate education to meet a child's individualized needs. LRE means that, to the maximum extent possible, children with disabilities are educated with children who have no disabilities. Recommendations for placements other than a general education classroom in the child's home school must be accompanied by a written rationale. (Eligibility requirements vary among local educational agencies.) There should be a description of the *extent* to which the child will receive educational services with nondisabled peers. Parents must be participating members of teams that make placement decisions.

- *Individual accommodations:* This section of an IEP describes the accommodations necessary to measure the child's academic achievement and functional performance on statewide and district-wide assessments. Any recommendation for alternate assessment measures must specify the tools to be used.

- *Initiation and duration of services:* The IEP must state the projected date for the beginning of services/modifications as well as the anticipated frequency, location, and duration of these services.

These seven categories comprise the basic structure of an IEP. Individual states or local educational agencies may impose additional requirements pertaining to format or content information such as formal or informal plans for transition to postsecondary or employment settings. These plans identify the accommodations/modifications needed by the student to successfully meet expectations within the setting.

Due Process

IDEA (2011) provides legal and procedural safeguards throughout the educational placement process, including timelines for completion of each step, parental notification and consent, and an appeal system to ensure due process for all parties involved. The parent or responsible party must be notified prior to any changes in a child's educational program. The due process system provides a formal mechanism for parents to protest decisions they consider inappropriate or unfair to their child.

Individualized Family Service Plan

In 1986, the federal mandate for a free and appropriate education was extended by enactment of PL 99-457 (Part H) to include infants and toddlers with special needs between birth and 3 years of age. Updated in 2011, Part C of this legislation is notable for its emphasis on the importance of early intervention.

This legislation requires the development of an **Individualized Family Service Plan (IFSP)**, which is similar to an IEP. It differs from the IEP in that its main focus is on the family as a unit rather than solely on the child. The written document must include the following components:

- *Statement of child's present level of development:* This section provides information on physical, cognitive, communicative, and social/emotional status.

- *Statement of family resources, priorities, and concerns:* This section includes a statement of the impact that the child's developmental delay has on family functioning. In addition, individual families can specify their desired levels of involvement in the intervention plan.

- *Major outcomes:* This section identifies the goals, criteria, procedures, and timelines anticipated to be achieved for the child and family.

- *Specific early intervention services:* This section provides a statement of the services necessary to meet the child's and family's unique needs. It should include the frequency, intensity, location, and method of service delivery.

- *Natural environment:* This section describes the environments in which services will be provided. The extent to which services will not be provided in authentic settings must be justified.

- *Service coordinator/provider:* The IFSP specifically identifies the individual from the profession most relevant to the needs of the infant and family. This case manager is responsible for the development of the IFSP and for implementation, coordination, and monitoring of all services. The SLP is frequently named as service coordinator for infants and toddlers whose primary developmental delay consists of communication or feeding/oral-motor impairments.

- *Transition plan:* This section outlines the procedures that will be employed to facilitate the transition to services provided under PL 108-446 if the child continues to need special services beyond age 2 years, 11 months.

In addition to the differences just outlined, this legislation extends eligibility to "at-risk" youngsters rather than restricting services to children with recognized disabilities. Moreover, these services can be provided through agencies outside the public school system (e.g., community agencies). PL 108-446 also contains provisions for home-based instruction as well as family education and counseling. The IFSP is reviewed every 6 months rather than annually.

504 Plan

Students who do not meet the eligibility requirements for an IEP often need some assistance to participate fully in general school settings. These students may be candidates for a 504 plan authorized through the Americans with Disabilities Act Amendments Act (2008). The **504 plans** specify accommodations that allow students to complete the same assignments as their peers without altering the content of tasks or tests. Examples of potential accommodations include the following:

Presentation:	Provide audio recording
	Provide materials in large print
	Reduce number of items per page or line
	Present instructions orally
	Provide on-task, focusing prompts
	Provide positive behavioral supports
Response:	Allow for oral responses
	Allow for answers to be dictated
	Permit responses to be given via computer
	Permit answers to be recorded directly into test booklet
Timing:	Allow frequent breaks
	Extend allotted time for test taking and assignments
Setting:	Provide preferential seating
	Provide special lighting or acoustics
	Provide space with minimal distractions
	Administer tests in small-group setting or private room
Test Scheduling:	Administer tests over several sessions or days
	Allow subtests to be taken in different order

Professional Correspondence

In addition to clinical treatment reports, SLPs often interact with other professionals and agencies through written correspondence. These documents may vary with respect to length, content, and format, but all professional correspondence should be written in a clear, concise manner with correct spelling, grammar, and punctuation. Typically, written correspondence involves authorizing the release of information, making referrals to other professionals, and acknowledging referrals from colleagues.

Health Insurance Portability and Accountability Act

HIPAA is the acronym for the Health Insurance Portability and Accountability Act of 1996. For detailed information on the major components of this legislation, refer to the U.S. Department of Health and Human Services website (https://www.hhs.gov/hipaa/index.html). The component that addresses standards for privacy of **protected health information (PHI)** is most relevant to discussion in this chapter. PHI is *individually identifiable* health information created, received, transmitted, and/ or maintained by health care entities. These standards, which became effective in 2003 and were updated in 2013, are designed to regulate the storage, transmission, and confidentiality of personal patient information, which may include the following:

- Information in a client's file

- Conversations with others about a client's care or treatment

- Information about the client contained in his or her health insurer's data system

- Billing information

Within our profession, HIPAA regulations are applicable to a variety of settings, such as a private practice, school, nursing home, hospital, clinic, and other milieus, including distance services. In general, providers may use PHI for treatment, payment, and health care operations without special permission from clients. Written consent from the client is required for marketing, fundraising, or research activities. If there is a need to share PHI beyond these parameters, the Privacy Rules provide guidelines for how reports should be "de-identified" in order to protect the patient/client. The following list of types of information that should be omitted is adapted from the U.S. Department of Health and Human Services website. Please refer to this website for more detailed discussion and rationales for the following de-identification items:

- Names

- Street address, city, county, precinct, zip code, and their equivalent geocodes

- Telephone and fax numbers

- Email addresses and internet protocol (IP) addresses

- Medical record or health plan numbers

- Social Security numbers

- Photographs or other images

Health care providers are required to provide clients with a written description of how confidential information will be handled. This **Notice of Privacy Practices (NPP)** should be reviewed, signed, and dated by the client/legal guardian prior to the initiation of services. Forms 2–1 and 2–2 show a sample NPP and acknowledgment statement. Forms 2–3 and 2–4 show a reproducible release of information authorization form and sample referral letter and acknowledgment form. Additional information and frequently asked questions (FAQs) on PHI can be found in Appendix 2–C on the companion website.

Form 2-1. SAMPLE NOTICE OF PRIVACY PRACTICES

NOTICE OF PRIVACY PRACTICES

As Defined by the Privacy Regulations of the
Federal Health Insurance Portability and Accountability Act of 2013 (HIPAA)
PLEASE REVIEW THIS NOTICE CAREFULLY

I. OUR COMMITMENT TO YOUR PRIVACY

The Hearing and Speech clinic at the University of Maryland is dedicated to maintaining the privacy of your protected health information (PHI). PHI is individually identifiable health information about you that relates to your past, present, or future physical or mental health or other condition, as well as any related health care services. This Notice of Privacy Practices provides you with the following important information: our obligations concerning your PHI, how we may use and disclose your PHI, and your rights with regard to your PHI.

A. OUR OBLIGATION   The Hearing and Speech Clinic has chosen to abide by federal and state laws requiring that the privacy of your PHI be maintained. By complying with these laws, we are required to provide you with this notice regarding our privacy practices, our legal duties, and your rights concerning your PHI. Except for student records and certain records the University creates or receives in its role as an employer, this Notice of Privacy Practices applies to all records containing your PHI that are created or retained by the Hearing and Speech Clinic. A copy of the Notice of Privacy Practices will be posted in a visible location in the Hearing and Speech Clinic waiting room at all times, and you may request a copy of the Notice at any time.

B. WE MAY USE AND DISCLOSE YOUR PROTECTED HEALTH INFORMATION (PHI) IN THE FOLLOWING WAYS (NOT ALL POSSIBLE SITUATIONS ARE COVERED)

- *For treatment, payment, and health care operations, to third-party business associates (e.g., billing services), for health-related services, to individuals involved in your care, under some circumstances for research purposes, when required or allowed by law, with your written authorization.*

II. YOUR RIGHTS REGARDING YOUR PHI

You have the following rights regarding your PHI, and you may request any of the following:

- *Confidential communications, restriction of communication to individuals otherwise permitted by law to inspect your PHI, inspection and copies of personal records, amendments to your PHI if you believe the information is incorrect or incomplete, a list of disclosures we have made of your PHI, and a copy of this Notice.*

III. IMPLEMENTATION, COMPLAINTS, AND QUESTIONS

A. IMPLEMENTATION   This Notice provides a general overview of our privacy practices. This Notice and our privacy practices are implemented in accordance with applicable University policies and procedures and the requirements of HIPAA and other federal and Maryland laws, as applicable.

B. COMPLAINTS   If you believe your privacy rights have been violated, you may file a complaint with the Hearing and Speech Clinic. All complaints must be submitted in writing. We will not retaliate against you in any way if you file a complaint with us.

IV. CONTACT INFORMATION

If you have any questions regarding this Notice or our health information privacy practices, please contact:

Director of Hearing and Speech Clinic: _____

Address: _____

E-mail: _____   Phone: _____

Form 2-2. SAMPLE ACKNOWLEDGMENT OF PRIVACY PRACTICES NOTICE

ACKNOWLEDGMENT OF RECEIPT
HEARING AND SPEECH CLINIC NOTICE OF PRIVACY PRACTICES

I acknowledge that I have received a copy of the University of Maryland Hearing and Speech Clinic's Notice of Privacy Practices.

_____   _____   _____
Printed Name   Signature   Date

- -

FOR INTERNAL USE ONLY

Client declined to provide signature for acknowledging receipt of privacy practices

_____
(Clinic staff signature and date)

Client was not able to provide signature for acknowledging receipt of privacy practices

_____
(Clinic staff signature and date)

Form 2-3. AUTHORIZATION FOR RELEASE OF INFORMATION FROM ANOTHER AGENCY OR PHYSICIAN

The following person has requested the services of our facility: _____.
We understand that this individual has been seen by you. Please forward any hearing, speech, language, medical, psychological, educational, or social records regarding this individual. Below is written authorization for the release of these records. Please send this information to the attention of _____ at the following address:

_____

_____

_____

Thank you for your cooperation.

This will certify that you have my permission to release information concerning

_____

(Client Name)

to the following facility: _____

Signature: _____ Date: _____

Form 2-4. AUTHORIZATION FOR RELEASE OF INFORMATION TO ANOTHER AGENCY OR PHYSICIAN

Name: _____ Date of Birth: _____

I hereby consent to the release of any and all hearing, speech, and language records concerning the above-named individual to:

Name/Agency: _____

Address: _____

_____

_____

_____

Signature: _____ Date: _____

Form 2-5. REFERRAL LETTER FORMAT

Date: _____

Name of Recipient: _____

Address: _____

Dear _____,

_____ is being referred to you for _____

_____.

He/she was seen at our facility for _____

_____ on/from _____.

His/her communication status is characterized by _____.

I am making this referral because _____

_____. Enclosed please find a copy of _____

_____, along with the client's written authorization for the release of this

information. If you have any questions, please contact me at _____

_____.

Sincerely,

_____

Signature and Title

Form 2-6. SAMPLE REFERRAL LETTER

April 25, 2023

Timothy Anderson, MD
866 Manor Drive
College Park, MD 20742

Dear Dr. Anderson,

Kevin Walters is being referred to you for a laryngoscopic examination. He was seen at our facility for a voice evaluation on April 24, 2023. His communication status is characterized by harsh voice quality, intermittent aphonia, and accompanying throat pain.

I am making this referral to verify Mr. Walter's medical status prior to the initiation of therapy services. Enclosed please find a copy of the diagnostic report, along with the client's written authorization for the release of this information. If you have any questions, please contact me at (301) 555-1212.

Sincerely,

Mary Ann Schilling, MS, CCC-SLP
Speech-Language Pathologist

Form 2-7. ACKNOWLEDGMENT OF REFERRAL FORMAT

Date: _____

Name of Recipient: _____

Address: _____

Dear _____,

    Thank you for referring _____ to our clinic.

He/she was seen for _____

on/from _____.

    I have enclosed a copy of my full report, including recommendations regarding future services.

If you have any questions, please do not hesitate to contact me at _____

_____.

    We appreciate your referral and look forward to continued collaboration with you.

Sincerely,

_____

Signature and Title

Form 2–8. SAMPLE REFERRAL ACKNOWLEDGMENT

April 27, 2023

Kitty Davidson, MD
31 Rose Lane
Kendall, FL 02113

Dear Dr. Davidson,

Thank you for referring Barbara Hawley to our clinic. She was seen for an initial speech and language evaluation on April 18, 2023.

I have enclosed a copy of my full report, including recommendations regarding future services. If you have any questions, please do not hesitate to contact me at (305) 555-1846.

We appreciate your referral and look forward to continued collaboration with you.

Sincerely,

Marian Kirley, MA, CCC-SLP
Speech-Language Pathologist

Additional Resources

A Guide to Clinical Assessment and Professional Report Writing in Speech-Language Pathology, Second Edition

Stein-Rubin, C., & Fabus, R. (2018); Slack Incorporated.

Stein-Rubin and Fabus wrote this guide with the intent of combining diagnostic protocols with report writing techniques to assist clinicians in report writing. It covers areas such as differential diagnosis, interview questions, and informal and formal assessment measures.

The SLP's IDEA Companion, Third Edition

A resource for goals and objectives that match the guidelines outlined in the Individuals with Disabilities Education Act (IDEA). Therapy goals link to the classroom curriculum, and appropriate benchmarks for students and levels of performance are determined using the baseline measures provided in the book. Classroom expectations are provided for grades K–12 in the areas of fluency, semantics, syntax, voice, word finding, pragmatics, phonological awareness, oral-motor skills, articulation, and narrative/expository writing.

Report Writing for Speech-Language Pathologists and Audiologists, Second Edition

This is a resource that describes all the necessary information to be included in reports of various types. There is information about referral acknowledgements, diagnostic evaluation reports, integrated diagnostic reports, treatment plans and reports, IEPs, and progress reports.

A Coursebook on Scientific and Professional Writing for Speech-Language Pathology, Fifth Edition

An interactive resource manual designed to help students, clinicians, and instructors master technical writing skills as well as professional writing skills. Includes worksheets of practice exercises for each topic.

Part Two

Providing Treatment for Communication Disorders

Chapter 3

Intervention for Articulation and Phonology in Children

This chapter focuses on the management of articulation and phonological disorders demonstrated by children. An **articulation** model emphasizes the motor component of speech, whereas a **phonologic** orientation stresses the linguistic aspect of speech production. Most articulation approaches focus on the incorrect production of individual phonemes, traditionally classified as substitution, omission, and distortion errors. In contrast, phonological approaches concentrate on rule-based errors that affect multiple speech sounds that follow a predictable pattern. The phonological system governs the ways in which sounds in a language can be combined to form words. Children with phonologically based problems demonstrate difficulty in applying sound-system rules, not necessarily in production of the sounds. These children do not simply possess an incomplete system of speech sounds; rather, their errors have logical and coherent principles underlying their occurrence.

Articulation disorders can be classified as functional or organic in nature. Articulation disorders are considered **functional** when no known pathology is causing the errors. Children with functional articulation disorders demonstrate speech production errors in the absence of any identifiable etiology. These children present with adequate hearing acuity and intellectual abilities and with no signs of significant structural abnormalities or neurological dysfunction. The specific errors displayed vary greatly from one child to the next and are not as readily predictable as those found in organically based disorders. **Organic** disorders result from known physical causes, such as cleft palate, neurological dysfunction, or hearing impairment. Some children may demonstrate both functional and organic deficits.

The information provided in this chapter is based on Standard American English. (See Appendix B on the companion website for International Phonetic Alphabet symbols.) It is imperative that clinicians take a child's cultural and linguistic background into account in determining whether the production of a given speech sound represents an error or a dialectal difference. (See Chapter 12 for more about multicultural and English-language learner treatment.)

Treatment Approaches

There are a variety of phonetic (i.e., articulation) and phonological (i.e., linguistic rules) approaches to intervention. Williams et al. (2010) identified 23 approaches that have been utilized in the treatment of speech sound disorders and Cabbage and DeVeney (2020) identified some considerations and approaches commonly used by speech-language pathologists (SLPs) in school settings. Some approaches place heavy emphasis on perceptual/sound discrimination (Cabbage & Hitchcock, 2022) while others focus mainly on sound production (DeVeney & Peterkin, 2022). Selected examples of classic and more recent remediation approaches are described in the following sections.

Traditional (Van Riper, 1978)

This phonetic approach to intervention is also known as the sensory-perceptual or motor-based approach. It relies on sensory training (i.e., auditory discrimination or "ear-training") either before or concurrently with speech production training to provide the client with an internal standard with which to compare correct versus incorrect productions of sounds. The typical sequence for training in the traditional approach involves (a) speech sound discrimination training, including identification, isolation, and bombardment of specific target sounds; (b) achieving phonetic placement of the articulators for the sound; (c) producing the sound in isolation; (d) producing the sound in nonsense syllables; (e) producing the sound in the initial, medial, and final positions of words; (f) producing the sound in phrases and sentences; and (g) producing the sound in conversational speech. It incorporates several teaching strategies, such as imitation, multisensory cues for phonetic placement and production, and successive approximation. For more detailed information on this approach, see Bauman-Waengler (2016) and Rvachew et al. (2004).

Motor Kinesthetic (Stinchfield-Hawk & Young, 1938)

This phonetic approach emphasizes development of correct movement patterns and requires the clinician to manipulate the articulators to facilitate sound production. This method is based on the assumption that it is possible to establish positive kinesthetic and tactile feedback patterns through direct manipulation of the client's articulators. As a result of the feedback, the client is helped to recognize and then to produce the movements of speech. In this approach, the basic unit of therapy is the isolated sound; only later are words and sentence patterns introduced and established. A more recent iteration of the motor-kinesthetic philosophy concept is PROMPT, which stands for Prompts for Restructuring Oral Muscular Phonetic Targets (Chumpelik, 1984). Originally developed for children with severe speech motor production difficulties, PROMPT is a multidimensional approach that incorporates three main domains: motor-sensory, cognitive-linguistic, and social-emotional. Speech production is facilitated through the use of tactile cues that focus on jaw height, labial/facial positioning, and mylohyoid posture for each sound/word (Grigos et al., 2010; Hayden et al., 2010). The program is highly structured, and therapists must be trained/certified through the PROMPT Institute (https://www.promptinstitute.com) in order to utilize this therapy approach. In summary, the motor-kinetic method also advocates for the use of tactile, kinesthetic, and proprioceptive cues to facilitate "motor maps" for production of individual speech sounds. For additional information and techniques, see Dale and Hayden (2013), Dodd and Bradford (2000), Sugden et al. (2019), Ward et al. (2014), and Yu et al. (2018).

Distinctive Features (McReynolds & Bennett, 1972)

Distinctive feature therapy is a phonological approach based on the theory that speech sounds can be defined in terms of articulatory patterns and acoustic properties. Each phoneme in a language consists of a bundle of binary features in which the presence or absence of these features is specified (e.g., +voicing/–voicing, +nasal/–nasal, +continuancy/–continuancy; Jakobson, 1968). Some phonemes, such as /t/ and /d/, differ by only one feature contrast—in this case, voicing. Other phonemes, such as /s/ and /g/, differ by many feature contrasts, including voicing, continuancy, placement, and stridency. Table 3–1 presents a complete list of the 11 distinctive features originally identified by Chomsky and Halle (1968). For the purposes of clinical application, however, sounds are usually analyzed according to three basic feature categories: place, manner, and voicing. This breakdown is illustrated in Table 3–2.

Table 3–1
Distinctive Feature Analysis Chart

Features	Consonants																								
	k	g	t	d	p	b	f	v	θ	ð	s	z	ʃ	ʒ	tʃ	dʒ	m	n	ŋ	l	r	h	w	j	ʔ
Vocalic	–	–	–	–	–	–	–	–	–	–	–	–	–	–	–	–	–	–	–	–	–	–	–	–	–
Consonantal	+	+	+	+	+	+	+	+	+	+	+	+	+	+	+	+	+	+	+	+	+	–	–	–	–
High	+	+	–	–	–	–	–	–	–	–	–	–	+	+	+	+	–	–	+	–	–	–	+	+	–
Back	+	+	–	–	–	–	–	–	–	–	–	–	–	–	–	–	–	–	+	–	–	–	+	–	–
Low	–	–	–	–	–	–	–	–	–	–	–	–	–	–	–	–	–	–	–	–	–	+	–	–	+
Anterior	–	–	+	+	+	+	+	+	+	+	+	+	–	–	–	–	+	+	–	+	+	–	–	–	–
Coronal	–	–	+	+	–	–	–	–	+	+	+	+	+	+	+	+	–	+	–	+	+	–	–	–	–
Voiced	–	+	–	+	–	+	–	+	–	+	–	+	–	+	–	+	+	+	+	+	+	–	+	+	–
Continuant	–	–	–	–	–	–	+	+	+	+	+	+	+	+	–	–	–	–	–	+	+	+	+	+	+
Nasal	–	–	–	–	–	–	–	–	–	–	–	–	–	–	–	–	+	+	+	–	–	–	–	–	–
Strident	–	–	–	–	–	–	+	+	–	–	+	+	+	+	+	+	–	–	–	–	–	–	–	–	–

Note. – Absence of feature. + Presence of feature. *Vocalic:* Oral cavity constriction is less than required for the high vowels /i/ and /u/. *Consonantal:* Marked constriction in the midline region of the vocal tract. *High:* Body of the tongue is raised above the neutral or resting position. *Low:* Body of the tongue is lowered below the neutral or resting position. *Back:* Body of the tongue is retracted from the neutral or resting position. *Anterior:* Point of constriction is farther forward than required for /ʃ/. *Coronal:* Tongue blade is elevated toward alveolar ridge/palate from the neutral position. *Voiced:* Vocal folds vibrate during sound production. *Continuant:* Partial constriction of oral cavity; sound can be sustained in a steady state. *Nasal:* Velum is lowered to allow sound stream to escape through the nose. *Strident:* Turbulent noise is created by rapid airflow released through a small opening.

Table 3–2
Place, Manner, and Voicing Chart for English Consonants

Manner	Place	Voiced	Voiceless
Stop	Bilabial	b	p
	Alveolar	d	t
	Velar	g	k
	Glottal	—	ʔ
Fricative	Labiodental	v	f
	Linguadental	ð	θ
	Alveolar	z	s
	Palatal	ʒ	ʃ
	Glottal	—	h
Affricate	Palatal	dʒ	tʃ
Glide	Bilabial	w	—
	Palatal	j	—
Liquid	Alveolar	l	—
	Palatal	r	—
Nasal	Bilabial	m	—
	Alveolar	n	—
	Velar	ŋ	—

The clinician selects a feature for training (e.g., continuancy) and presents syllable or word pairs that contrast presence with absence of the feature (e.g., /fo/ versus /po/). After establishing the feature contrast in auditory discrimination activities, the clinician moves therapy through the traditional speech production hierarchy from isolation/syllables through conversation. For more detailed information, see Blache (1989), Stevens and Hanson (2013), and Ball (2016).

Paired Oppositions—Minimal and Maximal (Weiner, 1981)

These phonologically based approaches target phonemic contrasts (errored versus correct) that signal differences in meaning between two words. No explicit instruction on articulatory placement or sound production is given. Instead, this approach emphasizes the use of the child's communication success or breakdown to teach target sound productions. Minimal opposition pairs differ in only one feature of sound production (e.g., *ban* versus *pan* differ only in voicing) and are generally used with children who demonstrate relatively fewer errors, primarily characterized by sound substitutions. Maximal opposition word pairs differ in several features (e.g., *sad* and *bad* vary in place, manner, and voicing) and are generally used with children who display a larger number of errors that also include omissions and distortions. Four major steps are commonly used with this approach: (a) client is introduced to pairs through pictures or objects; (b) client identifies picture/object named by clinician; (c) roles are reversed and client must request or label picture/object; and (d) client is rewarded by clinician's selection of correct stimulus or is given a chance to repair the communication breakdown caused by inaccurate sound production. Gierut (2001, 2007) has advocated for an intervention strategy to speech production that focuses on across-sound class generalizations to facilitate system-wide phonological change. Storkel (2022) recently discussed minimal, maximal, or multiple opposition approaches for speech sound disorders.

In this approach, targets selected for treatment based on complexity principles would include those more complex, later developing, and less stimulable (Storkel, 2018). For more detailed information on oppositions as an approach to treatment, see Barlow and Gierut (2002), Stoel-Gammon et al. (2002), and Wren et al. (2018).

Phonological Processes (Oller, 1975)

This phonological approach to intervention is based on the strategies used by young, typically developing children between 1½ and 4 years of age to simplify the production of an entire class of adult speech sounds (Hodson & Paden, 1991; Khan & Lewis, 2002). For example, young children frequently omit weakly stressed syllables in multisyllabic words (e.g., *ephant/elephant, jamas/pajamas*), reduce consonant clusters (e.g., *bue/blue, dek/desk*), assimilate consonants in words (e.g., *goggie/doggie, chichen/chicken*), and delete final consonants (e.g., *ba/ball, hou/house*). Children who persist in using these processes beyond the age of 4 years are frequently referred for speech-language services because their speech is now perceived as difficult to understand. Some children exhibit phonological processes that are not typical of normally developing children. These nondevelopmental processes include (a) backing, the substitution of sounds that are more posterior than the usual place of production (e.g., *koe/toe, mackiz/ matches, gipper/zipper*); (b) initial consonant deletion (e.g., *ouse/ house, amp/lamp, ellow/yellow*); and (c) glottal replacement, substitution of a glottal stop for a consonant (e.g., *boʔle/ bottle, chiʔen/chicken, miʔey/ mickey*). Table 3–3 describes the most common phonological processes exhibited by normally developing children. For more detailed information, see Baker and McLeod (2011) and Baker et al. (2018).

Cycles Approach (Hodson & Paden, 1983)

One of the better known phonological process intervention programs is the "cycles" approach, which is intended for children with highly unintelligible speech. The clinician identifies phonological patterns that are targeted for a designated amount of time (i.e., cycles lasting 5–16 weeks). A typical session sequence includes (a) auditory bombardment, (b) production training, (c) stimulability probes, and (d) take-home activities for generalization. After approximately 2 to 6 hr of direct intervention, the child is given time to internalize the pattern while the clinician introduces new targets. Thus, the child's progression through the program is not based on achieving a criterion level of mastery. Focus on the original target resumes later in the therapy program. Each cycle is repeated until the target pattern emerges in spontaneous speech. For more detailed information, see Rvachew et al. (1999), Stoel-Gammon et al. (2002), Hassink and Wendt (2010), and Hodson (2010).

Core Vocabulary (Dodd et al., 2010)

This approach focuses on functional outcomes in which consistency, as opposed to accuracy, is targeted. The speech-language pathologist (SLP) selects 50 to 70 "functionally powerful" words and targets up to 10 at once. Children learn to produce their best pronunciation of the words consistently, both in isolation and connected speech. It targets the ability to generate consistent plans for words; the ability to create a phonological plan is improved by providing detailed, specific feedback about a limited number of words. This approach relies heavily on systematic practice in a drill-like format.

Table 3–3
Selected Developmental Phonological Processes

Process	Definition	Examples
Suppressed by 3 years		
Assimilation (harmony)	A sound becomes similar to or is influenced by another sound in the same word	*guck/duck* *toat/coat* *doddie/doggie*
Final consonant deletion	Omission of the last sound in word	*be/bed* *fi/fish* *so/soap*
Syllable deletion	Omission of weak or unstressed syllable(s)	*nana/banana agator/alligator* *zert/dessert*
Suppressed after 3 years		
Cluster reduction	Omission of at least one consonant from a cluster	*top/stop* *mall/small* *net/nest*
Epenthesis	Addition of sounds in a word	*bulack/black* *sthoap/soap* *pulay/play*
Fronting	Substitutions are produced anterior to their usual place of production	*tome/come* *cats/catch* *dum/gum*
Metathesis	The order of sound segments is reversed	*aminal/animal* *flutterby/butterfly* *bakset/basket*
Stopping	Fricatives/affricates are replaced by stops	*tun/sun* *dat/that* *dump/jump*
Voicing/devoicing	Voiced consonants replace voiceless sounds in the initial position; in the final position voiced consonants become voiceless	*gup/cup* *doe/toe* *bet/bed*

Sources: Based on the works of Bauman-Waengler (2007), Bernthal et al. (2009), Hodson (2004), and Shriberg and Kwiatkowski (1980).

Metaphon (Howell & Dean, 1994)

This approach is more accurately labeled a "philosophy" rather than a program; it is designed to provide children with explicit information that will enable them to consciously reflect on the phonemic structure of language. Heavy emphasis is placed on the child's awareness/understanding of the detailed aspects of speech sounds (separately from word meaning) to facilitate accurate sound production. It utilizes a "word-pair" technique to highlight the salient differences between individual sounds in similar words ("deep/keep"). The clinician does not provide specific or corrective feedback regarding the accuracy of the child's tongue placement or manner of sound production. Instead, the environment is deliberately structured to give the child repeated opportunities to distinguish between effective and ineffective communication attempts.

Oral-Motor Considerations

Some children with speech impairments (particularly those with organically based disorders) may exhibit deficits in oral-motor function that affect the neuromuscular control and organization needed for the production of intelligible speech. These deficits may manifest themselves as **hyposensitivity** (reduced reactions to sensation); **hypersensitivity** (overly strong reactions to sensation); and weakness or incoordination of oral structures, including the jaw, tongue, lips, or palate. Please see Appendix D on the companion website for a schematic of the vocal tract structures discussed in this section. It is important to realize that speech is not an isolated act, but the product of a highly complex and synchronized oral-motor system. Oral-motor therapy for children with functional articulation disorders generally consists of a variety of tongue, lip, and jaw exercises. Most proponents of this approach subscribe to one or more of the following basic rationales: (a) speech is founded on earlier developing nonspeech motor patterns, such as sucking and chewing (Marshalla, 1985; Ruark & Moore, 1997); (b) reduced muscle tone in the oral-facial area results in limited strength of speech articulators (Robin et al., 1991); (c) normal movement and sensation significantly influence motor learning, a Piagetian construct (Piaget, 1951; Thelen & Smith, 1994); and (d) speech is a highly complex behavior that is more easily learned when broken into smaller components (Magill, 1998). However, controversy exists regarding this approach to intervention. The few controlled studies present correlational rather than causal findings and report no significant connection between nonspeech oral-motor exercises (NSOMEs) and speech sound production (Bunton, 2008; Clark, 2003; Love, 2000; Moore & Ruark, 1996; Nittrouer, 1993). See Forrest (2002), Lass and Pannbacker (2008), and McCauley et al. (2009) for a comprehensive discussion of the efficacy of oral-motor intervention for functional articulation errors. In 2015, Kent suggested that NSOMES may have more value with disorders such as obstructive sleep apnea and jaw hypermobility.

The authors of this book do not endorse the use of NSOMEs for any specific clients or groups of clients, especially those with speech sound disorders of nonorganic origin.

Treatment Efficacy and Evidence-Based Practice

Gierut (1998) reviewed 64 publications whose subject matter included intervention effectiveness for functional articulatory/phonological disorders in children. The summary includes mainly small sample studies that focused on the treatment of consonant sounds. In 2003, Weston and Bain conducted a meta-analysis of 41 peer-reviewed articulation and phonology studies. The studies included descriptive and experimental designs involving children from ages 3 to 8+ years. Similar conclusions were reached in both analyses: (a) intervention is generally effective in improving correct sound production and increasing speech intelligibility; and (b) no one treatment approach was identified as being more effective than any other. Other factors to consider include the following:

- Minimal pair treatment and cycles approach treatment generally result in phonological gains.

- Computerized instruction is an effective supplement to direct clinical intervention.

- Efficacy data are needed to determine the relative effectiveness of specific treatment procedures as well as their efficiency (i.e., time needed for completion of the therapy programs).

- Clinician and family variables may have an impact on outcomes and should be examined in treatment studies (e.g., level of clinical expertise, parental/family attitudes and motivation).

- Scheduling of treatment (i.e., session frequency and intensity) requires further study as a potential variable in treatment outcomes. However, more recent studies have begun to suggest that higher intensity delivery schedules are associated with improved outcomes (Hegarty et al., 2018; Kaipa & Peterson, 2016; Tyler, 2005; Wren et al., 2018).

In 2004, Law et al. conducted a meta-analysis of studies focusing on intervention for children with speech-language difficulties. Not surprisingly, the results indicated a significant effect favoring speech interventions compared with no treatment conditions. Courses of therapy lasting less than 8 weeks appeared to be less effective than longer programs. Finally, parent-administered interventions based on receptive auditory techniques (e.g., auditory bombardment) did not significantly affect speech sound production. In 2018, Wren et al. published a systematic review of interventions for speech sound disorders and found that there continues to be a relative lack of highly graded evidence for treatment effectiveness with any specific approach to speech sound disorders. An evidence-based practice (EBP) approach to treatment comprises three basic elements: (a) scientific research, (b) clinical expertise, and (c) client/family values. Because the existing literature on treatment efficacy does not clearly identify any gold standard approach to intervention for articulation/phonology deficits, the SLP's clinical judgment becomes the driving force in the EBP process. For this reason, clinicians often adopt a "what works" approach (Stanovich, 2000) to intervention that utilizes the best features of multiple approaches. For more information on SLPs' use of evidence-based practices, see Baker and McLeod (2011) and Hoffman et al. (2013).

Target Selection for Intervention Programming

Two primary approaches are used for choosing initial therapy targets for children with articulation/phonological disorders: developmental and nondevelopmental.

Developmental

In this approach, therapy targets are identified based on the order of acquisition in normally developing children. Table 3–4 provides a list of English consonants in the order of their emergence. Table 3–3, earlier in the chapter, outlines the most common phonological processes exhibited by young children.

Table 3–4
Age of Acquisition of English Consonants

Consonant	Poole (1934)	Templin (1957)	Prather et al. (1975)	Smit et al. (1990) Females	Males
m	3½	3	2	3	3
n	4½	3	2	3½	3
h	3½	3	2	3	3
p	3½	3	2	3	3
f	5½	3	2–4	3½	3½
w	3½	3	2–8	3	3
b	3½	4	2–8	3	3
h	4½	3	2	7–9	7–9
j	4½	3½	2–4	4	5
k	4½	4	2–4	3½	3½
g	4½	4	2–4	3½	4
l	6½	6	3–4	6	6
d	4½	4	2–4	3	3½
t	4½	6	2–8	4	3½
s	7½	4½	3	7–9	7–9
r	7½	4	3–4	8	8
tʃ	—	4½	3–8	6	7
v	6½	6	4	5½	5½
z	7½	7	4	7–9	7–9
ʒ	6½	7	4	—	—
θ	7½	6	4	6	8
dʒ	—	7	4	6	7
ʃ	6½	4½	3–8	6	7
ð	6½	7	4	4½	7

Note. Variability in reported ages of acquisition is partly due to the different criterion levels used across studies to determine mastery of each sound. Poole (1934) = 100%, Templin (1957) = 75%, Prather et al. (1975) = 75%, Smit et al. (1990) = 90%.

Nondevelopmental

In this approach, developmental norms are not used in the selection of target behaviors. Instead, the determining factors fall into two groups. One strategy is client specific and bases the selection of therapy objectives on several factors:

- Target(s) should be most relevant to a child or parent (e.g., a sound in the child's name).

- Target(s) should be most stimulable in a given child's error repertoire regardless of developmental sequence. It should be noted that several authors take the opposite view and recommend choosing the least stimulable sounds as targets for intervention. They suggest that stimulability is indicative of some degree of phonological knowledge, and these sounds may be likely to emerge naturally; in contrast, nonstimulable sounds would benefit most from targeted intervention. (For more detailed information, see Gierut et al. [1987]; McLeod & Baker [2016]; Rvachew [2005]; and Williams [2002].)

- Target(s) should be most visible when produced (e.g., /θ/ versus /g/).

The second nondevelopmental strategy is based on the degree of perceived deviance associated with a child's errors. This strategy can be applied to both articulation and phonological errors, as follows.

Articulatory

- Omission errors contribute most to unintelligibility, followed by substitutions, and then distortions.

- Errors in the initial position of words contribute most to unintelligibility, followed by medial, and then final.

- Errors that occur on the most frequent sounds in a language contribute significantly to unintelligibility.

Phonological

- Patterns of initial consonant deletion and glottal replacement of medial consonants tend to contribute significantly to listener perception of unintelligibility.

In addition to choosing therapy targets, clinicians must determine the most appropriate "goal-attack strategy" for each client (Fey, 1986). Several strategies can be utilized in the design of a client's therapy program: vertical, horizontal, and cyclical. The basic assumption of **vertical** training is that the best route to target mastery is through intense practice on a limited number of targets. If therapy is being programmed with a focus on motor learning, the clinician is encouraged to design session activities that provide the opportunity for a high rate of responses or **massed practice** (e.g., 150 target productions in 30 min). The clinician focuses on one or two targets until the client achieves some predetermined level of mastery, usually at the level of conversation. Therapy then moves on to the next target(s) identified in a hierarchical level of difficulty. This "deep" approach to intervention tends to be most appropriate for clients with relatively few articulatory/phonological errors.

In contrast to training deeply, a **horizontal** strategy attacks goals broadly. It assumes that simultaneous exposure to a wide variety of targets will facilitate a client's ability to produce phonemes or sound patterns. The clinician provides less intense practice on a larger number of targets, even within the same session. This strategy focuses on efficient generalization of target behaviors across the speech sound system and tends to be most appropriate for clients with multiple errors.

Clinicians may choose to combine aspects of the vertical and horizontal strategies into the **cycles** approach. Recall that instead of attacking therapy targets deeply or broadly, this strategy provides a client with practice on a given target for a predetermined amount of time, and then moves on to another target (Hodson & Paden, 1991; Sugden et al., 2018). This approach gives the client an opportunity to internalize the original sound or pattern while the clinician introduces the new target. Focus on the original target resumes later in the therapy program. This cycle is repeated until the target(s) emerges in spontaneous speech.

Example Profiles for Functional Articulation Disorders

This section presents three commonly seen profiles of childhood articulation problems. These examples have been designed to illustrate the selection of intervention targets as well as specific therapy activities and materials. Most of the chosen activities are easily implemented in either individual or group therapy settings.

For many children, it may be necessary to teach the phonetic placement of target sounds prior to the introduction of actual activities. Appendix 3–A on the companion website provides specific instructions for establishing the correct placement for consonants that are typically considered difficult to elicit.

The first profile describes a *young child with multiple errors.*

PROFILE 1: FUNCTIONAL ARTICULATION—3-YEAR-OLD

Jill is 3 years old and demonstrates the following articulation errors (error sound/intended target):

Initial	Medial	Final
d/g	d/g	ʃ/tʃ
j/l	w/r	-/s
b/v	f/θ	-/k
-/s	j/l	-/d
p/f	ʔ/t	s/f
b/m	j/n	-/ŋ
	-/s	

Blends   b/bl, f/fl, w/kl, t/sl, t/skw, fw/kr, b/br, d/dr, w/pr

Selection of Therapy Targets Using a Developmental Approach. Based on this child's chronological age, the errors to be targeted first are d/g, b/m, p/f, j/n, -/ŋ, because these are the earliest emerging sounds, as can be seen in Table 3–4. The second set of target sounds consists of -/k, -/d, and ʔ/t. The remaining errors would not be considered appropriate targets for intervention, because they emerge well beyond 3 years of age.

Selection of Therapy Targets Using a Nondevelopmental Approach. The errors to be targeted are /θ/, /v/, /m/, /f/, /g/, and /s/. The /θ/ and /v/ sounds were chosen despite developmental considerations, because Jill was highly stimulable for these sounds in isolation during the diagnostic session. The /m/ and /f/ sounds were selected because they are visible when produced, which facilitates learning of correct articulatory placement. The /f/ and /g/ sounds were included as beginning targets, because their status as initial-position errors make them significant contributors to Jill's overall unintelligibility.

Sample Activities

1. Modify a board game, such as Hasbro's Candy Land by requiring a child to produce a target sound in isolation, following the clinician's model, in order to move a game piece. Close approximations, rather than accurate productions, of the target phoneme may be acceptable in the very early stages of therapy. Once the child improves her performance by 30% to 50% over baseline measures, clinician models should be faded. Three consecutive spontaneous productions can then be required for the child to take a turn in the game.

2. Create a game with colored paper fish. Each fish has a picture on it designed to elicit a target sound in the desired position. Attach paper clips to the back of each fish, and give the child a "fishing pole" with a magnet on the end of its string. Have the child dangle the magnet over the fish. Instruct the child to respond by producing the stimulus item three times as she lands each fish. The difficulty level of the response can be programmed to vary from single words to lengthy sentences.

3. Assemble 25 4 × 4-in. squares of colored paper with one stimulus picture on each. One of the squares should be marked in a special way (e.g., with a star or a sticker). Cover one wall with the squares so that the stimulus pictures are facing the wall. Tell the child that she is going to pretend to be a detective who has to find the "magic square" in the dark. Hand the child a penlight, turn out the lights, and instruct her to aim the beam at the square that she thinks is the magic one. As each square is lit up, ask the child to produce the target item at the appropriate level of complexity.

4. Assemble the following materials to make two puppets: two glue sticks, two brown paper bags, yarn, two sets of paper cutouts of facial features, and other accessories such as earrings, mustaches, and eyeglasses. Collect 25 pictures containing the targeted therapy sounds and place them in a pile on the table. Explain that the clinician and child will construct puppets using the paper bags and other materials. The clinician selects one picture from the pile, models the correct production of the word, and then glues one feature/accessory to one of the bags. Instruct the child to select the next picture from the pile, produce the word correctly three times, and glue a feature/accessory on the other bag. Alternate turns until both puppets are completed.

The second profile describes a school-age child with *multiple articulation errors*.

PROFILE 2: FUNCTIONAL ARTICULATION—6-YEAR-OLD

Joe is 6 years old and demonstrates the following errors:

Initial	Medial	Final
j/l	j/l	j/l
	s/θ	s/θ
ʃ/tʃ	ʃ/tʃ	ʃ/tʃ
		-/d
ʃ/f	ʃ/f	s/f
b/v	b/v	
w/r	w/r	

Blends: s/sl, b/bl, k/kl, fw/fl, fw/fr, tw/tr, k/skw, fw/kr, t/st

Selection of Therapy Targets Using a Developmental Approach. Based on this child's chronological age, the errors to be targeted first are -/d, ʃ/f, b/v, and j/l, because these are the earliest emerging sounds as shown in Table 3–4. The second set of targets consists of the remaining sound and blend errors, because all of these are typically acquired by 6 years of age.

Selection of Therapy Targets Using a Nondevelopmental Approach. The errors to be targeted are /r/, /fr/, /fl/, and /θ/. The /r/ was chosen because it is one of the most frequently occurring sounds in English (Table 3–5). The /fr/ and /fl/ blends were selected because these are the only phonetic contexts in which Joe can correctly produce his otherwise misarticulated /f/ sound. The blends can provide a starting point for facilitating the correct production of /f/ as a singleton. Finally, the /θ/ was chosen because its articulatory placement is highly visible and is therefore relatively easy to approximate.

Sample Activities

1. Draw 10 pictures on a dry-erase board, each containing one instance of a target sound. Give the child a beanbag and tell him to hit one of the pictures. Instruct the child to produce the stimulus item at the appropriate level of complexity (e.g., single word, carrier phrase, sentence, narrative).

2. For a group activity, gather at least 20 pictures/objects that contain the target sound(s) and place them around the room. Give each child a "suitcase" (box) and tell them that the group is going on a trip. Say, "I'm going to Disney World. I'll take you too if you bring the right things in your suitcase." Have the children take turns retrieving stimulus items from around the room. They may place them in their suitcases upon correct production of the appropriate target sounds.

Table 3–5
Frequency of Consonant Occurrence in English

Sound	Cumulative Percentage	Percentage of Occurrence
n	12.0	12.0
t	11.9	23.9
s	6.9	30.8
r	6.7	37.5
d	6.4	43.9
m	5.9	49.8
z	5.4	55.2
ð	5.3	60.5
l	5.3	65.8
k	5.1	70.9
w	4.9	75.8
h	4.4	80.2
b	3.3	83.5
p	3.1	86.6
g	3.1	89.7
f	2.1	91.8
h	1.6	93.4
j	1.6	95.0
v	1.5	96.5
ʃ	0.9	97.4
θ	0.9	98.3
dʒ	0.6	98.9
tʃ	0.6	99.5
ð	<0.1	99.6

Source: Adapted from "Computer-Assisted Natural Process Analysis (NPA): Recent Issues and Data," by L. D. Shriberg and J. Kwiatkowski, 1983, *Seminars in Speech and Language, 4*(4), p. 11.

3. Assemble at least 20 pictures/objects that contain target sound(s) and place them on the table. Introduce a "shopping game" by presenting a carrier phrase such as, "I went to the food store and bought _____, _____, and _____." Have the child remove the corresponding pictures from the table. Then instruct the child to take a turn at making a shopping list by producing the same carrier phrase with three new food items chosen from the remaining picture stimuli. The type of store named in the carrier phrase can be varied to expose/reinforce the child's ability to organize lexical items into semantic categories (e.g., clothing, toys, pets). Each list can also be written on a dry-erase board or chart paper to emphasize the connection between writing, reading, and speaking. The activity can be easily adapted for small group sessions.

4. Write each verse of the following song on a sheet of paper. Place clip art or other icons above words containing a targeted sound (e.g., /θ/). Provide a microphone and arrange a spotlight using a flashlight in a darkened room. Explain that in this activity the child will pretend to be on stage. Teach the child to sing the song using any familiar melody.

I'd rather use a bathtub than a booth
I'd rather have a toothache than no tooth
I'd rather have a birthday than a wreath
I'd rather be an athlete than a thief

Refrain
Wouldn't you?
Yes I would!
Yes I would!

I'd rather use a thumbtack than a thorn
I'd rather have a thick one than a thin
I'd rather have some mouthwash than a bath
I'd rather be a Matthew than a Keith

Repeat refrain

The third profile describes an older school-age child with *persistent /r/ and /s/ substitution errors.*

PROFILE 3: FUNCTIONAL ARTICULATION—8-YEAR-OLD

Sammy is 8 years old and demonstrates the following errors:

Initial	Medial	Final
w/r	w/r	w/r
θ/s	θ/s	θ/s

Blends: Sammy has the same substitution pattern for all /r/ and /s/ blends.

Selection of Therapy Targets Using a Developmental Approach. A developmental approach for therapy target selection is not relevant in this case. The /r/ and /s/ sounds are typically acquired by 8 years of age; therefore, both would be considered appropriate therapy objectives.

Selection of Therapy Targets Using a Nondevelopmental Approach. The /s/ phoneme is selected as the primary therapy target because Sammy was stimulable for this sound in isolation. It is also considered a particularly relevant objective for Sammy, because /s/ is the first sound in his name.

Sample Activities

1. Draw a football field on chart paper with the yard lines (e.g., 10-yard line, 20-yard line, and so on) and end zones clearly delineated. Make a football from colored paper/cardboard and affix masking tape or other adhesive to the back. The therapist and child select team names. The child takes control of the ball at the 50-yard line because he represents the home team. Model stimulus items containing the target sound and instruct the child to repeat the stimulus item five times. He can move the football 5 "yards" toward his end zone for every correct response. If the child produces no correct responses, the clinician gets to move the ball 5 yards toward the other end zone. The difficulty level of this game can be modified in various ways: fading the therapist model, increasing the number of required responses, and increasing the length and complexity of the target response from isolation to complex sentences. This activity also works well in small-group sessions.

2. Design a game sheet with at least six or eight drawings of blank TV/movie screens. Instruct the child to name television shows containing the target sound. A correct production allows the child to draw or write something related to that show on one of the TV sets on the game sheet. For example, for the target sound /r/, the child may name shows such as *Rugrats, Max and Ruby, Ratatouille, Robin Hood,* and *Meet the Robinsons.* Once all of the screens are filled in, begin a guessing game in which the child is instructed to describe one of the shows/movies without using the title, and the therapist has to guess its name. All correct spontaneous productions of the target sound during this conversational task should be reinforced. If the child meets a predetermined criterion for accuracy of sound production, a paper "Emmy" can be awarded. Task difficulty can be increased to more complex levels by requiring the child to summarize a show/movie or describe one of its characters in order to fill in a blank screen on the game sheet. This activity is easily adapted for group sessions.

3. On slips of paper, write 25 single words containing the target sound /s/ in initial, final, or medial position. Fold slips of paper and place them in a container or pile them on the table. Affix a Hasbro NERF basketball hoop (or equivalent) to a therapy room wall at least 3 ft higher than the child's standing height. Explain that this game requires the child to select a slip of paper from the pile and produce a sentence using the word written on the slip. If the target sound is produced correctly, the child is allowed to crumple the paper slip and shoot it at the basketball hoop. If target sound /s/ is incorrectly produced, the slip of paper is returned to the pile or container. The game continues until the pile is depleted and all paper slips have been crumpled and shot.

4. Gather materials to play "detective," including a badge and a small notebook with pencil. Design several simple crime scenarios that contain multiple instances of the target sound. One example of a possible scenario follows:

> Sue is lying on the floor beside a windowsill in a sealed room. Scattered on the floor, there is water and broken glass. Simon is asleep on the sofa across the room. Mr. Soaps, a window washer, spots Sue and calls the police to report his suspicions.

Tell the child to play a detective and ask questions of the witness, Mr. Soaps (played by the therapist), to solve the crime. The child should be encouraged to ask questions that contain as many instances of the target sound as possible. To facilitate this, all questions could begin with, "Well, Mr. Soaps . . ." Appropriate questions for this scenario include "What sort of clothes was Sue wearing when you saw her?"; "How old is Simon?"; "Where do you suppose the broken glass came from?" (Solution: Sue is a goldfish, and Simon is a cat.)

Helpful Hints

1. Do not include more than one error sound in a stimulus word, phrase, or sentence during the initial stages of therapy.

2. Pay attention to the phonetic context of words that contain a child's target sounds. Certain consonant-vowel sequences may facilitate or impede correct production.

3. In some ways, the production of speech sounds is a motor skill like that of playing a piano. Therapy sessions that elicit the greatest number of sound productions will be the most effective in establishing correct production as an automatic behavior.

4. Children with persistent errors that appear to be functional should be evaluated for the presence of oral-motor difficulties.

5. Use books that contain target sounds as immersion activities. The books can be given to parents to use at reading time with their child. For our example child, Sammy, good choices include *Rotten Ralph* by J. Gantos, *Rain Makes Applesauce* by J. Scheer, *Miss Nelson Is Missing* by H. Allard and J. Marshall, and *My Mama Says* by J. Viorst.

6. It is important to counsel parents to respond consistently to the content of their child's utterances before pointing out speech errors or modeling correct productions. This is particularly relevant in the early stages of therapy to avoid frustration and other negative feelings.

Example Profiles for Phonological Disorders

Following are two profiles commonly seen in children with phonological rule problems. The first case depicts a process approach to intervention; the second case illustrates a modified distinctive feature strategy. These examples have been designed to illustrate the selection of intervention targets as well as specific therapy activities and materials. Most of the chosen activities are easily implemented in either individual or group therapy settings.

PROFILE 4: PHONOLOGICAL—5-YEAR-OLD

Gerry is 5 years old and demonstrates the following phonological processes:

- **Final consonant deletion**
  - -/s
  - -/v
  - -/p
  - -/d
  - -/k

- **Unstressed syllable deletion**
  - *tephone/telephone*
  - *way/away*
  - *tato/potato*
  - *amance/ambulance*

- **Cluster reduction**
  - -t/st
  - -m/sm
  - p-/pl
  - -k/sk
  - n-/nd

- **Fronting**
  - t/k
  - d/g

- **Voicing**
  - b/p
  - d/t
  - z/s
  - v/f

- **Initial consonant deletion**
  - -/k
  - -/l
  - -/h
  - -/p
  - -/t

- **Glottal replacement**
  - ʔ/t
  - ʔ/k
  - ʔ/g

Selection of Therapy Targets. The patterns to be targeted are final consonant deletion, fronting, voicing, and initial consonant deletion. The first five patterns in the preceding list are exhibited by typically developing children and are therefore considered developmental in nature. Final consonant deletion and fronting were targeted because these developmental processes are suppressed from children's speech production repertoires earlier than the other two (by 3 years of age). The last two processes occur much less frequently among typically developing children. Initial consonant deletion was selected as a therapy target because of its severe impact on intelligibility (Khan & Lewis, 2002; Leinonen-Davis, 1988; Yavas & Lamprecht, 1988).

Sample Activities

1. Cut out a large dinosaur (about 3 ft in length) with a very long, detachable tail (e.g., Tyrannosaurus rex) from poster board or colored paper and obtain a small paint bottle with a sponge top (bingo marker). Collect a pile of 25 pictures for the child to name. The names should be monosyllabic and contain a variety of singleton final consonants, including examples of his deletion errors as well as any that he might be able to produce spontane-

ously. Remove the tail from the dinosaur and explain to the child that words have sounds at the ends just like dinosaurs have tails. Instruct the child to select a picture from the pile and name it, making sure to put the ending sound on the word. Following each correct response, illustrate the parallel between the dinosaur's tail and the final sound of the word by allowing the child to reattach the dinosaur's tail and decorate it with one dot of sponge paint. The ultimate goal of this activity is to decorate the dinosaur's tail completely and attach it permanently for the child to take home. This activity can be used effectively up through the level of conversation and narration.

2. Create or collect a deck of picture cards for the game Go Fish, depicting pairs of identical words and minimal contrast words that incorporate the child's fronting errors. Recall that minimal pairs consist of two words that are identical except for a single distinctive feature or phoneme. This approach is designed to emphasize the concept that even small sound contrasts can signal differences in word meanings. Examples include *t*ap and *c*ap, *t*op and *c*op, *d*ate and *g*ate, pi*t* and pi*ck*, be*d* and be*g*. Begin the game by dealing three cards to each player and placing the remainder in a pile in the middle of the table. Explain to the child that the object of the game is to make pairs for all the cards in his hand with *identical* pictures by asking other players, "Do you have any _____?" A correct production allows the child to continue requesting cards. If the child uses a fronting error during a turn at requesting a card, he should be given the picture that corresponds to his actual, not intended, production. For example, if the child says "date" when attempting to match his picture of a gate, he will receive the card depicting a date on a calendar and therefore not obtain the match. The clinician should model the intended production for the child to imitate. A correct imitation is rewarded with the desired picture match, but the turn passes to the next player. The player who has the most pairs at the end of the game is the winner.

3. Gather pictures for the parenthesized words in the following sentences and arrange them on a table. Explain that the clinician will say a sentence with a word missing at the end. Instruct the child to finish the sentence by selecting the picture that sounds almost the same as a word in the sentence, except for using "voice on" or "voice off." The clinician reads one sentence at a time with particular emphasis on the italicized word. (Note: The clinician provides the child with a hint that the target word rhymes with one of the words in the sentence.)

   The *pig* is _____ (big).
   Put the *coat* on the _____ (goat).
   The *fan* is in the _____ (van).
   I *see* the letter _____ (Z).
   Put the *pin* in the _____ (bin).
   Don't *tip* over the _____ (dip).
   The *girl* has a _____ (curl).
   Sue likes the _____ (zoo).
   Dan is very _____ (tan).
   Go *down* to the _____ (town).
   He *came* to play the _____ (game).
   Put the *pack* on your _____ (back).

4. Cut out a minimum of 30 colored paper turtles that are approximately 8 in. in length. Two-thirds of the turtles should have their heads protruding out from their shells, whereas the heads of the remaining one-third should not be visible. Place the turtles in an obstacle course-like path around the room so that a child can hop easily from one turtle "stepping-stone" to another. Gather a deck of 20 pictures whose names begin with the child's initial consonant deletion errors. Prepare numerous slips of paper that instruct the child to perform one of the following: (a) hop forward one turtle, (b) hop forward two turtles, (c) hop backward one turtle, or (d) hop backward two turtles. Fold these paper slips and place them in a paper bag. Tell the child that to play the "turtle stepping-stone" game, she has to hop on the turtles and say some words. For each turn, she has to choose a slip of paper from the bag without looking and follow its instruction. As she lands on a turtle, the clinician holds up one card from the picture deck. If the child is on a turtle that has no head, she should name the picture three times without producing its initial consonant sound. If the turtle has a head, the word must be produced five times with its initial consonant sound present. The object of the game is to reach the final turtle on the obstacle course.

Note: It is important to remember that the focus of these activities is on phonological processes rather than the production of particular sounds. For this reason, in the early stages of therapy, the clinician should reinforce any responses that demonstrate a child's use of the targeted phonological process, regardless of the actual phoneme(s) produced. For example, during work on the final consonant deletion process, a child may be reinforced for producing "bat" or "bam" instead of his habitual "ba" when naming a picture of a bag.

PROFILE 5: PHONOLOGICAL—5-YEAR-OLD

Grace is 5 years old and demonstrates the following feature errors:

Manner Errors	Examples
Stops for fricatives:	zoo → /doo/, soap → /toap/
Fricatives for affricates:	porch → /porsh/
Glides for liquids:	right → /yight/

Place Errors	
Alveolars for velars:	tuptake/cupcake, det/get
Alveolars for palatals:	sue/shoe, trezure/treasure

Voicing Errors	
Voiced for voiceless:	gow/cow, doe/toe
Voiceless for voiced:	loose/lose, stofe/stove

For clarity, the examples in the preceding list reflect a single feature contrast between the error sound and the intended target. However, children frequently produce errors that differ from the target by two or more feature contrasts (e.g., *late* → /jet/ differ in both place and manner; *sip* → /gip/ differ in all three features).

Selection of Therapy Targets. The first set of therapy targets includes one error contrast from each of the three feature categories. The manner contrast of stop/fricative was selected because fricatives emerge earlier developmentally than the other two sound classes listed under this category (i.e., affricates and liquids). In addition, fricatives have a higher frequency of occurrence in English than affricates. The place contrast of alveolar/velar was chosen because palatals are acquired much later in the developmental sequence than velars. The voiced/voiceless contrast was included because this feature error generally occurs in word-initial position, which contributes heavily to perceived unintelligibility.

Sample Activities

1. Using masking tape, create a hopscotch grid with eight squares on the floor. Draw a long slide on a dry-erase board or piece of paper and obtain a spinner with numbers. Provide a doll or stuffed animal figure and tell the child that "Harry" uses different types of sounds when playing these two different activities. Demonstrate that Harry produces "short hopping" sounds (stops)—such as /b, p, d/—as he jumps on the hopscotch grid. Then demonstrate that Harry produces "long, sliding" sounds (fricatives)—such as /s, z, f, v/—as he goes down the slide. Check the child's grasp of the concepts involved by modeling alternating examples of each manner of sound production and asking the child to place Harry on the corresponding activity.

    Start with the hopscotch game and explain that the child will jump from the beginning to the end of the grid while holding Harry. The clinician models examples of stops (such as /t/ or /k/) when the child lands on each square. The child must produce three imitations of the stop before jumping to the next square. After completing the hopscotch grid, move on to the slide activity. Emphasize the feature contrast between stops and fricatives by reminding the child that Harry uses "long, sliding" sounds with this activity. Have the child use the spinner to determine the number of times Harry can go down the slide. The clinician models an example of a fricative sound with exaggerated duration (such as /fffff/ or /sssss/). Tell the child to place Harry at the top of the slide and move him down slowly while imitating the clinician's exaggerated production. Repeat as many times as indicated by the spinner and then have the child spin again for another turn. The clinician should model different fricatives for each turn. Allow the child four more turns with the spinner and then return to the hopscotch game to reinforce the targeted feature contrast.

    Once the child demonstrates mastery at this level, the clinician can introduce more complex stimulus items such as syllables and words.

2. Create a racetrack game board with starting and finishing lines that are connected by 20 squares. Provide a small race car game piece. Make a spinner with numbers, half colored green and half colored red. Tell the child that the race car moves forward when the spinner indicates a green number and backward with a red number. Explain that whenever the spinner points to a green number, the child will imitate the clinician's model of a "forward" sound (alveolar such as /d/ or /t/), while moving the game piece. If the spinner points to a red number, a contrasting "backward" sound (velar such as /g/ or /k/) will be modeled for imitation. A variety of sounds that highlight the alveolar/velar place contrast should be modeled throughout the game. The object of the game is to cross the finish line.

3. Make a 24-square bingo card (six rows of four squares) and place pictures/stickers of butterflies and bumblebees in alternating columns on the card. Collect a deck of 24 pictures for the child to name. One-third of the names should have voiced consonants in the initial word position (e.g., *boy, girl, duck, zipper, jump*) and the other two-thirds should have voiceless initial consonants (e.g., *soup, table, chair, cat, piano*). Provide 24 game tokens. Explain to the child that bumblebees and butterflies make two different kinds of sounds. The bumblebee uses sounds that buzz, like /zzzzz/, and the butterfly uses sounds that do not buzz, like /sssss/. Then select a picture card from the deck and hold it up. Instruct the child to name the picture and then to categorize the initial phoneme as a bumblebee or butterfly sound. If the child responds correctly to both parts, she is able to place a game token on one of the picture squares that corresponds to the sound category of the target word (i.e., bumblebee versus butterfly). The object of the game is to fill an entire column of squares with tokens.

4. Gather a plastic tablecloth and napkins for a pretend tea party and arrange them on a table in the therapy room. Collect 20 pictures of objects/animals that have easily identifiable front portions and back portions and cut them in half (e.g., train, horse, car, dog, snake, airplane, pencil, bus, giraffe, fish). Separate the front and back pieces into two piles. Briefly review that certain sounds are made in the front of the mouth (e.g., /p/, /t/), while others are made in the back (e.g., /k/, /g/). Practice a few examples of each with the child.

    Explain that the tablecloth and napkins need to be decorated in a special way for the tea party. Model a front or back sound in a consonant-vowel (CV) syllable and instruct the child to identify it as "front" or "back" and imitate three times. If identification and production responses are correct, the child picks a picture from the appropriate pile and pastes/tapes it to the tablecloth or napkins. Alternate CV models between front and back sounds until all picture pieces have been used as decorations.

Helpful Hints

1. When using a phonological processes approach, it is sometimes useful to teach the underlying concepts in nonspeech activities before moving to speech production tasks.

2. One consideration in the selection of phonological processes for therapy is the relative consistency of their use. Processes that a child demonstrates only occasionally may be more easily modified than those used on a consistent basis.

3. In the initial stages of distinctive feature therapy, selection of target sounds that differ by only a single feature may increase the likelihood of early success.

4. Distinctive feature theory predicts that generalization will most likely occur from trained phonemes to phonemes that share the same feature. Thus, it is important to regularly probe these untrained sounds to determine whether any have been acquired spontaneously and will not require subsequent intervention.

5. Clinicians may need to explain to parents that therapy for phonological disorders focuses on appropriate use of linguistic rules rather than acquisition of correct motor movements. This may eliminate a parent's confusion in the early stages of therapy when the clinician reinforces a seemingly incorrect response (e.g., *toat/boat* when targeting initial consonant deletion), when, in fact, the child is now using the correct rule.

6. Choosing two therapy targets that differ maximally from each other (e.g., /s/ vs /g/) can be a useful strategy for teaching the client to recognize/understand the concepts of place/manner/voicing.

Organic Articulation Disorders

Three pathologies associated with severe articulation problems in children are cleft palate, hearing impairment, and childhood apraxia of speech. The selection of initial therapy targets for organic disorders is based on a nondevelopmental approach, because the accompanying speech production deficits are the direct result of structural/neurologic anomalies and are not developmental in nature.

Cleft Palate

This is a congenital malformation of the palate and/or lip that results from the failure of oral structures to fuse at midline during the first trimester of pregnancy (4–12 weeks of gestation). A cleft can be unilateral (one sided) or bilateral. Clefts of the palate have substantially more severe effects on speech intelligibility than do isolated clefts of the lip. Management of children with clefts generally is carried out by an interdisciplinary team that includes an SLP. Although variations exist across settings, there is a basic timeline associated with cleft palate management. Following is one example of a typical timeline.

Within the first three weeks of life the child has his or her first evaluation in the clinic for
- Proper feeding
- Hearing
- Genetic counseling
- Dental/palatal impressions
- General counseling and support
- Social services to help with family or financial considerations

Between 0 and 3 months
- Dental splints for cleft palate children, if indicated
- Routine pediatric visits

At approximately 3 months of age
- Surgical repair of cleft lip

Between 3 and 12 months of age
- Dental splints for cleft palate children, if indicated
- One or two hearing/ear evaluations
- One speech evaluation

At approximately 12 months of age
- Surgical cleft palate repair
- Placement of ear tubes, if necessary

Between 12 months and 5 years

- Speech (if abnormal, speech therapy started through school, etc.)
- Hearing
- Dental
- Social/emotional development
- Possible palate repair revision, if speech suboptimal

Between 5 and 7 years

- Prepare primary teeth orthodontically for surgical bone graft of cleft before permanent teeth erupt
- Continue speech assessment
- Consider first surgical revision/refinement of lip and/or nose

Surgical repair of labial clefts is completed at approximately 3 months of age or earlier; palatal repairs generally occur before the child's second birthday (Kummer, 2018; Peterson-Falzone et al., 2001). Pharyngeal flap procedures are considered secondary surgical interventions and involve joining a flap of soft tissue from the posterior pharyngeal wall to the palate, creating a bridge that partially occludes the velopharyngeal space. This procedure is performed primarily for the purpose of facilitating velopharyngeal closure during speech. Speech therapy may begin before surgical repairs are completed but is primarily provided following surgical intervention. Some authors recommend a 3-month postsurgical recovery period before therapy is initiated or resumed. See Peterson-Falzone et al. (2016) for detailed discussion of the SLP's role in treating cleft palate speech.

The most significant speech problem associated with cleft palate is **velopharyngeal incompetence (VPI)**. VPI is the inability to close off the oral cavity from the nasal cavity during speech due to inadequate velar movement (Peterson-Falzone et al., 2006). This results in audible nasal emission of air, hypernasal resonance, and articulation errors. Audible nasal emission occurs when air flows at an excessive rate through the nasal passages, creating turbulence and generating distracting noise during speech. This leakage of air results in reduced oral breath pressure for the production of pressure consonants (i.e., fricatives, affricates, and plosives). **Hypernasal resonance**, or hypernasality, occurs when the balance between oral and nasal resonance shifts to such a degree that speech is perceived by listeners to be "nasal." This phenomenon is particularly noticeable during the production of vowels, especially when the degree of mouth opening is restricted.

In misarticulations related to VPI, the most frequent errors occur on fricatives, affricates, and plosives. The most common types of errors demonstrated by cleft palate speakers are distortions and omissions, with occasional substitutions in the form of glottal stops and pharyngeal fricatives. In general, the provision of therapy is appropriate only for children who have velopharyngeal (VP) competence or questionable/marginal incompetence, as determined by the cleft palate team (Kuehn & Moller, 2000; Pamplona et al., 2004). Therapy focusing solely on oral direction of the breath stream is not usually recommended for children who demonstrate clear evidence of VPI. It may lead to elevation of the larynx and result in voice disorders. Recent studies indicate that better outcomes may be more strongly associated with a therapy approach that focuses on linguistic/phonological aspects of speech sound production than approaches that heavily emphasize motor aspects of speech production (Alighieri et al., 2020). Literature on dosage effects of intervention for cleft palate speech is limited. However, a recent study by Alighieri et al. (2021) investigated the effects of a "high" versus "low" intensity therapy schedule:

- high intensity = five 1-hr sessions per week over two weeks

- low intensity = single 1-hr session per week over 10 weeks

Results indicated that participants who received the high intensity intervention demonstrated equal, and in some cases, even superior progress in only two weeks compared to the participants who received therapy on the low intensity schedule.

Following is a profile of the speech sound errors in children with cleft palates:

- The most frequent errors occur on fricatives and affricates, followed by plosives.

- Distortions and omissions are the most common error types, followed by substitutions.

- Singleton fricatives and affricates are most likely to be distorted.

- Consonants in blends are most likely to be omitted.

- Glottal stops tend to be substituted for plosives.

- More misarticulations occur on voiceless consonants than their voiced cognates, especially in young children.

- Most errors occur in the final position, followed by medial and initial positions, respectively.

Example Profile

Following is a typical profile for a child with cleft palate. This example has been designed to illustrate the selection of intervention targets as well as specific therapy activities and materials. The chosen activities are easily implemented in either individual or group therapy settings. Each activity is identified with a specific intervention technique/strategy.

PROFILE 6: CLEFT PALATE—4-YEAR-OLD

Eddie is 4 years old, has undergone successful palatal repair, and demonstrates adequate VP closure in nonspeech activities. His speech is characterized by audible nasal emission of air, hypernasality, and the following articulation errors:

	Initial	Medial	Final
Distortions	s, z, ʃ k, g, p, b	s, z, ʃ f, θ, k, g	s, z, ʃ f, θ, k, g
Omissions	-r/pr*	-l/pl*	s-/st*
Substitutions	n/d	ʔ/p, ʔ/b, ʔ/d, ʔ/t	ʔ/p, ʔ/b, ʔ/d, ʔ/t

*Consonant blends are consistently reduced to singletons in all positions and, therefore, are too numerous to list individually.

Selection of Therapy Targets. The five main goals of speech therapy with children with cleft palate are (a) correct articulatory placement, (b) achieve light articulatory contacts, (c) attain a greater mouth opening, (d) decrease hypernasal resonance quality, and (e) promote more anterior placement of articulatory production (Golding-Kushner, 2000; Kummer, 2008). Given these goals, the errors to be targeted for intervention are /p/, /b/, /s/, /θ/, /k/, /g/, /t/, /d/, and vowels. The first four sounds were chosen to decrease Eddie's tendency to move frontal articulatory placements to the back of the vocal tract. The /k/, /g/, /t/, and /d/ as well as /p/ and /b/ were selected because pressure consonants are the most effective vehicles for demonstrating light articulatory contact (less forceful movements of oral muscles). Vowels were included because they are the most appropriate targets for encouraging increased or exaggerated mouth opening as a means of improving the balance between oral and nasal resonance.

Sample Activities

Promote Anterior Placement of Speech Production

1. Compile a set of 20 pictures that are clear demonstrations of the concept of front versus back (e.g., train, dog, car, house, horse, truck) and cut them in half. (In addition, decorate a blank sheet of paper with 25 drawings or stickers of balloons without strings for later use.) Shuffle the pictures and place them face down on the table. Tell the child that this is a memory game in which he and the clinician will take turns selecting pictures, one at a time, to try to match the pairs that represent the front and back of each object. The child is instructed to identify each picture piece as it is uncovered (e.g., "This is the front of a train"). Each correctly matched pair is given to the player who found both pieces. The player with the most pairs at the end of the game is the winner.

   Once it is established that the child understands "front/back" in relation to everyday objects, explain that this concept also applies to his mouth. Tell him that some sounds are made at the front of the mouth, like /p/ and /t/, and others are made at the back, like /k/ and /g/. Sit with the child in front of a mirror and model the anterior placement of simple syllables (i.e., /pa/, /bæ/, /so/, /θi/). Engage the child in a "Simon Says" game in which he has to imitate sounds made by the clinician. For each correct production, the child may draw a string under one balloon on the prepared sheet. The object of the game is to fill the sheet with strings on all of the balloons.

Light Articulatory Contact

2. Obtain two puppets with easily manipulable mouths. Introduce the puppets to the child. Explain that one uses very hard (forceful) movements of his mouth when he talks, while the other uses gentle (light) movements. The clinician's speech and hand movements should demonstrate forceful versus light contacts as the explanations are given. To ensure the child's understanding of the basic concept, model several exaggerated examples of both articulatory contact types and have the child point to the puppet that uses that speech pattern. Once the child can reliably discriminate between "hard" and "gentle," hide both puppets in a bag or box, and instruct the child to close his eyes and pull one out and place it on his hand. The clinician provides a model of the type of contact used by the chosen puppet at the syllable level. Models should focus on pressure consonants in the initial position (e.g., /ka/, /gu/, /ti/, do/, /pa/, and /bæ/). The child is then required to imitate the clinician's stimulus and should be encouraged to use appropriate hand and mouth movements simultaneously. Return the puppet to its hiding place, and repeat the activity for 20 or more trials. The level of response

complexity can be increased from imitative to spontaneous and also can be programmed to vary from syllables to lengthy sentences.

Increased Degree of Mouth Opening

3. Draw or attach two pictures of frogs to a dry-erase board. One should be depicted as having an exaggerated open-mouth posture, whereas the other frog's mouth is only slightly opened. Instruct the child to throw a beanbag at either of the frogs. The clinician should model a vowel production with the degree of mouth opening that corresponds to the frog that is struck by the beanbag. The child is required to imitate the clinician's model five times for another turn at the game. The vowels /a/, /æ/, /o/, and /e/ are good candidates for the initial phase of training.

Accurate Articulatory Placement

4. Cut out a 12-in. circle from poster board to use as a "pizza." Use a marker to draw lines dividing the pizza into eight equal slices. Affix three to five small pieces of Velcro to each slice. Gather 24 to 40 small pictures containing targeted therapy sound(s) and attach Velcro strips to each. Explain that the child will decorate the pizza with picture "toppings." Instruct the child to name a picture with emphasis on the target sound. If production is correct, the child can place the topping on the pizza. Repeat this sequence until all toppings have been used.

Helpful Hints

1. Children who show only glottal and pharyngeal places of articulation should have therapy to assess the adequacy of fricative and plosive production before any pharyngeal flap surgery is considered.

2. If the child has questionable VPI, delay training of /k/ and /g/ to avoid the tendency to adopt compensatory movements.

3. Children with cleft palates often have persistent dental anomalies that may result in *lateralization* of fricatives and affricates that is not amenable to articulation therapy.

4. In general, speech therapy should be initiated at the earliest possible age to take advantage of sensitive periods in speech development.

5. Self-monitoring skills in children with nasality problems may be strengthened with the use of biofeedback devices such as the Oral & Nasal Listener (SuperDuper, Inc.), the Nasometer II (KayPentax Corporation), and See-Scape (Pro-Ed). These devices detect nasal emission/resonance and display this information visually or auditorily. The child uses the displayed information to monitor and eventually control velopharyngeal function.

6. The therapeutic process for children with oral-facial anomalies must frequently address the emotional well-being of the child and the family as well as the symptoms of the physical defect.

7. Parents of infants with clefts may require gentle but firm encouragement to engage in natural smiling and vocal interactions with their babies. Parents may need guidance to see beyond the obvious craniofacial defect to bond successfully with their child.

8. Clinicians treating children with cleft palates should be prepared to make referrals to parent support groups or to counseling professionals who have expertise in the area of birth defects.

Hearing Impairment

Hearing impairment refers to a significant loss in auditory acuity. There are two major types of hearing impairments: conductive and sensorineural. A **conductive**, or peripheral, hearing loss refers to a disruption in the mechanical transmission of sounds from the external auditory canal to the *cochlea* or inner ear (Martin & Clark, 2019). Conductive losses do not exceed 60 dB HL (decibel hearing level) and generally are amenable to medical treatment. A common cause of conductive hearing loss in young children is otitis media, an inflammation in the middle ear. A **sensorineural** loss involves a deficit in the neural transmission of sound impulses through the cochlear hair cells or the auditory nerve. Losses of this type usually do not respond to medical treatment and are generally irreversible. A disruption that occurs simultaneously in both pathways is termed a *mixed* hearing loss.

The degree of loss can range in severity from mild to profound. The majority of children with hearing losses are typically labeled hard of hearing (loss of <80 dB HL) and can derive significant benefit from articulation therapy. Children who are profoundly hearing impaired or deaf (loss of >80 dB HL) experience great difficulty acquiring intelligible speech even with intervention. In general, greater degrees of hearing loss result in more severe disruptions of speech development. It is important to note, however, that a loss as mild as 10 dB HL to 15 dB HL may be handicapping in the classroom setting with an ambient noise level of 25 dB to 35 dB. Deficits in speech production may not be marked if the hearing loss is unilateral rather than bilateral. Table 3–6 outlines the effects of different degrees of hearing loss on children's speech production abilities.

Speech intelligibility is also significantly affected by several other factors, including age of onset, configuration of hearing loss, age of identification, and degree of linguistic complexity (Martin & Clark, 1996; Radziewicz & Antonellis, 2008). With regard to amplification, important factors include the age at which appropriate amplification is fitted, the type and amount of habilitation, and the consistency of device use. Age of onset is a particularly critical factor. Children who are born with or sustain significant hearing losses prior to the critical language learning period (before age 3 years) will have more severe articulation deficits than children whose losses occurred later in life.

Following is a list of the most common types of speech errors exhibited by children with hearing impairment. The first four are characteristic of children whose hearing losses fall in the moderate range. Children who have profound hearing impairment or deafness will likely display all of the following behaviors:

- Omission of final consonants

- Substitution of voiced consonants for voiceless

- Substitution of stops for nasals, fricatives, and affricates

- Omission of consonants in blends

- Omission of initial consonants

- Substitution of schwa for other vowels (neutralization)

- Insertion of schwa into words or added to the ends of words

- Substitution of vowels for other vowels

- Nasalization of vowels

Educational Approaches

There are three basic approaches to instruction for children with hearing impairment: oral, manual, and total communication. **Oral** programs emphasize spoken language as the primary mode of communication through the use of strategies such as speech reading, amplification, auditory training, and explicit speech-language instruction. A commonly used oral approach is **auditory-verbal therapy**. Auditory-verbal therapy aims to improve the spoken language abilities of a child with hearing impairment to the level of a child with typical hearing by developing his or her listening skills independent of other cues such as speech reading and gestures (Brennan-Jones et al., 2014; Jackson & Schatschineider, 2014; Lim et al., 2018). Many authors suggest music as a beneficial addition to therapy programming for individuals with hearing aids and cochlear implants due to the perceptual similarities to the fundamental frequencies and rhythms found in verbal speech. See Torppa and Huotilainen (2019) for a systematic review of studies in this area. **Manual** programs focus on the earliest possible acquisition of a linguistic system, generally via American Sign Language (ASL), finger spelling, and/or manually coded English systems. **Total communication** is a philosophy that encourages any combination of modalities (e.g., speech, writing, signing, gestures, and facial expressions) that is effective in facilitating an individual child's acquisition of language. Recently, a **bilingual/bicultural** model of education has been implemented for children with significant hearing loss. In this approach, children

Table 3–6
Effects of Hearing Loss on Articulation Development

Degree of Loss	Characteristics
Slight (16–25 dB HL)	No noticeable difficulty in relatively quiet listening environments
Mild (26–40 dB HL)	Occasional difficulty with voiceless consonants, vowels and voiced consonants generally intact
Moderate (41–70 dB HL)	Some difficulty with sounds characterized by low intensity, high frequency, or short duration (e.g., final consonant omission, distortion of fricatives and affricates)
Severe (71–90 dB HL)	Significant difficulty in consonant production, with additional confusion of voiced/voiceless consonants and omission of consonants in blends
Profound (91 dB HL)	Global speech production impairment with the addition of neutralization or greater (schwa), substitution, addition, and nasalization of vowels as well as the omission of initial consonants

Sources: Adapted from "Phonological Substitution Processes of a Hard-of-Hearing Child," by D. K. Oller and C. A. Kelly, 1974, *Journal of Speech and Hearing Disorders, 39*, pp. 65–74; *An Investigation of the Intelligibility of Speech of the Deaf* (*Genetic Psychology Monographs* (pp. 289–392), by C. V. Hudgins and F. C. Numbers, 1942, Provincetown, MA: Journal Press; "Articulation of the Deaf," by E. H. Nober, 1967, *Exceptional Child, 33*, pp. 611–621; and "Uses and Abuses of Hearing Loss Classification," by J. G. Clark, 1981, *ASHA, 23*, pp. 493–500.

are exposed to ASL as their first language for communication and learn English in the school setting to develop reading and writing skills. Lively debate continues regarding the educational, social, and cultural impact of these different approaches. For comprehensive discussion on this topic, see Knoors and Marschark (2018). The most recent advance in rehabilitation for children with deafness is the use of **cochlear implants (CIs)**. The following discussion represents the most current data available at the time of this edition. Because state-of-the-art knowledge in this area is evolving rapidly, clinicians are encouraged to seek out additional, updated information.

Unlike a traditional hearing aid, a CI directly stimulates surviving auditory nerve fibers. One component of the device is a body-worn processor that highlights speech signals and minimizes background noise. These signals are routed first to a receiver implanted in the mastoid bone. Then the signals travel to an array of electrodes implanted in the cochlea, which transfers the sound to the auditory nerve (Niparko, 2009). The CI devices currently approved by the U.S. Food and Drug Administration (FDA) for implantation in children as young as 12 months of age provide multichannel stimulation and continue to evolve technologically. Children implanted at younger ages generally make greater and more rapid strides in vocal development and speech production than those implanted later in life (Dunn et al., 2014; Ertmer & Goffman, 2011; Ruff et al., 2017). A more recent development is the bilateral implantation of CIs. In a 2007 meta-analysis, Schafer et al. examined the relative effectiveness of bilateral and bimodal stimulation (i.e., two cochlear implants versus one cochlear implant and one hearing aid) and recommended bimodal stimulation as the first-order treatment approach for children who can derive benefit from hearing aid use in the nonimplant ear. Two research studies of adults (Gifford et al., 2018; Yawn et al., 2018) found less clear evidence for the effectiveness of one approach versus another. For additional information on bilateral cochlear implants, see Lammers et al. (2014), Peng et al. (2019), Välimaa et al. (2018), and Sarant et al. (2018). Historically, the cochlear implant literature suggested that five important factors are associated with improved speech production skills: age at implantation, years of device use, nonverbal intelligence, oral communication as primary mode after the implant, and number/placement of active electrodes with a wide dynamic range (Chin et al., 2003; Geers, 2002; Kirk et al., 2002; Robbins, 2017; Svirsky et al., 2004; Tobey et al., 2003). However, a more recent study on the relationship between speech intelligibility and cochlear implants (Ruff et al., 2017) suggests that a short duration of postlingual deafness may have a stronger correlation with better speech production than other factors. Within a social model of disability, clinicians are encouraged to identify structural barriers that may hinder the individual from obtaining full benefit from therapy services. Barriers may include low socioeconomic status (SES), poor insurance coverage, and lack of family education regarding hearing impairment, among other factors (Noblitt et al., 2018).

Example Profile

Following is a typical profile for pediatric hearing loss. This example has been designed to illustrate the selection of therapy targets as well as specific therapy activities and materials. The chosen activities are easily implemented in either individual or group therapy settings.

PROFILE 7: HEARING IMPAIRMENT—7-YEAR-OLD

Sherry is 7 years old, with a congenital moderate-severe bilateral sensorineural hearing loss. She is fitted with binaural hearing aids and demonstrates the following errors. These errors are illustrative of the misarticulations of children with this degree of hearing impairment.

1. Omission of final consonants
   - -/s
   - -/z
   - -/t
   - -/d
   - -/k
   - -/g
   - -/tʃ

2. Substitution of voiced for voiceless consonants
   - v/f
   - b/p
   - d/t
   - g/k
   - ð/θ

3. Substitutions of stops for nasals, fricatives, and affricates
   - d/n
   - g/ŋ
   - t/s
   - d/z
   - d/tʃ
   - t/ʃ

4. Substitution of schwa for other vowels*
   - ə/æ (hat)
   - ə/ɛ (bet)
   - ə/ʊ (boot)

*Errors of this type may not be found in all children with this degree of hearing loss.

Selection of Therapy Targets. The errors to be targeted are -/s, -/z, -/t, -/d, ə/æ, ə/ɛ, ə/ʊ, v/f, b/p, and ð/θ. Final consonant omissions and schwa substitutions were identified as priorities because these error types have a significant negative impact on perceived speech intelligibility. The four deletion errors listed (-/s, -/z, -/t, -/d) were chosen because, in the word final position, these sounds also function as plural and tense markers. The ə/æ, ə/ɛ, and ə/ʊ were included because these three substitutions have highly contrastive lip configurations that facilitate differential production. The voiced/voiceless confusion is an appropriate initial target, because two of the three critical characteristics of these phonemes (i.e., place and manner) are already present in the child's repertoire, thus increasing the likelihood of early success in therapy. The v/f, b/p, and ð/θ confusions were selected because they are highly visible, which eliminates the need for placement cues and allows training to focus solely on voicing. Production of /ʃ/ also was included as a therapy target because it is the initial sound of Sherry's name. This sound will be programmed at the sentence level, because Sherry demonstrates relatively consistent production at the level of isolated words.

Sample Activities

Final Consonant Production

1. Draw three "speech flowers" on large pieces of paper, each with a distinct rounded center and 10 petals (similar to daisies). From colored paper, cut 30 loose flower petals that are the same size as the drawn petals, and place them in a pile on the table. Write a different consonant-vowel (CV) syllable on every petal and a different final consonant in the three flower centers. The combination of each CV syllable with the final consonant should constitute a real word (e.g., fa + t = *fat*; be + t = *bet*, and so on). Explain to the child that the activity

will focus on the production of final sounds in words. Provide a glue stick or other adhesive. Instruct the child to pick a petal from the pile and fit it in an empty petal on the drawing. The clinician then glides a finger from the top of the petal to the flower center as the child produces the syllable plus final sound and forms a real word. After five correct productions of the target word, the child may glue the petal to the flower. Repeat this sequence until all the CV petals have been attached. The completed flowers can be used for home practice. (This activity can also be used to facilitate language awareness by using rhyming stimuli.)

Contrastive Lip Configurations for Vowel Productions

2. Draw three faces on separate pieces of paper or poster board, each depicting distinctly different mouth configurations corresponding to the target vowels. The mouth posture representing /æ/ should be drawn with an exaggerated lowering of the mandible. The /ɛ/ should depict clear lip retraction (similar to a smile), and the /ʊ/ drawing should display a pursed, rounded lip position that is slightly opened. For each vowel sound, gather or prepare 10 picture cards representing common monosyllabic words, for a total of 30 cards (e.g., *cat, bag, pen, bed, boot, shoe,* and so on). Draw three stacked circles on the blackboard in preparation for a Snowman game. Place the three face cue cards on the table, and put the shuffled card deck face down in front of the child. Explain the rules of Snowman (similar to traditional Hangman) and emphasize that the game will focus on correct vowel production. Begin the game by having the child turn over the top card of the deck and place it next to the corresponding face cue card. Instruct the child to produce the correct vowel in isolation, making sure to match mouth configuration to the corresponding face, and then name the card five times. Each incorrect production allows the clinician to fill in one part of the snowman drawing. The object of the game is to deplete the picture deck before the snowman is completed.

Voicing Contrast

3. With masking tape on the floor, create an outline of a mountain range with at least six peaks. Provide a small toy train or other vehicle, and tell the child that the train is going on a long journey up and down the mountain peaks. The clinician introduces a voiced/voiceless cognate pair (e.g., v/f) and instructs the child to produce the voiced sound while moving the train *up* the mountain and to produce the voiceless sound as the train is moved *down* the mountain. Instruct the child to monitor voice onset and offset by placing her free hand on her throat (tactile cue) throughout the journey. Repeat this activity with each target cognate pair.

Production of /ʃ/

4. Engage the child in a hand-clapping or jump rope activity using the following chant. Explain that the chant emphasizes correct production of the /ʃ/ in lots of different words. Teach one verse at a time to control task difficulty level. Use pictures and/or written words as needed.

*Sh*eila the fi*sh*, fi*sh*, fi*sh*
*Sh*e had one wi*sh*, wi*sh*, wi*sh*
To have a bowl, bowl, bowl
Without a hole, hole, hole

*Sh*e called up Jo*sh*, Jo*sh*, Jo*sh*

Who said, Oh go*sh*, go*sh*, go*sh*

Do you have a ga*sh*, ga*sh*, ga*sh?*

Or a red ra*sh*, ra*sh*, ra*sh?*

*Sh*e said, Oh *s*ure, *s*ure, *s*ure

Quite an eyesore, sore, sore

My bowl was sma*sh*ed, sma*sh*ed, sma*sh*ed

When the table cra*sh*ed, cra*sh*ed, cra*sh*ed

Jo*sh* said, Let's ru*sh*, ru*sh*, ru*sh*

Or the water will *gush, gush, gush*

Get the *mesh* net, net, net

So you stay wet, wet, wet

*Sh*eila the fi*sh*, fi*sh*, fi*sh*

Was plopped in a *dish, dish, dish*

And said, Oh *sheesh, sheesh, sheesh*

I thought I'd be qui*ch*e, qui*ch*e, qui*ch*e

After a while, while, while

*Sh*e began to smile, smile, smile

At first slugg*ish, ish, ish*

*Sh*e now goes swi*sh*, swi*sh*, swi*sh*

Helpful Hints

1. Cued speech can be a helpful tool for teaching place, manner, and voicing in the initial stages of therapy for children with hearing losses greater than 85 dB HL. (For more information and specific techniques, see Cornett [1967] and the National Cued Speech Association website.)

2. Try to incorporate alternative sensory modalities (i.e., visual, tactile, and so on) in the early stages of each therapy task. These cues can be faded out as soon as they are no longer required to elicit a target sound.

3. For school-age children whose hearing losses also result in language impairments, select stimulus words that are related to the classroom curriculum (e.g., spelling words, science vocabulary).

4. Always ensure that the child's amplification system is in working order during therapy sessions to maximize residual hearing capabilities. Good sources for tips regarding troubleshooting hearing aids are Hull (2009) and the ASHA Audiology Information Series website.

5. Auditory trainers are often used in the classroom environment to facilitate the child's ability to monitor his or her own speech production as well as that of the teacher. Auditory trainers are high-fidelity systems in which the speaker's voice is fed into a microphone, amplified,

and then directed to the child through a receiver. These devices make it possible for the child to receive speech input with minimum background noise (a high signal-to-noise ratio). One widely used system consists of a microphone/transmitter worn by the teacher, which broadcasts directly to an FM receiver worn by the child. Anderson and Goldstein (2004) and J. Martin (2013) provide informative discussions regarding the relative benefits of various listening devices.

6. As counselors, clinicians may be asked to provide information regarding a child's academic aptitude and recommendations for appropriate educational placement. For more information on counseling skills for working with the hearing impaired population, see Scott (2018).

7. Clinicians should anticipate that some children may demonstrate confusion or fear when experiencing sound input for the first time (via devices such as hearing aids and cochlear implants). Comfort with sound stimulation and auditory awareness develops gradually.

8. Given that the number of children with cochlear implants is steadily increasing, SLPs need to develop an ample repertoire of strategies for facilitating auditory perception and speech production skills. Practical clinical ideas can be found in Ertmer (2005).

Childhood Apraxia of Speech

Childhood apraxia of speech (CAS) is a speech-motor planning disorder characterized by a reduced ability to volitionally sequence movements of the articulators for speech in the absence of paralysis, incoordination, or weakness of the oral musculature (dysarthria). (See Appendix 3–B on the companion website for normative data on diadochokinetic rates for children.) CAS is thought to result from neurologic dysfunction, although currently no definitive evidence of specific brain pathology exists. There is much controversy in the literature as to whether CAS constitutes a discrete clinical entity (e.g., American Speech-Language-Hearing Association, 2007a; Highman et al., 2013; Lewis et al., 2004; McCauley & Strand, 2008; Murray et al., 2015; Shriberg et al., 1997a, 1997b, 1997c). Three characteristics have been identified as hallmark indicators of CAS: (a) vowel errors or distortions may be present, (b) speech production errors are highly inconsistent, and (c) prosodic disturbances are evident, particularly in the appropriate use of stress patterns. This profile of characteristics is generally not observed in children with other articulatory or phonologic disorders. In a recent series of articles, Shriberg and colleagues (2017) argue that the presence of a between-word pause of more than 150 msec ("pause marker") can be used as a reliable diagnostic indicator for the presence of CAS.

Following is a list of additional speech production characteristics that have been associated in the literature with CAS:

- The repertoire of phonemes is extremely restricted.

- A reduced ability to imitate sounds modeled by others, especially at the multisyllabic level, is present.

- Omission errors predominate; substitution, distortion, addition, prolongation, and metathetic errors (transposition of sounds) also occur.

- A higher percentage of errors in sounds requiring complex oral movements (e.g., fricatives, affricates, consonant clusters) is present.

- Struggling or groping movements of the oral musculature are present.

- The number of errors increases as the length and complexity of utterances increase.

- The ability to sequence phonemes in words/phrases and diadochokinetic tasks is reduced.

- More recently, it has been suggested that CAS symptoms include deficits in speech perception and often in literacy-related skills as well.

In general, these children demonstrate receptive language abilities that are significantly superior to their speech production skills and may exhibit an accompanying oral apraxia. Children with CAS can be highly unintelligible; at the most severe levels, these children may be categorized as nonverbal, meaning the near absence of oral expressive output. They frequently demonstrate awareness of and frustration with their reduced ability to communicate. CAS is noted for its resistance to remediation. That is, CAS does not respond easily to traditional articulation techniques. In fact, there is little scientific support for the effectiveness of therapy approaches for CAS (McCabe et al., 2017; Thomas et al., 2018).

The literature describes several therapy approaches for children who demonstrate CAS (Morgan et al., 2018). **Integral stimulation** (Milisen, 1954a, 1954b) utilizes a hierarchical cueing procedure that begins with a high level of support characterized by production of simple utterances spoken slowly and simultaneously by both client and clinician accompanied by visual and tactile cues. The simultaneous production is gradually faded, and cues are provided until they are no longer needed. The client then produces delayed repetitions of increasingly complex stimulus items. **Dynamic temporal and tactile cueing (DTTC)** is a variation of the integral stimulation approach and is described by Strand (2020). It retains the same hierarchical structure as just described, but it also allows the SLP to use tactile prompts/cues to facilitate correct jaw and lip positions for the initial articulatory configuration. Proprioceptive processing is maximized by having the child maintain the postures for several seconds. Also, DTTC incorporates production of simple consonant-vowel-consonant (CVC) target words, which are slowed down by elongation of the vowel to provide more time to achieve correct phonetic placement. In addition, some approaches target prosodic variables (e.g., loudness, pitch) rather than phoneme production (Ballard et al., 2010).

More recently, McCabe et al. (2017) demonstrated the efficacy and effectiveness of Rapid Syllable Transition (ReST) as an intervention for CAS. It is based on the premise of neuroplasticity and incorporates principles of motor learning as key elements of programming. Intervention is divided into two main phases, training and practice, and focuses on three major components of speech sound production: (a) beats—lexical stress; (b) smoothness—transitions between speech sounds; and (c) speech sounds—consonant and vowel combinations. This approach utilizes nonsense words as a means to concentrate on speech motor patterns without the distraction of word meaning.

Another suggested approach for implementing therapy for children with CAS was presented by Strode and Chamberlain (2006). Their hierarchy of overlapping steps is based on the principles of motor learning and gradually increases the complexity of the speech task while continuing to utilize repetitive drill and significant cueing:

Level 1: Stabilize existing vowels and consonant sounds

Level 2: Sequence established vowels and consonants in CV and VC syllables

Level 3: Teach new vowel and consonant sounds

Level 4: Produce CVCV and VCVC syllable sequences (emphasis on using established CV and VC syllables from Level 2)

Level 5: Close established CV and VC syllables with an established consonant sound to produce CVC words

Level 6: Produce multisyllabic words from stabilized sounds, syllables, and CVC words

Level 7: Produce consonant clusters and blends in words

Level 8: Produce phrases and sentences (sequencing syllables to form phrases and sentences begins as early as Level 2)

Regardless of the specific approach used, a set of basic factors to be considered in developing treatment programming for this population includes the following:

- Progress in therapy is slow and marked by poor retention and poor generalization of therapy targets across treatment sessions.

- Although repeated practice is an integral component of therapy for all types of articulation disorders, it is important to provide intensive, systematic drill for children with CAS in order for them to master the necessary speech-motor patterns. The random (versus massed) practice advantage observed in the non-speech-motor learning literature may not extend to treatment for CAS (Maas & Farinella, 2012).

- Based on the first two factors, sessions that are shorter and more frequent may be helpful in facilitating generalization and avoiding speech-system fatigue (Edeal & Gildersleeve-Neumann, 2011).

- Children with CAS have great difficulty learning articulatory patterns through auditory input alone. For this reason, the use of visual and tactile cues is essential for establishing these sensory-motor patterns.

- Remediation should include an early emphasis on improving children's ability to monitor their own speech production, particularly through tactile and/or kinesthetic modalities (e.g., concentrate on how sounds "feel" and where the tongue is during movement sequences).

- Intervention should incorporate a focus on the melody and rhythm patterns of connected speech.

- Children with CAS often demonstrate accompanying language difficulties. Further, a comprehensive approach to intervention programming for CAS should incorporate consideration of a child's speech perception abilities (Spencer et al., 2022).

- For children with extremely unintelligible speech, it may be necessary to use assistive technology (e.g., augmentative/alternative system) to provide the child with a functional means of communication. This option may be temporary in nature or serve as the child's long-term communication mode.

There is relatively little support in the literature for most therapy approaches to CAS. A few metaanalyses/systematic reviews have been conducted and have not reported definitively strong conclusions regarding treatment efficacy for specific approaches in the areas of CAS.

Example Profile

Following is a typical profile of a child with CAS. This example has been designed to illustrate the selection of intervention targets as well as specific therapy activities and materials. The chosen activities are easily implemented in either individual or group therapy settings.

PROFILE 8: CHILDHOOD APRAXIA OF SPEECH—3-YEAR-OLD

Billy is almost 3 years old and presents with unintelligible speech. His phoneme repertoire is limited to four consonant sounds /b, m, t, d/, which he substitutes for several other sounds. He sometimes produces the same CV syllables for many different words (e.g., /ba/ for *ball, table, telephone, door,* and *paper*). In addition, Billy demonstrates a significant number of omission errors (sounds and syllables), which occur in all word positions (e.g., /tə/ for *truck*, /ət/ for *dog*, /oh/ for *open*). Billy also demonstrates occasional vowel errors characterized by the substitution of schwa for other vowels, especially diphthongs.

Selection of Therapy Targets. The primary areas to be targeted are self-monitoring of speech production, restricted phoneme repertoire, and limited speech-sound-sequencing abilities. The self-awareness skills selected for remediation include tongue-tip elevation, tongue lateralization, tongue protrusion/retraction, lip pursing, and lip retraction, because these movements are highly visible. (Children who demonstrate an accompanying oral apraxia may find these tasks very frustrating.) The phonemes /p/ and /f/ were chosen as targets to be added to Billy's consonant repertoire for several reasons. These sounds appear early developmentally, are highly visible, and are sufficiently different from one another to avoid confusion during training. In addition, these consonants are voiceless and therefore require the mastery of one less feature for correct production than do voiced sounds. The complexity level selected for work on sequencing skills was reduplicative CV and VC syllables in which the consonant and vowel remain constant across syllables. The phonemes identified for use in the sequencing tasks were /b, m, t, d/, because these sounds are already present in Billy's consonant repertoire at the single-syllable level.

Sample Activities

Self-Monitoring

1. Gather two sets of 5 to 10 items of varying texture, size, shape, and temperature (e.g., ice, tongue depressor, straw, warm liquid, rubber toy). Encourage the child to use each of the objects in a set to engage in oral-exploratory play. Imitate each of the child's play behaviors using the objects in the second set. Establish the child's conscious awareness of oral-motor sensations by commenting on what the child is doing and how it makes the mouth feel. Promote expansion of the number and variety of oral-motor play movements demonstrated by the child. This task is most effective when used as a warm-up activity at the beginning of a therapy session to heighten self-awareness as a building block for monitoring of the child's own speech production.

Visual Cueing and Massed Practice

2. Sit next to the child in front of a large mirror. Tell the child that he is going to play a "clown" game and show him a clown hat and wig made from colored paper and yarn. Instruct the child that this game involves taking turns making funny faces in the mirror. The clinician takes the first turn by putting on the clown hat and modeling a target tongue or lip movement. Have the child imitate the target movement a minimum of five times to earn a chance to be the clown. (In the early stages of therapy, it may be necessary to reinforce any voluntary oral-motor movement that occurs in response to the clinician's stimulus.) Explain

that it is now the child's turn to wear the hat and make a funny face for the clinician to imitate. Repeat this sequence with other oral-motor movements that are absent from the child's repertoire. This activity also works well as a warm-up procedure at the beginning of a session (5–10 min) and may be repeated at intervals throughout the session to reinforce targeted motor patterns. (Refer to the "Oral-Motor Considerations" section at the beginning of this chapter for additional information.)

Intensive Short Drill

3. Gather four large sacks (pillowcases, trash bags, grocery bags, and so on), fill each one with at least five objects whose names begin with a target sound (avoid blends), and attach the sacks to the wall. For example, objects for the target sound /p/ might include pencil, puzzle, paint, puppet, and pot. Give the child a beanbag and tell him to throw it at one of the sacks. The clinician removes the sack that was hit from the wall and tells the child to close his eyes and pick one object at a time from the sack. The clinician holds the object next to his or her mouth and models the target phoneme in isolation for the child to imitate five successive times. When the sack is empty, take a short break. Then, give the child the beanbag and start the game again.

Intonational Contour

4. Cut an egg carton in half lengthwise, turn it upside down, and color or paint each of the six protruding sections a different color. Hide the last three sections from the child's view by covering them with a piece of aluminum foil or other material. Obtain a large plastic dinosaur or other animal with a large mouth opening and collect at least 25 marbles. Explain to the child that he is going to play a game in which he has to sing silly sounds in exactly the same way as the clinician to earn a chance to feed marbles to the very hungry dinosaur. The clinician then "sings" a string of three reduplicative CV syllables that are constructed from the identified consonant targets /b, m, t, d/. The clinician produces these strings with a distinctive intonational contour pattern, while simultaneously tapping the egg carton protrusions to pace each CV syllable as it is "sung." Intonational contour patterns might include rising/falling intonation, primary stress on a particular syllable, and increased/decreased loudness on initial/medial/final syllables. Instruct the child to imitate the clinician's syllable sequence using the same intonational pattern and pacing cues as the clinician. Following the successful imitation of at least three different sequences, the child is allowed to feed a marble to the dinosaur. Continue this activity using varied combinations of phonemes and intonation patterns until the dinosaur has eaten all the marbles. The level of difficulty can be modified by increasing the number of syllables in the reduplicative CV/ VC strings or by introducing nonreduplicative syllable strings.

Note: This activity represents a simplified adaptation of melodic intonation therapy (Sparks et al., 1974), in which rhythm and intonation patterns are used to facilitate speech output.

Helpful Hints

1. Oral-motor movements can be used to facilitate articulatory placement for the acquisition of new consonants. For example, after work on tongue-tip elevation, you can add voice to it to produce /l/.

2. Capitalize on an acceptable speech-motor pattern at the moment of its production, when the experience is most recent and vivid in the child's mind. Have the child repeat the utterance immediately for multiple trials to reduce the probability that the articulatory gesture will fade.

3. Early therapy should focus on a child's ability to produce *accurate* responses. As the child improves, the focus can be shifted to *speed* of response by requiring rapid automatic production of the accurate articulatory movements.

4. Rhymes and songs can be used as stimulus materials to facilitate oral-motor sequencing abilities for children who can produce sentence-length utterances.

5. For children at the single-word level, it may be helpful to introduce words that contain reduplicative syllables (e.g., *mama, bye-bye, night-night, dada*). Such utterances highlight the rhythm of speech and can provide a transition to other bisyllabic words (e.g., *cookie, allgone, open*).

6. Given that children with CAS may demonstrate intact language comprehension skills and normal intelligence, there are two commonly occurring counseling issues: (a) the child may be significantly frustrated by the inability to intelligibly convey his or her ideas and thoughts, and (b) parents may inaccurately perceive the inconsistent nature of their child's poor speech production as an indicator of laziness or lack of motivation.

7. Clinicians should make every effort to ensure that therapy remains a positive experience for the child, because intervention with this disorder consists largely of repetitive drill.

8. Incorporating an emphasis on variations in prosody at all stages of therapy can contribute to improved overall intelligibility of speech in children with CAS.

9. Clinicians interested in facilitating parent/family understanding of this disorder are encouraged to consult the series of "Letters to the parent of . . ." by Hall (2000a, 2000b, 2000c, 2000d), which explains the nature, causes, and treatment of CAS in clear, simple language.

Conclusion

This chapter has presented basic information, protocols, and procedures for intervention for articulation and phonology at an *introductory* level. This information is intended only as a starting point in the reader's clinical education and training. For in-depth coverage of this area, the following readings are recommended.

Articulation and Phonology

Bernthal, J. E., Bankson, N. W., & Flipsen, P., Jr. (2020). *Articulation and phonological disorders: Speech sound disorders in children* (8th ed.). Pearson.

Bleile, K. (2017). *The late eight* (3rd ed.). Plural Publishing.

Marshalla, P. (2011). *Carryover techniques (in articulation and phonological therapy)*. Marshalla Speech and Language.

Peterson-Falzone, S., Trost-Cardamone, J., Karnell, M., & Hardin-Jones, M. (2016). *The clinician's guide to treating cleft palate speech* (2nd ed.). Mosby Elsevier.

Rvachew, S., & Brosseau-Lapre, F. (2016). *Developmental phonological disorders: Foundations of clinical practice* (2nd ed.). Plural Publishing.

Strode, R., & Chamberlain, C. (2006). *The source for childhood apraxia of speech.* LinguiSystems.

Oral-Motor Dysfunction

Alexander, R., Boehme, R., & Cupps, B. (1998). *Normal development of functional motor skills: The first year of life.* Therapy Skill Builders.

Marshalla, P. (2004). *Oral motor techniques in articulation and phonological therapy.* Marshalla Speech and Language.

Morris, S. E., & Klein, M. D. (2000). *Pre-feeding skills: A comprehensive resource for mealtime development* (2nd ed.). Psychological Corp.

Additional Resources

Articulation

Apraxia Uncovered: Seven Stages of Phoneme Development
The *Apraxia Uncovered* book shows how to develop consonants and vowels by using information from articulation, phonology, and oral-motor methodologies. It presents a systematic plan of phoneme development for children who have apraxia and other severe expressive speech disorders.

Artic Chipper Chat
Sixty different game boards, each filled with sound-loaded pictures. Students pick a question card and search their boards for the correct picture answer. As they answer questions, they fill up their boards with magnetic chips. The game focuses on 12 different sounds, targeting the initial, medial, and final position and/or combinations.

Artic Shuffle
Fifty-two different pictures per deck to give students tons of articulation practice by playing Go Fish, Crazy Eights, or a memory-type board game. Students match suits, numbers, and face cards so there is no need for picture pairs. Ten card decks cover 12 sounds plus sounds in blends.

Carryover Techniques in Articulation and Phonological Therapy
This resource book provides an overview of the research on carryover and generalization. The author includes a discussion of various factors that can affect carryover, including personality traits and behavior modification. The book also includes tips, methods, and activities that can be used in therapy to promote carryover of skills.

Easy Does It for Apraxia and Motor Planning
This program includes techniques from traditional articulation therapy and phonology therapy and emphasizes developing sound sequencing skills and closed syllables in tasks of increasing complexity.

Eliciting Sounds: Techniques and Strategies for Clinicians, Second Edition
This resource provides SLPs with multiple strategies to use with clients to elicit a targeted phoneme. The book contains sections on each consonant and vowel sound. It also includes sections on common errors, dialectical variations, stimulability, and articulation screening.

50 Quick-Play Articulation Games
More than 50 creative, fun, interactive games on reproducible sheets for ages 5 to 10. Games target these sounds in all positions: *p, b, m, k, g, t, d, f, v, sh, ch, j, s, z, r, l, l* blends, *r* blends, *s* blends, and voiced and voiceless *th*. There are 50 path games, 15 card games, 11 noncompetitive games, plus a *Make Your Own Game* path and a *Target the Stars* motivational sheet.

40,000 Selected Words
This resource has compiled word lists for each consonant sound of the English language in each word position. It also divides words into lists based upon syllable number. SLPs can use this book to find target word stimuli to use with both children and adults.

No-Glamour Articulation
This book provides over 11,500 pictures, scenes, words, and sentences for articulation practice. Picture cards are organized by word position as well as syllable number. The stimuli can be used for drills, reading tasks, or to expand language and transition articulation skills to conversational levels.

Photo Articulation Library—Complete Kit
This consists of 1,085 real-life photos arranged by sounds and word positions, 350 cards in each set, suitable for all ages. Twenty-seven categories include events, communication, actions, games and toys, occupations, transportation, and more, organized by consonants, vowels, and word position.

The Source for Childhood Apraxia of Speech
This resource provides tips for clients who are resistant to therapy, have developmental delays or autism, or are very young. It contains comprehensive information on the neurologically based disorder as well as goals and techniques to facilitate both speech and language skills simultaneously.

Webber Articulation Cards (Sets I, II, and III)
Decks of cards with colored pictures designed to elicit 15 target phonemes in all word positions; duplicate cards are included to make the decks suitable for many children's card games.

Phonology

Giant Book of Phonology
This spiral-bound book contains reproducible pictures to practice phonological processes with target words, phrases, and sentences.

Say & Glue Phonology and Artic Fun Sheets
This workbook provides cut and paste activities per target phonological process or speech sound. The worksheets can then be used at home for practice and there is a parent letter included in the book.

Silly Sets: Minimal Pairs for Maximum Progress

This card deck contains 100 3 × 5-in. cards color coded by phonological process, including stopping, fronting, and final consonant deletion. The cards have illustrations on one side and text on the other side. The deck also includes ideas for games and activities.

Sourcebook of Phonological Awareness Activities: Children's Core Literature; Children's Classic Literature

These books include training materials to be used in conjunction with popular books such as *The Hungry Caterpillar (Core version) and Charlotte's Web (Classic version)*. They also introduce the concept of phonological awareness and its relationship to reading skills.

Webber Phonology Cards

Decks of cards with colored pictures designed to target eight phonological processes, including stopping, gliding, fronting, final consonant deletion, and cluster reduction. There are duplicate cards included to make the decks suitable for many children's card games.

Introduction to Language Intervention for Children and Adolescents

Chapters 4 and 5 focus on the treatment of childhood language disorders. Childhood language disorders affect a diverse group of children who present with differing profiles of language impairment. Intervention with this population is the subject of an enormous amount of literature that covers the age span from infancy through adolescence. To organize this body of information in a manner that is clinically useful for the reader, this section of the book begins with overview material that is germane to the entire range of child language disorders. Chapter 4 then presents specific intervention information for children from birth through the preschool years. Intervention information for school-age children and adolescents is the subject of Chapter 5.

The information in these chapters is provided as a general guideline regarding language acquisition and treatment. The relative applicability of this material will depend on a host of factors, including the sociocultural background of any particular client and family.

A **language disorder** can be defined as the abnormal acquisition, comprehension, or use of spoken or written language. This includes all receptive and expressive language skills. The disorder may involve any aspect of the form, content, or use components of the linguistic system. Children with language disorders are a heterogeneous population in several respects, including the following:

- *Primary versus secondary disorder:* For some children, the reduced ability to acquire language is their primary deficit in the relative absence of impairment in other developmental areas. For other children, the language deficit occurs in association with other impairments (e.g., intellectual disabilities).

- *Developmental versus acquired:* Developmental language disorders are present from birth or occur prior to the onset of typical language acquisition. Acquired disorders involve the loss or interruption of language function due to illness or trauma.

- *Delayed versus aberrant/unusual acquisition:* Children with delayed language proceed through the same sequence of acquisition as typically developing children but at a substantially slower rate. In contrast, children with aberrant language development demonstrate acquisition patterns that are atypical and diverge significantly from the normal developmental sequence.

- *Range of severity:* The severity of language deficits can range along a continuum of mild to profound impairment.

Classification of Language Disorders

A disorder can involve both the comprehension and production of language. Language **comprehension** (receptive language) refers to the ability to derive meaning from incoming auditory or visual messages. Language **production** (expressive language) involves the combination of linguistic symbols to form meaningful messages. Language disorders are generally classified according to the major components of the linguistic system: semantics, morphology, syntax, pragmatics, and phonology.

Semantics involves the meaning of individual words and the rules that govern the combinations of word meanings to form meaningful phrases and sentences. Impairments in this subsystem can take the form of reduced vocabulary and depth of word knowledge, restricted semantic categories, word-retrieval deficits, poor word-association skills, limited word-definition skills, and difficulty with figurative (nonliteral) language forms such as idioms, metaphors, and humor.

Morphology involves the structure of words and the construction of individual word forms from the basic elements of meaning (i.e., morphemes). Deficits in this component are manifested as difficulties with inflectional markers such as plurals, past tense, auxiliary verbs, possessives, and so on.

Syntax involves the rules governing the order and combination of words in the construction of well-formed sentences. Syntactic deficits are characterized by problems with simple and complex sentence types such as negatives, interrogatives, passives, and relative clauses as well as occasional word-order difficulties.

Pragmatics involves the rules governing the use of language in a social context. Pragmatic impairments can include a reduced repertoire of communicative intentions, poor shared/joint attention, reciprocal turn-taking difficulties in conversation, an inability to repair messages that are not understood by the listener, and difficulty with narrative discourse such as storytelling and personal narratives.

Phonology involves the particular sounds (i.e., phonemes) that make up the sound system of a language and the rules that govern permissible sound combinations. (For a discussion of phonological impairments, see Chapter 3.)

Language disorders can affect the development of basic language skills and/or higher order *meta*linguistic knowledge in any of the previously mentioned components. In addition to language deficits, children may demonstrate certain associated behavioral characteristics, the most common of which are defined in Table I–1.

Relationship Between Oral Language and Literacy

It is now recognized that speech-language pathologists (SLPs) play a significant role in the acquisition of literacy. Literacy involves the development of reading and writing skills. From a basic perspective, reading consists of two component processes: word recognition and comprehension. Word recognition includes decoding and reading fluency. Decoding is the ability to assign sound–letter correspondences to printed symbols (the alphabetic principle), whereas reading fluency refers to the speed, accuracy, and automaticity of reading words and connected text. Comprehension involves the ability to derive meaning from printed text at the word, phrase, sentence, or text level. Writing involves the acquisition of spelling and the ability to compose text at the sentence level and beyond. Spelling is the ability to construct words using the conventional orthography (i.e., written symbols) of a given language, and composition is the formulation of coherent units of connected language, including narrative and expository texts.

Table I–1
Behavioral Characteristics Associated With Language Disorders

Behavior	Definition
Inattention	Impairment of concentration characterized by difficulty with completing tasks, attending to details, following through on instructions, and tuning out distracting stimuli
Impulsivity	The abrupt performance of actions without sufficient deliberation or consideration of the consequences
Hyperactivity	An excessively high level of activity accompanied by a reduced ability to inhibit the activity volitionally
Attention Deficit Disorder (ADD)	Disorder characterized by one or more of the above features: inattention, impulsivity, or hyperactivity
Perseveration	Inappropriate and often involuntary continuation of a motor or verbal response when it is no longer relevant
Echolalia	Excessive and developmentally inappropriate repetition of the speech of others, generally with the same intonation; may be immediate or delayed; may be communicative or noncommunicative

Oral language serves as the basis for the development of reading and writing skills, beginning with the period known as *emergent literacy*, which extends from birth through the preschool years. **Emergent literacy** is a child's increasing awareness of the world of print and an understanding of the functions of literacy. During the preschool period, children develop foundational knowledge about print through everyday, naturally occurring experiences in their home and preschool/day care environments. These experiences prepare them for the formal literacy instruction (learning to read and write) that begins in the early elementary school grades. For this reason, emergent literacy skills are considered the developmental precursors to children's achievement of skilled reading and writing.

Of the oral language skills studied thus far, metalinguistic awareness is the area that has been most closely linked to literacy acquisition. **Metalinguistic awareness** is the explicit knowledge of and ability to manipulate aspects of the linguistic system independently of the meaning conveyed by the message. Phonological awareness is a metalinguistic skill that involves manipulation of the sound structure of language through tasks such as rhyming, blending, and segmenting of words, syllables, or phonemes. In particular, a child's control of sounds at the phoneme level (*phonemic awareness*) is highly predictive of decoding and spelling skills. A common example of a phonemic awareness task is asking a child to say a word such as *fat* and then to say it again without the /f/. In turn, acquisition of decoding skill leads to subsequent improvement of phonemic awareness ability. (Note: *Phonics* is the written language counterpart to this ability and focuses on sound–letter correspondences.) Children and adolescents with language and learning impairments demonstrate considerable difficulty with phonemic awareness tasks. There is evidence that these children can benefit from direct phonological awareness instruction (Pfost et al., 2019; Torgesen et al., 1994).

Table I–2
Scope and Sequence for Phonological Awareness Intervention

Phonological awareness skills

1. Rhyming/alliteration
2. Blending
3. Segmenting
    a. Categorization (e.g., Which one begins with a different sound: *feet, five, soup, fat?*)
    b. Deletion (e.g., Say *trip* without the /t/.)
    c. Substitution (e.g., Replace the /m/ in *man* with /f/.)
    d. Manipulation (e.g., Say the word *stop*. Now move the /s/ to the end of the word and say it again.)

Task mode

1. Matching (e.g., Show me the one that rhymes with *hat*.)
2. Elimination (e.g., Show me the one that does not rhyme with the other two words.)
3. Judgment (e.g., Do *hat* and *bat* rhyme?)
4. Production (e.g., Tell me a word that rhymes with *hat*.)

Stimuli level for segmenting/blending

1. Sentences into words
2. Words into syllables (Compound words such as *blackboard* are easier than noncompound words such as *finger*, because each syllable is a common word.)
3. Syllables into phonemes such as "c-a-t" (Polysyllabic words and/or consonant clusters increase task difficulty.)

Phoneme class for segmenting/blending

Continuant sounds, such as fricatives and nasals, are easier than noncontinuant sounds, such as stops. (Continuants are longer in duration and acoustically more discrete; they can be produced in isolation and emphasized by overarticulation.)

Sources: Adapted from *Phonemic Awareness in Young Children*, by M. J. Adams, B. R. Foorman, I. Lundberg, and T. Beeler, 1998, Baltimore, MD: Paul H. Brookes Publishing; "Promoting the Awareness of Sounds in Speech: An Initial Report of an Early Intervention for Children with Speech and Language Impairments," by F. P. Roth, G. A. Troia, C. K. Worthington, and K. A. Dow, 2002, *Applied Psycholinguistics, 23*, pp. 535–565; "Promoting Awareness of Sounds in Speech (PASS): The Effects of Intervention and Stimulus Characteristics on the Blending Performance of Preschool Children with Communication Impairments," by F. P. Roth, G. A. Troia, C. K. Worthington, and D. Handy, 2006, *Learning Disability Quarterly, 29*, pp. 67–88.

Intervention in this skill area is most effective when delivered in conjunction with training on the alphabetic principle and results in measurable gains in reading and spelling (Torgesen & Davis, 1996). See Table I–2 for scope and sequence information on phonological awareness instruction, organized in a progression from least to most difficult.

Other aspects of oral language that are associated with literacy development are vocabulary knowledge, word retrieval, and morphological awareness (Adlof & Hogan, 2019). Vocabulary size during the toddler years appears to be related to a child's ability to accurately decode single words in the first and second grades (Scarborough, 1998; Scarborough & Dobrich, 1990). Once a child reaches the middle elementary school years, the focus of reading shifts away from decoding or word recognition and vocabulary size becomes predictive of reading comprehension skill (Baker et al., 1998; Stanovich, 1986). With regard to word retrieval, naming accuracy is predictive of current and future decoding skill, whereas naming speed has been found to be strongly related to reading comprehension (Scarborough, 1998; Wolf, 1984, 1991). Morphological awareness is linked to both word reading and reading comprehension, as it reflects a child's familiarity with the meanings of words and their parts (e.g., prefixes, suffixes) as well as the ability to apply this knowledge to decipher the meaning of written words and text (Carlisle & Goodwin, 2014). Importantly, deficits in vocabulary and word retrieval are among the most common characteristics of language impairment throughout childhood and adolescence.

Role of the Speech-Language Pathologist (SLP) in Literacy

The traditional scope of practice for SLPs has evolved over the past several years to incorporate more emphasis on literacy-related issues. Accordingly, in 2000, the American Speech-Language-Hearing Association (ASHA) developed a position statement, guidelines, and several other documents to address the roles and responsibilities of SLPs in serving children and adolescents with reading and writing difficulties. These documents clearly indicate that "SLPs play a critical and direct role in the development of literacy for children and adolescents with communication disorders . . . " (p. 1) and are based on the following premises:

- Oral language is the basis for the acquisition of reading and writing.

- There is a reciprocal relationship between oral and written language in that each builds on the other.

- Children and adolescents with oral language deficits often have difficulty acquiring the ability to read and write (and vice versa).

- Reading and writing deficits can involve any of the subsystems of language: phonology, morpho-syntax, semantics, and pragmatics.

- SLPs have knowledge of typical and atypical patterns of language development as well as experience in assessment and intervention for children and adolescents.

- Literacy development requires an interdisciplinary approach in which SLPs participate collaboratively with other professionals, families, and students.

The ASHA guidelines also identify the various roles and responsibilities that SLPs may undertake to foster literacy development. These include, but are not limited to, the following:

- *Prevention:* Promote opportunities to participate in oral and written language experiences that facilitate literacy (e.g., shared book reading, alphabet/letter exposure, adult modeling of reading and writing).

- *Identification:* Provide screening/early detection of children with or at risk for reading and writing problems as a result of oral language difficulties.

- *Assessment:* Evaluate reading and writing abilities in relation to oral language skills, using a comprehensive battery of norm-referenced and descriptive measures.

- *Intervention:* Implement evidence-based instruction for reading and writing problems that emphasizes the reciprocal relationships between oral language and literacy and utilizes curricular subject matter.

- *Other roles:* Collaborate/advocate for effective language-based literacy practices in general and special education settings, promote family involvement in literacy activities, and advance the knowledge base regarding the relationship between oral language and literacy through clinical research and continuing education.

For more information on the role of SLPs in literacy, refer to ASHA's Scope of Practice (2016) and ASHA's Practice Portal on the topic of Written Language Disorders.

Theoretical Models of Intervention

There are different theoretical orientations to language intervention. These arise, in part, from different philosophies about the nature of normal language acquisition and differing viewpoints regarding the application of normal language acquisition to children with language disorders. Theoretical models differentially stress the primacy of cognitive, linguistic, or behavioral variables (e.g., Chomsky, 1965; Piaget, 1954; Pinker, 1989, 1996; Skinner, 1957; Vygotsky, 1962). Other models propose an integrative/connectionist approach and incorporate elements of several philosophies (Bates & MacWhinney, 1987; Bruner, 1974; MacWhinney, 2001, 2004). Still others use computational analyses (statistical probabilities) to make predictions that quantify the ease of acquisition of linguistic constructions (Hsu et al., 2011). Regardless of theoretical perspective, intervention practices should be informed by evidence. Clinicians implement effective strategies and procedures in conjunction with their own judgment and knowledge acquired through professional experience.

These models lead to different strategies of language intervention. In general, a behavioral orientation results in a nondevelopmental approach to therapy. Language targets may be selected without consideration of prerequisite skills, and behaviors are taught solely through the use of stimulus–response–consequence procedures. In contrast, other models are associated with developmental strategies in which target selection is determined by known sequences of acquisition, whether cognitively, linguistically, or pragmatically based. (See Appendix 4–A for major developmental language milestones.) For most children who present with a profile of delayed language, a developmental treatment strategy is generally utilized. A nondevelopmental approach may be adopted for atypical patterns of language acquisition (e.g., children with severe-profound intellectual impairment).

In an article that focuses on different treatment factors, Paul (2017) reviews the data available for clinician-directed approaches versus client-centered approaches. Within clinician-directed approaches, the SLP selects the stimuli and utilizes formats such as drill and discrete trials. There is research evidence to support using this type of approach to elicit new language skills, although the evidence for carryover and generalization may not be as strong (Eisenberg, 2014; Reichow, 2011). Client-centered approaches are considered more natural. The client takes the lead in interacting with the chosen stimuli, and the SLP responds using techniques such as recasts, expansions, and parallel talk to indirectly target language skills (Cirrin et al., 2010; Cleave et al., 2015; Paul, 2017). In addition, SLPs may use aspects of both approaches when designing therapy in order to promote language growth (Cable & Domsch, 2010; Mulhern et al., 2017).

Treatment Efficacy/Evidence-Based Practice

Two comprehensive reviews have examined peer-reviewed studies on evidence-based practice (EBP) in the area of child language (Carson et al., 2022; Walker et al., 2020); see Table 1–4 in Chapter 1 for an evidence-rating hierarchy). The overall findings indicate that language intervention is effective for preschool, kindergarten, and first-grade children, especially in the areas of phonology, expressive vocabulary, simple syntax/morphology, and phonological awareness. Rinaldi et al. (2021) reported similar results in their study of preschool children through 8 years of age. None of these studies included information on high-quality studies of language intervention for older children and adolescents.

Significant gaps in the professional literature were identified by these investigations; the gaps include the following:

- Studies on receptive language

- Experimentally controlled studies

- Studies of relative effectiveness of different treatment approaches for the same therapeutic targets

- Studies on higher order language skills (e.g., figurative language, narrative discourse)

- Studies on pragmatic language skills

- Studies examining intervention characteristics (e.g., duration, dosage, delivery model)

- Investigations of the effects of language intervention with general/special education curriculum

- Studies of maintenance of treatment effects

Cirrin et al.'s (2010) work focused on the effect of different service-delivery models (e.g., pull-out, classroom based, indirect consultation) on speech-language intervention outcomes for students of elementary school age. Their systemic review of evidence-based studies published during the past 30 years and found that only five studies met the review criteria and addressed the effectiveness of service-delivery models. Even within this small sample, results were mixed, revealing large gaps in our knowledge of the relative effectiveness of different service-delivery models. Phillips et al. (2016) developed and conducted a language intervention program (20 min/day, over 12 weeks) for 3½ to 4-year-old children at significant risk for language impairment and school difficulties. Children were randomly assigned to an experimental group or a control group that maintained the children's routines/business as usual group. The experimental group received direct instruction on syntactic and semantic aspects of the linguistic system. Results indicated that the linguistic instruction was effective; children in the experimental group evidenced significant gains and moderate language effect sizes in comparison to the control group. Lowe et al. (2018) were interested in vocabulary interventions specific to adolescents with language disorders and conducted a systematic review of 14 databases and 1,320 studies (age range 11–17 years). Results indicated that several approaches were effective, but that a phonological–semantic model was most effective for older children.

Kamhi (2014) argues there often is a disconnect between the findings of efficacy research and clinical practice implementation. Two examples are *treatment intensity* and *distributed practice*. Most efficacy studies suggest that a higher dose of instruction (e.g., four 50-min sessions/week) will result in better learning outcomes than a lower dose (e.g., two 30-min sessions/week; Bellon-Harn, 2012). Yet, evidence shows that "more is not always better." Studies suggest that many children show learning plateaus and threshold effects for early reading intervention (e.g., Denton et al., 2011), expression of communicative intentions (Fey et al., 2013), and print referencing instruction (McGinty et al., 2011). Beyond a point, the quantity or quality of the intervention has little effect on language and literacy outcomes. Another example involves *massed practice* versus *distributed practice*. Research findings on *spacing effects* (long intervals between learning episodes) show that distributed learning resulted not only in short-term gains but also in better retention of newly learned behaviors. In fact, Yoder et al. (2012) suggested that the spacing and distribution of teaching episodes may have a greater influence on learning outcomes than treatment intensity. Taken together, these findings demonstrate the need for further study of the instructional elements that impact language learning and development.

There also are a number of smaller studies that examine the value and benefits of specific treatment protocols. For example, a growing body of emergent literacy literature indicates that read-alouds, shared/interactive book reading, and print referencing are efficacious approaches for at-risk preschool children with and without language impairments and can be used successfully in home-based programs (e.g., Grolig, 2020; Justice et al., 2010; Justice et al., 2011; Pelatti et al., 2013).

A final topic of discussion in this section is *central auditory processing (CAP)*. This refers to the perceptual processing of auditory stimuli in the central nervous system. There are three major sets of skills which are of importance: auditory discrimination (differentiating one acoustic signal from another), temporal processing (identifying gaps between signals, identifying the ordering of signal presentation), and binaural processing (sound localization, sound lateralization). Deficits in the CAP system can be difficult to differentiate from impairments in higher order domains such as language and cognition, particularly within the context of behavioral testing without additional electrophysiologic measures to substantiate the neurophysiologic deficits. Richard (2013) proposed a three-tiered continuum for thinking about the relationship between CAP and language.

- Central auditory processing: Neural representation of acoustic signals as they travel through the auditory nerve pathways.

- Phonemic processing: The individual analyzes sound patterns in order to discriminate, segment, and blend relevant acoustic features.

- Linguistic processing: Meaning is attached to the acoustic signal.

Central auditory processing disorder (CAPD) remains a topic of ongoing debate due to a variety of factors such as variability of symptoms, lack of definitional clarity, and lack of consensus regarding best practices in remediation (de Wit et al., 2016). From a clinical perspective, it is necessary for SLPs to remain informed about developments in this evolving topic area to provide up-to-date programming for clients. The ASHA Practice Portal can provide useful information in this area.

Chapter 4

Intervention for Language in Infants and Preschool Children

Intervention With Infants (Birth to 3 years)

During this early developmental period, the infant masters the cognitive, social, motor, and communicative behaviors that underlie the acquisition of the linguistic system. (On the companion website, see Appendix 4–A for major developmental language milestones, Appendix 4–B for gross and fine motor skills milestones, Appendix 4–C for stages of cognitive development, Appendix 4–D for gesture development, Appendix 4–E for vision development milestones, Appendix 4–F for stages of feeding development, Appendix 4–G for stages of play development, Appendix 4–H for a developmental toy list, and Appendix 4–I for example lessons from the "Promoting Awareness of Speech Sounds" [PASS] program.) In this view, language is one aspect of the baby's developing system and requires the clinician to look across developmental systems when planning and implementing language interventions. This perspective also promotes a collaborative team-based approach rather than a series of fractured interventions by the speech-language pathologist (SLP), occupational therapist (OT), physical therapist (PT), and other professionals.

Some children are "late talkers," who between 18 to 30 months demonstrate good language comprehension skills along with good social, thinking, and play skills but show late emerging expressive language (vocabulary) skills. It is important to differentiate these children from children who are at risk or are identified with a developmental language disorder. It is generally agreed that early intervention is crucial for infants who do not demonstrate these prerequisite skills within the typically expected time frame (Ward et al., 2020). Early intervention also is critical for children who are considered at risk for developing language difficulties due to factors such as prematurity, low birth weight, family history, medical complications, and so on (e.g., Dawson & Bernier, 2013; Diamond et al., 2013; Guralnick, 1997, 2011, 2012, 2013; Paul & Roth, 2011). For at-risk children, intervention can be provided indirectly through monitoring of developmental progress or directly through infant stimulation and family enrichment programs. Some programs extend this focus to the concept of prevention, in which attempts are made to reduce or eliminate the risks and conditions that ultimately may result in communication disorders. Intervention provided during the first two years of life is thought to be extremely productive, because it capitalizes on the rapid neural growth and learning potential of the young brain.

American Speech-Language-Hearing Association (ASHA) Early Intervention Guidelines

According to the American Speech-Language-Hearing Association (ASHA, 2008), **early intervention (EI)** refers to a broad range of services, including the following:

- Prevention

- Screening

- Evaluation and assessment

- Planning, implementing, and monitoring intervention

- Consultation with and education for team members, including families and other professionals

- Service coordination

- Transition planning

- Advocacy

EI is characterized by a primary emphasis on family involvement and education (Ingber & Dromi, 2010; Wilcox & Woods, 2011). A family-centered approach addresses the child's needs within the sole relevant context for the child—the family unit. This model acknowledges the cultural, social, economic, and values or belief factors that may affect family dynamics. EI services promote children's participation in their natural environments, which can include home- or center-based settings (Banerjee & Luckner, 2014; Caesar, 2013). Although the term *natural environment* has often been assumed to refer to a child's home, it actually encompasses all settings and individuals with whom the child has regular contact. With infants and toddlers, more than with any other single age group, the clinician will likely work in an interdisciplinary, interprofessional, or transdisciplinary model of service delivery. In an interdisciplinary model, each team member functions within his or her specific discipline and shares information with other team members through established channels such as team meetings. On interprofessional teams, two or more individuals with different expertise work together as a collaborative unit and share information with one another on a continuous basis through informal and formal channels. In contrast, members of a transdisciplinary team cross traditional professional boundaries. They receive training in other disciplines and interchangeably provide services as needed by the child and family. These collaborative approaches to intervention are highlighted in Part C of the Individuals with Disabilities Education Act (IDEA, 2011) and emphasize the need for a team of professionals to be involved in the Individualized Family Service Plan (IFSP) process (Paul & Roth, 2011).

The goal of EI is the development of basic skills thought to be critical to successful speech, language, and communication learning. Repeated, interactive exposure to **authentic learning experiences in natural environments** and **modeling/stimulation** are the primary therapy strategies for infants. (Additional strategies relevant to this population are presented later in this chapter.) The main therapy targets for infant intervention programs comprise the following prelinguistic and early language skills.

Prelinguistic and Early Language Therapy Targets

Localization

Infants demonstrate awareness of sounds in their environment by turning toward and visually searching for the source of a sound. This auditory–visual association marks the beginning of an infant's conceptual grasp of cause–effect relations.

A clinician can enhance the localization behaviors of an infant by presenting a sound stimulus (e.g., rattle or other noisy object) outside the baby's visual field. This stimulus will require an observable head turn for the baby to locate the sound source. If this response is not observed, the clinician can gently turn the infant's head toward the sound to reinforce the auditory–visual association. The following developmental sequence can be used as a guideline for the appropriate response level for a given infant.

3 to 4 months: Primitive attempt to turn head

4 to 7 months: Localization to side only

7 to 13 months: Localization to side or below

13 to 21 months: Localization to side, below, or above

21 to 24 months: Direct localization to any angle

Joint/Shared Attention

A shared focus underlies successful communication. Joint attention between an adult and infant highlights the relationship between the adult's utterances and the objects, actions, or concepts they represent (Fredman, 2017; Siposova & Carpenter, 2019). In this context, the adult and infant are focused on the same referent in the environment (e.g., a rattle). According to Bruner (1977), joint visual attention is the prerequisite for all subsequent communication. One effective method for facilitating joint attention or shared reference is to place an attractive or noisy object in front of the infant, look at it, and comment on it. The adult may point to the object, shake it, or gently turn the infant's head to encourage eye contact with the object. Sometimes, it may be necessary to follow the infant's gaze to a particular object and then point to and label it to promote joint visual regard.

Mutual Gaze

This eye gaze pattern is a characteristic of early communicative development in which the infant and caregiver look at each other during social interactions. It is thought to form the basis for attachment/bonding between infant and caregiver (Lloyd & Masur, 2014; Rollins et al., 2021; Rossetti, 2001) and serves as a basic building block for later development of the important skill of turn taking in conversation (Owens, 2014). Immediate parental response to the infant's initiation of eye contact increases the baby's motivation to communicate and ultimately results in more frequent and varied interactions (Zero to Three, 2012). Establishment and maintenance of mutual gaze with infants can be enhanced when adult eye contact is accompanied by smiling and other facial expressions, touching, and novel or entertaining vocalizations.

Joint Action and Routines

Joint action between an adult and infant occurs in play sequences known as sound–gesture games or routines such as peekaboo, patty-cake, or "I'm gonna get you." A **routine** is a prepackaged or ritualized exchange between an adult and an infant. It has a definite structure with a clearly marked beginning, middle, and end, with clearly specified positions for appropriate vocalization or verbalization. This structure allows for the anticipation of events and increases the potential for successful adult–child interaction. It ensures that each partner knows what to expect from the other, thus making the order of events highly predictable. Ratner and Bruner (1978) point out that the semantic content of the mutual play is highly restricted and within the conceptual repertoire of the child. It is generally believed that the regularity and invariance of these routines allow the infant to make his or her first attempts at "cracking the linguistic code" and acquiring the first words (Ferrier, 1978; Newson, 1979). Many investigators also believe that these routines facilitate turn-taking behavior and role shifting in dialogue, both important building blocks of conversational exchanges.

Clinicians can initiate these playful routines in therapy and select the target response for an infant based on the following typical acquisition sequence for young children:

- At approximately 6 months, infants show enjoyment and pleasure (i.e., change in facial expression or body posture) when a parent initiates a sound–gesture routine.

- By 7 months, the infant anticipates the game when the adult produces the verbal component alone (independent of any gesture).

- The 8- to 9-month-old baby initiates as well as participates in the game (e.g., crawls behind the door and peeks his head out while smiling).

For slightly older babies, the clinician can utilize the "picture-book-reading routine" (Ninio & Bruner, 1978) with the baby seated next to or on the adult's lap. Select an enjoyable picture book and follow this sequence:

Adult: Say "Look" (attentional vocative) and point to picture

Child: Touches or looks at the picture (response)

A: Say "What are these?" (query)

C: Vocalizes, smiles, or names the picture (response)

A: Say "Yes, that is a _____" or "No, that's not a _____, it's a _____" (feedback)

Gestures

Children's development of gestures between 9 and 18 months of age lays the groundwork for their further communication and language learning (Caselli et al., 2012; Goldin-Meadow et al., 2007; Rohlfing, 2019). The types of gestures used during this 16-month period predicts language ability 2 years later (First Words Project, 2021; Watt et al., 2006). This developmental period often is referred to as "16 Gestures by 16 Months" to emphasize that infants should be using at least 16 gestures by the time they are 16 months of age and should be acquiring two gestures each month. Appendix 4–D on the Companion Website outlines the types of gestures and typical age of acquisition.

Vocalizations

The first year of life is characterized, in part, by rapid physical growth and neuromuscular maturation. As a result, the infant gains increasing control over the speech mechanism and exhibits significant expansion in the quality and variety of vocalizations. Infant vocalizations proceed through a series of predictable developmental stages, as outlined in Table 4–1.

Expansion of an infant's vocal repertoire can be promoted by increasing the frequency, variety, or quality of the vocalizations produced by the infant. The clinician can stimulate vocalization by talking to the infant, singing, humming, cuddling, tickling, or playing sound–gesture games such as peekaboo. Clinicians may also imitate the infant's vocalization in a playful manner to initiate a repetitive imitative exchange. Action-identification tags are playful sounds that infants enjoy listening

Table 4–1

Stages of Vocal Development in Infancy

Age	Behavior	Description
0–2 months	Reflexive	Undifferentiated crying and vegetative sounds (e.g., coughing, burping, sighing)
2–4 months	Cooing	Vocal signs of pleasure, primarily vowel and vowel-like sounds
4–6 months	Laughter	Sustained combination of cooing and crying features to produce audible "ha ha ha"
	Vocal play	Exploration of mouth with tongue, producing sounds such as squeals, growls, lip smacking, raspberries, and clicks
	Early babbling	Self-initiated sound play; combines stop consonants with vowels to produce isolated CV or VC syllables (e.g., /bo/ or /ok/)
6–8 months	Reduplicative babbling	Series of CV or VC syllables each identical to the other and frequently initiated with a /ə/ (e.g., /ədadada/)
8–10 months	Nonreduplicative babbling	Consonants and vowels may differ from one syllable to the next within a single string (e.g., /bawada/)
10–12 months	Jargon	Conversational intonation contours are imposed on longer strings of sound combinations; real words may be interspersed
	Protowords	Invented sound sequences that are used consistently to refer to a specific item or event (e.g., /na/ used to mean "Give [object] to me")

Sources: Adapted from "Stages of speech development in the first year of life," by R. Stark, in G. Yeni-Komshian, J. Cavanaugh, & C. Ferguson (Eds.), Child phonology: Vol. 1. Production (pp. 73–92), 1980, Academic Press; by G. Yeni-Komshian, J. Cavanaugh, & C. Ferguson (Eds.), New York, NY: Academic Press.

to and may attempt to reproduce, such as the motor sound ("vroom"), cow sound ("moo"), telephone ("ring-ring"), dog barking ("ruff ruff"), or car horn ("beep beep").

Communicative Intentions

The meaning that a speaker wishes a message to convey is known as a **communicative intention**. At about 9 months of age, infants discover intentional communication and begin to express their communicative intentions through gesture and vocalization (Table 4–2). Requests and statements are among the earliest communicative intentions to emerge. Requests represent the infant's intentional use of a listener as an agent or tool in achieving some end (e.g., a desired object). Statements are the infant's attempts to direct an adult's attention to some event or object in the environment. As children begin to acquire an initial vocabulary, they express communicative intentions through single-word utterances (Table 4–3). Evidence suggests that the *rate* of preverbal communication in young children with developmental delays is a strong predictor of later vocabulary usage (Brady et al., 2004; Calandrella & Wilcox, 2000; McCathren et al., 1999). The *frequency* of intentional communication

Table 4–2
Preverbal Communicative Intentions

Intention	Descriptive Example
1. Attention seeking	
a. To self	Child tugs on adult's jeans to secure attention.
b. To events, objects, or other people	Child points to airplane to draw adult's attention to it.
2. Requesting	
a. Objects	Child points to toy animal that he wants.
b. Action	Child hands book to adult to have story read.
c. Information	Child points to usual location of cookie jar (which is not there) and simultaneously secures eye contact with mother to determine its whereabouts.
3. Greetings	Child waves "hi" or "bye."
4. Transferring	Child gives mother the toy that he was playing with.
5. Protesting/rejecting	Child cries when mother takes away toy. Child pushes away a dish of oatmeal.
6. Responding/ acknowledging	Child responds appropriately to simple directions. Child smiles when a parent initiates a favorite game.
7. Informing	Child points to wheel on his toy truck to show mother that it is broken.

Sources: Categories are adapted, in part, from "The Acquisition of Performatives Prior to Speech," by E. Bates, L. Camaioni, and V. Volterra, 1975, *Merrill-Palmer Quarterly, 21,* 205–224; "Basic Modes of Social Interaction: Their Emergence and Patterning During the First Two Years of Life," by S. Escalona, 1973, *Merrill-Palmer Quarterly, 19,* 205–232; *Learning How to Mean: Explorations in the Development of Language,* by M. A. K. Halliday, 1975, London, UK: Edward Arnold; "Analysis of Intentional Communication of Normal Children from the Prelinguistic to the Multi-word Stage," by A. Wetherby, D. Cain, D. Yonclas, and V. Walker, 1988, *Journal of Speech and Hearing Research, 31,* 240–252.

is also predictive: Higher rates of nonverbal intentional communication during the preverbal stage are associated with better language outcomes 1 to 2 years later (Paul & Roth, 2011; Watt et al., 2006; Woynaroski et al., 2014).

Intervention in the area of communicative intentions may be aimed at (a) increasing the number of different types of intentions a child can understand or express and/or (b) increasing the variety of forms (e.g., vocalization, gesture, word) understood or used to express a given intention. To elicit specific communicative intentions, the clinician should provide facilitating environments in which the intentions are obligatory or at least highly likely to occur (Paul et al., 2018; Roth, 1999; Spekman & Roth, 1984). Following are examples of facilitating environments for selected intentions:

Requests for action: Introduce toys that cannot be operated without assistance from the clinician, such as a windup toy or an electric toy car.

Place highly desirable toys where child cannot gain access to them without assistance from the clinician.

Table 4–3

Communicative Intentions Expressed at the Single-Word Level

Intention	Definition
1. Naming	Common and proper nouns that label people, objects, events, and locations.
2. Commenting	Words that describe physical attributes of objects, events, and people, including size, shape, and location; observable movements and actions of objects and people; and words that refer to attributes that are not immediately observable such as possession and usual location. These words are not contingent on prior utterances.
3. Requesting object	
a. Present	Words that solicit an object that is present in the environment.
b. Absent	Words that solicit an absent object.
4. Requesting action	Words that solicit that an action is to be initiated or continued.
5. Requesting information	Words that solicit information about an object, action, person, or location. Rising intonation is also included.
6. Responding	Words that directly complement preceding utterances.
7. Protesting/rejecting	Words that express objection to ongoing or impending action/event.
8. Attention-seeking	Words that solicit attention to the child or to aspects of the environment.
9. Greetings	Words that express salutations and other conventionalized rituals.

Sources: Adapted from "Is Early Pragmatic Development Measurable?" by P. S. Dale, 1980, *Journal of Child Language, 8,* 1–12; "A Pragmatic Description of Early Language Development," by J. Dore, 1974, *Journal of Psycholinguistic Research, 3,* 343–350; *Learning How to Mean: Explorations in the Development of Language,* by M. A. K. Halliday, 1975, London, UK: Edward Arnold.

	Present incomplete or broken materials such as puzzles with missing pieces or paints without brushes.
Requests for: information	Introduce novel or enticing toys for which the child is likely to request a label or information regarding its function, operation, or construction, such as a transformer, spinning top, or a talking book.
Attention-seeking:	Pretend not to hear the child so that he or she must use the clinician's name, raise vocal pitch or intensity, or move closer to the clinician.

Nonsymbolic Play and Symbolic Play

Children learn through play and often practice their new acquisitions in play. Infants gain experience in how both receptive and expressive language function by participating in play sequences. In addition, play is the most important context for the development of social communication skills and the natural context for early language learning (Creaghe & Kidd, 2022; Creaghe et al., 2021; Quinn & Kidd, 2022). In early types of play, children use objects for their intended purposes (functional play) or engage in exploratory play, such as dropping, mouthing, or transferring objects, and do not require the use of symbolic agents. Additional examples of functional play include activities such as running, filling and emptying receptacles, driving toy cars, and water play. Later, symbolic forms of play emerge, where the child substitutes objects or events for other objects/events. Examples include pretending to talk on the telephone or using a stick as a sword. (See Appendix 4–G on the Companion Website for stages of play development.)

Following are some suggested themes and activities for facilitating play, arranged developmentally:

- Exploring common objects such as blocks, rattles, spoons, pots, and pans through banging, mouthing, manipulating, and visual inspection

- Using toys appropriately, such as a busy box or Fisher-Price See 'n Say

- Pretending to act out familiar single actions such as eating, sleeping, and drinking

- Manipulating a doll to perform familiar activities such as kissing, dancing, and waving bye-bye

- Pretending to act out sequences of familiar actions such as pouring liquid into a cup, taking a sip, and then spilling the liquid onto the floor

- Using dough or clay to create "pretend" food such as hot dogs or pancakes

- Using miniature people, cars, or dishes to act out daily routines such as taking a bath, going to the store, or having a birthday party

Initial Vocabulary/First Lexicon

Infants begin to understand a few familiar words between 6 and 8 months of age. Production of first true words occurs around the first birthday. Early vocabulary development can be stimulated at the receptive and/or expressive level (Bloom, 2000; Storch & Whitehurst, 2002; Tomasello, 2003; Wasik & Iannone-Campbell, 2012). Beck et al. (2013) identified three levels, or tiers, of vocabulary development (Table 4–4).

Intervention aimed at the facilitation of a child's *receptive* vocabulary generally consists of repeated presentation of a target word as well as the use of gestures and exaggerated/varied vocal intonation patterns to highlight salient aspects of an object or event. Following are two sample activities that can be used to stimulate comprehension of early vocabulary for a 12- to 24-month-old child with a language impairment:

- Engage the child in play with a large, lightweight ball. Demonstrate and say the following to the child:

  "Can you *throw* the ball to me? Put two hands over your head and throw it to me. That's right, let go and *throw* it over here. Great, you did it."

  "Now can you *drop* the ball? I'll drop it first and then you drop it again. Let me see you *drop* the ball. Good job."

  "Let me see you *kick* the ball. *Kick* the ball with your foot. *Kick* the ball as hard as you can. Good for you, you kicked the ball."

- Engage the child in play using a surprise box such as Playskool's Busy Poppin' Pals. Say to the child:

  "Can you find Monkey's *banana*? Guess what? I see a *banana* right here. Do you see Monkey's *banana*? That's not Monkey, that's Panda. Point to Monkey's *banana*."

Table 4–4
Definitions of Tier 1, Tier 2, and Tier 3 Vocabulary Words

Tier 1	Common, everyday words that most children know before entering school.
Tier 2	Academic vocabulary words that are used across all topics and content areas, yet are not a part of students' everyday social language. Examples include *require, analyze, evaluate, conceal, concentrate.*
Tier 3	This tier consists of low-frequency, subject-specific vocabulary words that are most commonly taught within a subject area or field of study (e.g., *volcano, legislature, migration, circumference, aorta*).

Source: Adapted from *Bringing Words to Life: Robust Vocabulary Instruction*, by I. L. Beck, M. G. McKeown, and L. Kucan, 2013, New York, NY: Guilford Press.

Table 4–5
Grammatical Classification of the First 50 Words Produced

Grammatical Function	Percentage of Vocabulary	Examples
Nominals	50	*milk, dog, car*
Action words	11–14	*give, do, up, bye-bye*
Modifiers	14–19	*mine, no dirty*
Personal/social	10	*no, please*
Functional	4	*this, far*

Sources: Adapted from "Early Lexical Development: Comprehension and Production," by H. Benedict, 1979, *Journal of Child Language, 6,* 183–200; "Structure and Strategy in Learning to Talk," by K. Nelson, 1973, *Society for Research in Child Development Monographs, 38* (1–2 Serial No. 149), (Reprinted in part in Mussen, Conger, & Kagan, *Readings in Child Development and Personality* [3rd. ed.], New York, NY: Harper & Row, 1975).

The early *expressive* vocabularies of young children are not arbitrary (Lee, 2011). Initial lexicons are highly selective because children communicate about the social and physical events that are within their conceptual grasp and immediate environment. A grammatical classification of a typical initial lexicon is presented in Table 4–5. Expressive vocabulary growth is charted in Table 4–6.

Researchers also agree that children's early vocabularies express a basic set of semantic functions or intentions (Bloom, 1973; Brown, 1968; Nelson, 1973). Strategies for facilitating the acquisition of early lexical items are frequently based on semantic function rather than agrammatical classification. Three main considerations in the selection of target vocabulary are (a) words that can be used in many different contexts during the child's daily activities; (b) words that are important to the child, such as names of significant others or types of favorite foods or toys; and (c) words that represent dynamic rather than static states, especially referents that can be acted on or manipulated directly by the child such as a ball or a spoon, rather than a tree or a wall. Following are suggested contexts/activities that can be used to stimulate different types of semantic intentions at the single-word level.

Table 4–6
Expressive Vocabulary Growth

Age	Number of Words
15 months	4–6
18 months	20–50
24 months	200–300
3 years	900–1,000
4 years	1,500–1,600
5 years	2,100–2,200

Source: Adapted from "Developmental and Stylistic Variation in the Composition of Early Vocabulary," by E. Bates, V. Marchman, D. Thal, L. Fenson, and P. Dale, 1994, *Journal of Child Language*, 21, 85–123.

Existence/naming: Introduce a container filled with interesting objects and reveal them to the child one at a time.

Nonexistence: Expose an attractive object to the child and then hide it from view.

Recurrence: Initiate a desirable activity and then stop.

Action: Engage the child in an activity such as making pudding that will elicit a number of different actions (e.g., open, pour, stir, mix).

Possession: Place a combination of the child's and clinician's belongings in a box, pull them out one at a time, and sort into separate piles.

Locative: Engage the child in play with trucks or cars using props such as a Little People Racing Garage Ramp or Rev'n Sounds Race Track that encourage changes in location.

Rejection: Offer objects or activities that are known to be unappealing to the child.

Denial: In a playful manner, intentionally misname objects or body parts that the child already knows.

One evidence-based strategy to promote simultaneous development of receptive and expressive vocabulary is reading books together. Clinicians should regularly engage in shared book reading with their young clients and encourage parents to read books to their children. (See the section on emergent literacy later in this chapter for more information.) Ideal books for infants include things to touch, language that repeats over and over again, and colorful pictures of objects and words to match.

The following case example illustrates several of the main principles of EI for infants and toddlers.

PROFILE 1: EARLY INTERVENTION—18-MONTH-OLD

Mina is an 18-month-old girl from a bilingual family (Spanish is her first language [L1]). Mina has a complex medical history of prematurity and seizures and is at significant risk for delayed language. She understands a few English words and uses vocalizations and gestures to communicate. In addition to SLP services, Mina is receiving PT, OT, and physician care through the county health department. The parents have a relatively good grasp of English, their second language (L2), but a language barrier remains. For example, they have difficulty understanding the specific nature of her language delay and the likelihood that Mina will continue to have language-learning problems. Their English-language comprehension also interferes with their ability to understand the SLP's initial suggestions for stimulating language and communication at home and in daily activities. Both parents work outside the home, and Mina is cared for by her grandmother (who only speaks L1) during the day. The family wants to know how to interact more effectively with their daughter in everyday situations and provide Mina with opportunities to interact more frequently with other children. They are also interested in learning more about the development of language/communication and reasonable expectations for their daughter at different stages of development.

Clinical Strategy. As part of the interprofessional EI team, the SLP initiated a family-centered approach that includes several areas of focus:

- The clinician refers Mina to an infant–toddler social interaction group at the county health department that is staffed by members of the EI team.

- The clinician also makes biweekly home visits with Mina's family to demonstrate behaviors for encouraging adult–child interactions (e.g., modeling, expansions) and directly engages Mina's family in the planning and implementation of these activities. The clinician consults with the family to select recommended developmentally supportive play activities and routines, toys, and books that Mina would likely enjoy that are consistent with the family's culture and interests to increase family–child engagement and build Mina's communication skills.

- The clinician recommends that the family participate in an ongoing support group for families of children with significant handicaps, which are coordinated by EI professionals at the county health center. These sessions provide information on early development, stress the importance of adult–child interactions in facilitating language learning, and offer ways to increase positive and relaxed adult–child engagement, because several of the family members expressed difficulties relating to their children with delays.

To ensure coordination of services across disciplines, the EI team meets regularly with one another and with the family. The SLP's main role is to provide information about language intervention targets, with expressive vocabulary being a primary focus. She also describes the cues/prompts/strategies that were most and least successful in stimulating Mina's vocabulary. The team discusses how the target vocabulary and strategies will be incorporated by the teacher of the interaction group, in OT and PT sessions, and at home. The SLP emails a weekly updated log of goals, strategies, and Mina's progress to the team, and updates the hard-copy binder that she maintains for the family and the teacher. At the end of each week, the EI team logs on to the web-based forum or chat site at a designated time to share updates, concerns, and next steps. (Mina's family requested that the SLP attend these weekly meetings on their behalf because of their work schedules.)

As children approach the third birthday, a **transition plan** is developed for those youngsters who are going on to other services. The transition plan is typically prepared at the last IFSP meeting before the transition occurs. It includes the steps needed to prepare the child and family for the new setting. It also outlines the steps for preparing the professionals who will be providing the special education services at the new setting.

Helpful Hints

1. Clinicians may want to incorporate some of the main characteristics of *motherese*, or child directed speech, in their speech to young children. These include exaggerated intonation, short utterance length, simple vocabulary and syntactic structures, frequent repetition of utterances, and talking about topics in the "here and now."

2. Clinician (CL) responses to child (CH) utterances should be framed in a way that encourages the exchange to continue and keeps the child in the interaction (sometimes referred to as **turnabouts**). For example:

   CH: dat?

   CL: Kitty cat. What does it say?

   versus

   CH: dat?

   CL: It's a kitty.

3. Clinicians can maximize the effectiveness of intervention activities by selecting toys and materials that are developmentally supportive for a particular child. (See Appendix 4–H on the Companion Website for a developmental toy list.)

4. Clinicians need to be aware that many infants with communication impairments may exhibit concomitant impairments in other areas. Intervention programs must accommodate the infant's overall developmental profile. For example, tactile stimulation often elicits abnormal primitive reflexes in children with cerebral palsy and can significantly interfere with therapeutic programming.

5. Clinicians should be prepared to address skepticism of other professionals and families/caregivers regarding the merits of language intervention with infants and very young children.

6. The clinician can provide families with the treatment steps that are followed and address their concerns and questions.

7. Although not a replacement for traditional therapy, parent input as members of the EI team is important. A parent's behavior affects the child's ensuing behavior, and the parent's

behavior is also influenced by the child's previous behavior. Changing the behavior of one inherently changes the behavior of the other, and these bidirectional exchanges with parents facilitate children's language learning.

Intervention With Children (3 to 5 years)

During this developmental period, children acquire the major portion of the linguistic system. This period is characterized by rapid growth in vocabulary. After the age of 18 months, children add approximately 9 to 10 new words to their lexicons each day, or 3,000 words per year (Graves, 1986). Average utterance length continues to increase, and the acquisition of syntax has its onset as children begin to impose word order on their two-word combinations. Morphological forms emerge and become solidified, although complete mastery is not attained until the early elementary school years. This developmental period also is marked by children's ability to understand and produce a variety of simple and complex sentence forms. In addition, children in this age range demonstrate substantial development in the area of emergent literacy through exposure and interaction with print. See Tables 4–7 through 4–15 for a review of mean length of utterance (MLU) stages, two-word semantic intentions, acquisition of grammatical morphemes, auxiliary verb development, negation development, question development, sentence-type comprehension progression, hallmarks of literacy development, and the developmental stages of early writing.

Table 4–7
Stages of Mean Length of Utterance (MLU) Development

Stage	MLU (morphemes)	Approximate Age
I	1.0–2.0	18–24 months
II	2.0–2.5	2–2½ years
III	2.5–3.0	2½–3 years
IV	3.0–3.5	3–3½ years
V	3.5–4.0	3½–4 years

Source: Adapted from *A First Language*, by R. Brown, 1973, Cambridge, MA: Harvard University Press.

Table 4-8
Two-Word Semantic Relations

Relation	Examples
Agent + action	Daddy eat, mommy drive
Action + object	Eat cookie, throw ball
Agent + object	Daddy shoe, grandma hat
Attribute + entity	Big doggie, pretty lady
Possessor + possession	Daddy car, baby bottle
Recurrence	More juice, more cookie
Nonexistence	No bed, allgone milk
Demonstrative + entity	This cup, that doggie
Entity + location	Daddy chair, toy floor
Action + location	Go home, sit horsie

Sources: Adapted from *One Word at a Time: The Use of Single-Word Utterances Before Syntax,* by L. Bloom, 1973, New York, NY: The Hague Mouton; *A First Language,* by R. Brown, 1973, Cambridge, MA: Harvard University Press; "Production of utterances and language acquisition," by I. Schlesinger, in D. Slobin (Ed.), The ontogenesis of grammar (pp. 63–101), 1971, Academic Press.

Table 4-9
Brown's 14 Grammatical Morphemes: Order of Acquisition

Morpheme	Example	Stage
Present progressive -*ing* (no auxiliary verb)	Daddy sleeping	I–II
In/On	Doggie on table	II
Regular plural -*s*	Me have two shoes	I–III
Irregular past	Drank, came, fell, broke, ate	I–IV
Possessive 's	Daddy's chair	I–IV
Uncontractible copula (used as main verb)	This is hot.	II–IV
Articles (*a/the*)	Open the door.	II–V
Regular past -*ed*	Mommy walked the dog.	I–Post V
Regular third person -*s*	Mommy works.	I–V
Irregular third person	Does, has	II–Post V

Table 4–9
continued

Morpheme	Example	Stage
Uncontractible auxiliary	The doggie was running.	II–Post V
Contractible copula	He is tall.	II–Post V
Contractible auxiliary	Daddy is coming home.	II–Post V

Source: Adapted from *A First Language*, by R. Brown, 1973, Cambridge, MA, Harvard University Press.

Table 4–10
Auxiliary Verb Development

Category	Form/Examples	Stage
Contracted form of *is*	's	Early II
Forms of *to be*	is, am, are, was	Late II
Early infinitives (catenatives)	hafta, gonna, wanna	Late II
Early modals	can, do, may, will	Stage III on
Subjunctive modals	could, would, should, might	Stage III on
Mood of obligation modals	should, must, have to	Stage IV on
Perfective	have ... -en	Stage V or later
Double expansion of auxiliary	has been, might have	Stage V or later

Table 4–11.
Development of Negation

Mean Length of Utterance Stage	Form	Example
I	Negative + utterance	No drink; not hungry
	Utterance + negative	Mommy no; doggie not
II–III	Subject + negative + main verb	Me no drink; he not sit
	Unanalyzed *don't/can't* (not true auxiliary forms)	Don't hit; You can't go
III–IV	Subject + auxiliary + negative + main verb	He is not running; Mommy cannot go

Sources: Adapted from *The Acquisition of Negation* (Unpublished doctoral dissertation), by U. Bellugi, 1967, Harvard University, Cambridge, MA; *Early Language* (The Developing Child), by P. A. DeVilliers and J. G. DeVilliers, 1979, Cambridge, MA: Harvard University Press.

Table 4–12
Development of Question Forms

Mean Length of Utterance Stage	Form	Example
I		
Yes/no	Rising intonation	Me go? See hole?
Wh-	What NP doing?	What daddy doing?
	Where NP going?	Where mommy going?
	Wh-word + NP	What that?
II–III		
Yes/no	Rising intonation in longer utterances	You see red ball?
Wh-	Wh-word + sentence	Who you draw in book?
III–IV		
Yes/no	NP and auxiliary verb	Can I go? Do you see me?
	Inversion of subject	
Wh-	Wh-word + subject NP + auxiliary + main verb	Why he can ride?
IV–V		
Yes/no	Remains the same in longer utterances	Should I throw it over there?
Wh-	Wh-word + auxiliary verb + subject NP + main verb	Why can he ride?

Note. Wh-words emerge in the following sequence: (a) what, where; (b) who; (c) when, how, and why, in variable order. NP = Noun phrase.

Sources: Adapted from "Syntactic regularities in the speech of children," by E. Klima & U. Bellugi, in J. Lyons & R. J. Wales (Eds.), Psycholinguistics papers (pp. 183–207), 1966, Edinburgh University Press; "Categories of first syntax: Be, be+ing, and nothingness," by V. Valian, in J. M. Meisel (Ed.), The acquisition of verb placement: Functional categories and V2 phenomena in language development (p. 401–422), 1992, Kluwer.

Table 4–13
Developmental Sequence of Sentence Comprehension

Syntactic Structure	Example	Age of Comprehension Between 75% and 90%
Simple imperative	Stop!	4–6 to 6–0
Negative imperative	Don't touch the stove!	5–6 to 7–0
Active declarative		
Regular noun and present progressive	The girl is walking.	3–0
Irregular noun and present progressive	The deer are running.	6–6 to 7–0
Past tense	The dog chased the cat.	5–6 to 7–0+
Past participle	The lady has spoken.	6–0 to 7–0+
Future tense	She will play the piano.	7–0 to 7–0+
Reversible	The man kisses the lady.	6–6 to 7–0+
Perfective	Daddy has been working.	7–0+
Interrogative		
Who	Who is on the bed?	3–0
What	What do we wear?	3–6 to 5–0
When	When do you sleep?	3–6 to 5–6
Negation	The man isn't swimming.	5–6 to 7–0+
Reversible passive	The dog is chased by the cat.	5–6 to 6–0
Conjunction		
If	If you're a teacher, point to the dog.	7–0+
Then	Look at the third animal, then point to the dog.	7–0+
Neither/nor	Show me the one that is neither the ball nor the dog.	7–0+

Source: Adapted from "Index of Productive Syntax," by H. Scarborough, 1989, *Applied Psycholinguistics, 11,* 1–22.

Table 4–14
Hallmarks of Literacy Development

Stage	Description
Early Emergent	Awareness of some print conventions (e.g., front versus back of books; left–right directionality of writing; words versus pictures) Shows sustained interest during book reading Recognizes familiar environmental print (e.g., logo for fast food restaurant) Engages in random drawing and scribbling
Later Emergent	Pretends to read and write Demonstrates a sense of "story" (i.e., beginning/middle/ending) Recognizes and produces predictable language patterns of familiar stories Attempts to write letters using scribbles and wavy lines
Early Beginning Reader	Attempts to read words by matching each letter to its corresponding sound (early decoding) Begins to develop a sight-word vocabulary that consists of highly familiar words Attempts to write words using primarily beginning and ending letters
Later Beginning Reader	Decodes familiar print easily; may struggle with new material Demonstrates large sight-word vocabulary Engages in self-correction during reading and writing Spells most familiar words accurately Shows awareness of writing conventions such as punctuation
Independent Reader	Reads fluently and focuses on understanding the meaning of text Uses text-based strategies such as predicting, summarizing, re-reading, and paraphrasing Demonstrates consistent use of spelling rules and writing conventions such as punctuation, paragraphing, and topic versus supporting sentences

Source: Adapted from "Assessing the literacy of young children: The case for multiple forms of evidence," by T. Salinger, in S. B. Neuman & D. K. Dickinson (Eds.), Handbook of early literacy research (pp. 390–418), 2001, Guilford Press.

Table 4–15
Developmental Stages of Early Spelling

Stage	Description/Example
Drawing	Child scribbles using wavy and circular lines
Pre-phonemic	Random combination of pictures, squiggles, letters, and numbers with no connection between letters and sounds (e.g., Az4Esu7)
Semi-phonemic	Writes one to three letters to stand for a word (e.g., P = piano, PTE = pretty)
Phonetic/letter name	Spells words the way they sound (e.g., LETL = little, EGL = eagle)
Transitional	Within-word patterns include vowels in each syllable (e.g., EGUL = eagle)
Conventional	Basic rules of spelling are mastered (e.g., EAGLE = eagle)

Sources: Adapted from "Explorations in Spelling: Foundations for Learning and Teaching Phonics, Spelling, and Vocabulary, by D. Bear and S. Templeton, 1998, *The Reading Teacher, 52,* 222–242; "A Retrospective on Invented Spelling and a Look Forward," by J. R. Gentry, 2000, *The Reading Teacher, 54,* 318–332.

Treatment Approaches for Infants, Toddlers, and Preschoolers

There are a variety of approaches to language intervention, most of which can be implemented with children across a wide range of ages and stages of development. These approaches emphasize the provision of intervention in naturalistic contexts. This means that children/students are engaged in authentic, meaningful activities that are functionally linked to their daily activities. Although not a replacement for traditional therapy, parent input is important to the therapeutic process (Te Kaat-van den Os et al., 2017). Not all children are likely to be referred for and receive language intervention; bias can exist. In a preliminary study, Wittke and Spaulding (2018) identified two bias factors: (a) children from higher socioeconomic status (SES) families and (b) teachers who perceive the children's specific language impairment (SLI) as having poor executive functioning skills. Several basic remediation approaches are described in the following sections. They can be used in combination and are appropriate for a variety of service models, including Response to Intervention (RTI), other collaborative approaches, and small-group/individual therapy.

Focused Stimulation (Fey, 1986)

In this approach, the clinician provides concentrated exposure to a target form in a variety of contexts (e.g., individual words, embedded in sentences or short stories). The clinician preselects a linguistic target and produces it in high concentration throughout natural and meaningful adult–child interactions. Because the focus is on comprehension, the child is not required to produce the linguistic form. This approach can encompass a wide variety of targets, including vocabulary, grammatical morphemes, and syntax.

Incidental Teaching *(Hart & Risley, 1974; Hart & Rogers-Warren, 1978)*

This is a naturalistic approach that encourages a child to initiate communication by arranging the environment to increase the likelihood that the child will produce a verbal or nonverbal intervention target. The child's successful communicative attempts are rewarded through natural consequences, such as a requested object or event. The clinician also responds to the child's communicative attempts with requests for expansion or elaboration. Variations of incidental teaching include milieu language teaching (Kaiser & Warren, 1986) and time-delay approaches (Halle et al., 1979).

Floortime/Developmental, Individual Difference, Relationship Based *(DIR; Greenspan, 1998)*

This approach to intervention focuses on building the foundations of social, emotional, and intellectual capacities in young children rather than targeting isolated behaviors or skills. It encourages socially appropriate, child-initiated interactions with emphasis on developmental milestones, individual differences, and the relationship between the child and others in the environment. A critical component of this model is family engagement.

Family Centered *(Manolson, 1985; Schopler & Reichler, 1971)*

This approach trains parents and other caregivers to foster the development of language and communication in naturalistic contexts such as the home setting (Heidlage et al., 2020). The SLP functions in an indirect or educational capacity with family members, helping them become the "change agents" for their child. These programs may focus on improving the child's communication skills and/or improving the adult family members' ability to engage in mutually reinforcing communicative interactions with their child.

Selective Mutism (SM)

Children with selective mutism (SM) have the ability to talk, but they do not talk in certain situations (Kearney & Rede, 2021). For example, some children will remain silent in school but will talk in other settings, such as at home, where they are more relaxed. According to the *Diagnostic and Statistical Manual of Mental Disorders, Fifth Edition* (DSM-5; American Psychiatric Association, 2013), these children are 5 years old or younger, often are anxious, are very shy, exhibit a blank stare, and show body rigidity (Muris & Ollendick, 2021). The precise cause of SM is unknown, but there is agreement among most researchers and clinicians that these children with SM suffer from an anxiety disorder such as social phobia. The anxiety interferes with their willingness to talk in public situations. Some of these children may also have speech or language problems that compound their fear of speaking. SLPs can work with these children to make talking comfortable in more and more situations using the following techniques (Cohan et al., 2006; Pionek et al., 2002; Zakszeski & DuPaul, 2017):

- **Stimulus fading:** Encouraging child to begin talking with someone with whom they are relaxed and then gradually adding less familiar people as conversational speakers.

- **Shaping:** Gradually introducing more sophisticated means of expression. As an example, for a child who communicates through pointing, the SLP may introduce a gesture, pair the gesture with a word, and prompt the child to mouth the word before saying it.

Essentially, treatment for this complex condition is based on a foundation of gentle, systematic desensitization and should be undertaken in collaboration with an appropriate mental health professional. More detailed information on treatment of SM can be found in ASHA's Practice Portal resources.

Emergent Literacy Intervention (Birth Through Preschool Years)

Rich home literacy and oral language environments provide a foundation for the expectations of the school environment (Carroll et al., 2019; Terrell & Watson, 2018). The overall goal of emergent literacy intervention is to promote oral- and print-knowledge skills that are associated with the ability to successfully learn reading and writing skills. This goal addresses the significant reciprocal relationship between early intervention and academic achievement. SLPs may play a variety of direct and indirect roles in this area of intervention. Clinicians can work directly on providing emergent literacy intervention to children with identified communication disorders. Indirect roles encompass collaborative consultation with others, professional staff development, parent/community education, and curricular policy recommendations regarding the critical nature of emergent literacy skill acquisition for all children. From an RTI/multitiered perspective, all areas of emergent literacy skill can be integrated into Tiers 1, 2, or 3.

There are several other components of emergent literacy, each of which can be used as an avenue to increase a child's print knowledge. Following are five main areas, accompanied by instructional guidelines (Roth & Baden, 2001).

Shared Book Reading and Sense of Story

- Engage in dialogic reading. It is important to ask questions throughout the reading activity about what has been read and what might happen next. (See Whitehurst et al., 1994; Whitehurst & Lonigan 1998; and Dowdall et al., 2020 for helpful guidance on the use of this technique).

- Expose the child to quality literature that is developmentally supportive with respect to complexity and content. A variety of text genres should be incorporated into intervention, including fictional narratives/stories (FNs), informational text (IT), and poetry. Fictional narratives are about make-believe characters and events and have clearly marked beginnings, middles, and endings. ITs convey facts about the natural or social world on topics such as science and geography (Duke & Bennett-Armistead, 2003) and are generally written one fact at a time/per page. Some children, such as second language learners, find IT easier than stories; often, stories have storylines and illustrations that are unfamiliar in other cultures and languages. Also, ITs typically have large, realistic photographs, illustrations, labeled pictures, tables of content, graphs, glossaries, and diagrams that provide visual support to English-language learners. Inclusion of IT as part of preschool intervention/instructional goals is paramount to high-quality preschool education to prepare children, especially those at risk for or with diagnosed language impairments, for the curricula and language demands of elementary school (Deshmukh et al., 2022; Pentimonti et al., 2010; Yopp & Yopp, 2012).

- Select predictably patterned stories with repetitive themes and well-developed plot structure.

- Direct the child's attention to the printed words rather than focusing solely on the pictures. Engage in *print referencing*, an interactive reading style in which adults highlight specific aspects of print in storybooks and other genres (e.g., alphabet or informational books) verbally with comments and questions and nonverbally through gestures and tracking print while reading.

- Encourage the child to recount familiar experiences that occur routinely in daily life (e.g., scripts), such as grocery shopping or getting dressed.

- Encourage the child to recount personal event narratives, which are event sequences experienced by someone else (e.g., Daddy cooking dinner).

Phonological Awareness

- Recite fingerplays (e.g., "Itsy-Bitsy Spider" and "I'm a Little Teapot").

- Sing songs and chants (e.g., "This Old Man" and "Teddy Bear, Teddy Bear").

- Engage in alliteration and rhyming (e.g., "dad, dad, stick, stad").

- Point out words that begin with the same sound.

- Say simple words such as "cat"; have the child think of one or two words that start with the same initial sound.

Application of phonological awareness instruction is clearly demonstrated in a program such as **Promoting Awareness of Speech Sounds (PASS**; Roth et al., 2012). PASS is a comprehensive and explicit phonological awareness curriculum that was originally designed for preschool children who may be at risk for literacy problems, including children with speech and language impairments or other learning disabilities. PASS also can be used with typically developing preschoolers and early elementary-aged children with and without disabilities. PASS consists of three instructional units—rhyming, blending, and segmentation—that can be used together or in isolation, depending on a child's current phonological performance profile.

In each unit, there are a series of highly structured lessons based on a developmental sequence of learning objectives: each lesson follows an identical format of opening activity, guided instruction, and closing activity. Each lesson can be taught in approximately a half hour, and the program is designed so that two to three lessons per week will permit a youngster to complete all three units in approximately 6 months. Evidence-based practices are embedded in the scripted lessons, and the program provides assessment/progress-monitoring procedures and forms. All lesson stimuli and materials are included, as are nine children's books such as *Mouse Mess* (Riley); *Polar Bear, Polar Bear, What Do You Hear?* (Martin); and *Dogs Don't Wear Sneakers* (Numeroff). PASS is intended to be used in conjunction with letter–sound correspondence training, because phonemic awareness instruction has the most impact on early reading when accompanied by alphabetic principle training.

PASS has demonstrated efficacy and effectiveness with several child populations, including preschool children with and without speech and language disabilities, preschool children at risk for literacy difficulties, and children who are English-language learners (ELLs). Further, research findings show that this instructional program is effective when implemented in several different contexts: as a whole-class activity, in small-group instruction, in one-on-one instruction, and in tier-based models of instruction, such as RTI (e.g., Roth et al., 2002; Roth et al., 2006; Roth et al., 2009).

Three lessons are presented in Appendix 4–I on the companion website that represent different levels of task difficulty:

- The rhyming lesson demonstrates a receptive task at the level of matching and recognition: choosing two pictures that rhyme from a set of three.

- The blending lesson utilizes a yes/no judgment task in which a child is given a word phoneme by phoneme (e.g., b-a-t) and then a whole word. The child is required to indicate whether the whole-word version is the same as or different from the unblended version.

- The segmentation lesson requires a child to produce a word using its individual sounds (e.g., when given the word "bat," the correct response is "b-a-t").

For additional information on the relationship between phonological awareness training and literacy, see Pfost et al., 2019.

Alphabetic Letter Name and Sound Knowledge

- Program instruction hierarchically in the following order: letters in which the sound represents the beginning of the letter name (e.g., b, p); letters in which the sound represents the end of the letter name (e.g., f, l); and, finally, letters in which the sound is not related to the letter name (e.g., w, y). (*Note:* The order in which alphabetic letters are introduced varies across curricula. The order presented here is one example.)

- Call attention to the way letters are formed by the mouth (e.g., lip rounding for /w/ or tongue tip elevation for /t/).

- Call attention to the sounds that each letter makes (e.g., "em" is the letter's name, whereas /mmmm/ is the sound it makes).

Adult Modeling of Literacy Activities

- Provide frequent opportunities for the child to observe adults engaged in reading and writing in natural contexts (e.g., preparing a grocery list, following written instructions to assemble a toy).

- Engage the child as a "helper" in everyday activities (e.g., hunting for items in a catalog or following a simple recipe to prepare a favorite food).

- Engage the child in interaction with various kinds of written materials (e.g., menus, shopping lists, recipes, books)

Experience With Writing Materials

- Provide materials that permit children to write by themselves (e.g., pens, pencils, markers, crayons, rudimentary keyboarding).

- Facilitate all forms of writing (e.g., drawing, scribbling, basic letter formation). (See Table 4–14 on literacy development for the stages of writing development.)

- Encourage child to dictate a "story" given visual stimuli (e.g., wordless picture books, cartoon frames).

Example Profiles

Following are two typical profiles of preschool children with language disorders. These examples have been designed to illustrate the selection of intervention targets as well as a variety of service models, specific therapy approaches, activities, and materials. Most are easily implemented in either individual, small group, or classroom settings.

PROFILE 2: PRESCHOOL—3-YEAR-OLD

Austin is a 3-year, 1-month-old male child who presents with moderate delays in receptive and expressive language skills. Birth and developmental history are unremarkable, and hearing acuity is within normal limits. The results of a recent speech-language evaluation indicate that Austin's language comprehension abilities approximate the 24-month level, whereas expressive language skills fall at the 18- to 20-month level. Numerous articulation errors also were noted. Family members and the preschool teacher report that Austin is a socially interactive child who understands simple directions and communicates mainly through single words and occasional gestures.

Selection of Therapy Targets. The areas to be targeted are the comprehension of two-step commands, production of action + object utterances, and comprehension of early developing wh- questions. These targets were selected for two primary reasons: (a) these behaviors represent the next logical steps in the normal developmental sequence and (b) they are highly relevant to the majority of Austin's daily activities. In addition, shared book reading was selected as an instructional focus to enhance the development of emergent literacy.

Sample Activities

Following Directions

1. Gather 20 common objects with which the child is familiar. Develop a list of 10 two-step commands, each containing four linguistic elements in verb + object (V + O) constructions (e.g., "*Give me the car and push the spoon*"). Place three objects at a time on the table in front of the child. Verbally present the corresponding two-step command, and encourage the child to perform each part as it is spoken. If the child is successful, repeat the same stimulus but instruct the child to refrain from responding until the entire two-stage command has been presented. Following are sample commands:

   Pick up the cup and give me the shoe.

   Throw the spoon and wave bye-bye to the doggie.

   Give me the cup and push the car.

   Drop the spoon and point to the ball.

   Give me the brush and pick up the shoe.

   Push the doggie and throw the ball.

   Open the book and drop the cup.

   Close the box and give me the car.

   Hug the doggie and bang the spoon.

   Pick up the block and close the book.

Two-Word Utterances

2. Develop a list of 20 two-word action + one object utterances containing vocabulary words that are already part of the child's spontaneous expressive repertoire. Try to develop sets of two or three utterances that are topically related to one another to provide a meaningful context. Examples include the following:

open juice	*throw ball*
pour juice	*kick ball*
drink juice	*roll ball*
open book	*wash baby*
read book	*brush hair*
close book	*kiss baby*

Gather toy replicas of each of the objects and any other toy props that may be required to perform the action sequences (e.g., for the utterance, "pour juice," a juice container and a cup will be needed). Place the objects in a large bag or pillowcase. Shake the bag to solicit the child's attention. Instruct the child to close or cover his eyes and to pull one of the objects from the bag. Depending on the child's abilities, either label the object or ask the child to name it. Then ask the child to perform one of the actions on the object (e.g., "Open the juice") and say, "What are you doing?" or "What's happening?" Following the child's correct production of the target utterance "open juice," reinforce the response with a comment, such as "I like the way you opened the juice so carefully," or an expansion, such as "You opened the juice." Then ask the child to perform another action with the same object (e.g., "Pour the juice"). Repeat the same training sequence with the other action + object combinations. If the child does not produce a verbal response or responds with a single-word utterance (e.g., "open"), model the target two-word utterance and repeat the item. After two unsuccessful attempts with a given utterance, model the target response and proceed to the next item.

Understanding Wh- Questions

3. Obtain a theme toy such as a farm, house, car wash, airport, or hospital and four toy people that can serve as a "mommy," "daddy," "sister/brother," or "baby," based on the composition of the child's family. Place the theme toy (e.g., house) on the floor in front of the child, and put the "family" in front of the house. To ensure understanding of the lexical items, ask the child to point to each of the locations in and around the house and the family members when named. Examples of locations include the following:

kitchen	patio
bedroom	stairs
bathroom	laundry room
den/family room	backyard
basement	dining room

Instruct the child to place one of the people in a location about the house (e.g., "Put mommy in the living room") and say, "Who is in the living room?" Following the child's correct response, query the child, "Where is mommy?" Reinforce a correct response with a comment, expansion, or other scaffolding utterance. If the child responds incorrectly to either or both of the wh- questions, provide a prompt such as "Who? Mommy. That's who is in the living room. Mommy." Then ask, "Who is in the living room?"

Shared Book Reading

4. Select a simple story from children's literature (e.g., The Three Bears) to read to the child. Throughout the reading of the book, engage the child in the PEER picture-book-reading routine (Burns et al., 1999):

> P = *Parent*/adult initiates exchange about the book (e.g., "What are the three bears doing?")
>
> E = Parent/adult *evaluates* child's response (e.g., "Yes, Papa Bear is tasting the porridge.")
>
> E = Parent/adult *expands* child's response (e.g., "And what is Momma Bear doing?")
>
> R = Parent/adult *repeats* initial question to check child's comprehension (e.g., "What are the three bears doing? Do you remember?")

PROFILE 3: PRESCHOOL—5-YEAR-OLD

Keisha is a 5-year, 7-month-old female child who demonstrates a mild receptive language delay and a moderate expressive impairment. Birth and medical history are unremarkable except for chronic middle ear infections during the first 2 years of life. At present, Keisha exhibits normal hearing acuity bilaterally. Her current communicative status is characterized by a 6- to 9-month delay in most areas of language comprehension. Her language production abilities are more impaired, approximating the 3- to 3½-year level and consisting primarily of three-word utterances that tend to be telegraphic in nature (e.g., "It my book"; "Daddy sleeping bed"). Keisha's pragmatic use of language is essentially age appropriate, and her speech intelligibility is judged to be good.

According to her kindergarten teacher, Keisha seems to understand most classroom activities but experiences a great deal of difficulty with emergent literacy skills, such as sound–letter correspondence.

Selection of Therapy Targets. The areas to be targeted are the auxiliary verb *is*, regular plural -*s*, and rhyme recognition. This auxiliary form was chosen for two reasons: (a) the progressive -*ing* form is already occasionally observed in Keisha's spontaneous speech and (b) the productive use of this auxiliary form would significantly decrease the telegraphic quality of her utterances. The plural marker -*s* was selected because Keisha grasps the concept of plurality but lacks the means for coding this information linguistically. Finally, rhyme recognition was targeted because it is a basic phonological awareness skill that contributes to early reading success. The SLP and the classroom teacher will work together to reinforce these learning objectives in the classroom setting.

Sample Activities

Present-Progressive-Tense Marker

1. Collect 20 pictures or drawings of single agents performing various actions, and attach each picture to an index card or other durable surface. Appropriate actions may include the following:

eating	kissing
drinking	reading
sleeping	hugging
laughing	painting
crying	washing
kicking	driving
throwing	swimming

Cut basic shapes of laundry items (e.g., shirts, pants, socks) out of colored paper, and mark an X on several of them. Loosely attach one picture card to the back of each laundry item cutout. String a clothesline between two chairs and hang the cutouts on the line with clothespins. Explain that the laundry items will be removed from the line one at a time. As the child removes an item from the line, the clinician models an appropriate sentence incorporating the *is____ing* construction (e.g., "The boy is swimming"; "He is sleeping") and instructs the child to imitate it. Following a correct response, the child can remove the picture card from the cutout to look for an X on the back of the laundry item. If an X is found, the child receives a sticker or other reinforcer. Repeat this sequence for all 20 action pictures.

Plurals

2. Gather materials including paper, marker, small paint bottle with sponge top (i.e., bingo marker), pictures or drawings of 10 single and 10 multiple objects, index cards, and a Colorforms kit. Using the marker, make a 20-square bingo board template (four rows of five squares each) on a large piece of paper. Laminate the pictures to the index cards and stack them randomly in a deck. Instruct the child to select the top card from the deck and name it three times. Remind the child that plural *s* must be added to the end of a word whenever more than one object is pictured (e.g., shoes). If all three productions are correct, the child uses the bingo marker to place a dot in one of the squares on the bingo board. Each time a row of five dots is completed, the child is given a Colorform piece. After the final row is completed, the child is allowed to create a picture using all of the accumulated Colorform pieces.

Rhyme Recognition

3. Write the numbers 1 to 10 on 3 × 5 in. index cards. Construct a list of 20 word-rhyme pairs, two of which rhyme with each number (adapted from B. Baden, personal communication, March 1994). Examples of rhyme pair stimuli are as follows:

1 = sun-done ton-won	6 = kicks-fix mix-sticks
2 = clue-blue shoe-moo	7 = heaven-leaven Evan-Kevin
3 = see-knee tree-free	8 = date-gate wait-mate
4 = store-pour sore-wore	9 = dine-line fine-mine
5 = dive-hive chive-drive	10 = men-pen then-den

Review the concept of rhyming with the child by explaining that rhymes are words that end in the same way. Give some examples of words that do and do not rhyme (e.g., hat-bat, shoe-blue, map-cap, cat-cow, top-tall), explaining why each does or does not rhyme. Place the number cards in a row on the table or floor in front of the child. Ask the child to name each of the numbers aloud. Explain that the clinician will say words that rhyme with or sound like the numbers on the cards. Instruct the child to listen carefully as the clinician says each rhyme pair and to hold up or point to the corresponding rhyming number. For example, the clinician says "store-pour," and the child holds up the number 4. Following a correct response, say, "That's right, store-pour-four all rhyme with each other." Instruct the child to repeat the verbal sequence.

Note: A variation of this activity is to substitute color words for number words with children who have reliable color word vocabularies.

Helpful Hints

1. It may be useful to teach the agent + action and action + object semantic relations sequentially, because it generally provides an easy transition into three-word utterances (i.e., agent-action-object constructions).

2. Clinicians can encourage families to engage children in activities to promote emergent literacy. These may include the following:

   - Reading aloud to a child who is in a comfortable position. Ideal features in books for children at this age range include objects to identify, language that repeats and has rhymes, and activities that are highly familiar to the child.

   - An adult reads a story and has the child draw a picture to go with it.

   - Have the child plan a party for four to six people. Look in the food section of the newspaper for ideas of what to serve.

   - Adult and child look through newspapers and clip out articles about events in different parts of the world and attach each article to its location on a map or globe.

   - Clinicians can recommend play activities that parents can use at home to encourage attention to and experience with writing, such as making letters in sand or soap and tracing letters in sand or paint.

   - Create a "sound-activity" calendar to promote phonological awareness skills. Each day on the calendar identifies a short, fun activity that families can easily incorporate into daily activities (e.g., On Monday, "Tell me three words that start with the sound /b/"; on Tuesday, "Do *bat* and *cat* rhyme?"; on Wednesday, "What would the word *cupcake* sound like if we didn't say the *cup* part?"; on Thursday, "Guess the word I'm trying to say *ba...na...na*"; on Friday, "Which word doesn't belong: *make, take, boot*?"). These can be repeated several times throughout the day in a wide variety of contexts (e.g., bath time, grocery store, car trip).

3. It may be more effective to repeat or expand a child's utterance than to directly correct the child's form.

4. Encourage parents to use daily activities (e.g., putting away toys; put clothes in hamper) to practice one- and two-step instructions. Model activity as needed, and provide praise for a job well done.

5. Many of the language and communication activities in *RTI in Action: Oral Language Activities for K–2 Classrooms* (Roth et al., 2010) are appropriate for preschool children.

6. Parents of children with severe language impairments often overestimate their child's level of ability, particularly in the area of language comprehension. Effective counseling may require that the clinician carefully guide parents to a more realistic perception of their child's true language skills.

7. SLPs can collaborate with others—including teachers, counselors, coaches, and family members—to understand SM and to determine fruitful strategies for interacting with the child.

8. In their 2018 tutorial, Terrell and Watson offer a "toolbox" of strategies, techniques, and activities that SLPs and parents can use to help children develop emergent and early literacy skills.

9. Pair the introduction of a new vocabulary word with its print version to promote the development of emergent literacy skills.

Conclusion

This chapter presented basic information, protocols, and procedures for intervention for early childhood language disorders at an *introductory* level. This information is intended only as a starting point in the reader's clinical education and training. For more in-depth coverage of this area, the following readings are recommended:

Owens, R. E. (2014). *Language disorders: A functional approach to assessment and intervention* (7th ed.). Allyn & Bacon.

Paul, R., Norbury, C., & Gosse, C. (2018). *Language disorders from infancy to adolescence. Listening, speaking, reading, writing, and communicating* (5th ed.). Elsevier.

Additional Resources

Language Strategies: For Little Ones (Grades K–1), for Children (Grades 2–5), and for Older Students (Grades 5–8)
These resources contain a series of curriculum-based lessons that focus on language comprehension, oral expression, and story grammar knowledge. The reproducible lessons reinforce listening, questioning, categorizing, sequencing, reasoning, and vocabulary skills. Each unit integrates whole-language philosophy, classroom curriculum concepts, literature-based intervention techniques, and strategies for self-prompting.

Literacy-Based Speech and Language Therapy Activities
This book was written to provide SLPs with the rationale and the resources needed to incorporate books and literacy elements into speech therapy sessions. It covers sections on the research behind literacy-based intervention, guidance for preparing for literacy-based sessions, and suggestions for templates and activities to use in sessions. The book also includes several book lists organized by age/grade, therapy goals, and curriculum topics.

Look Who's Listening

For ages 3 and up, this includes 10 auditory games in one. Included are auditory skill card decks to target auditory discrimination, auditory memory, and auditory integration. Students take turns listening carefully, following card directions, rolling the die, and placing tokens on the game board.

Preschool Vocabulary Cards: Actions, Concepts

These age-appropriate cards can be used to expand younger clients' receptive and expressive vocabularies as well as help them make requests and construct sentences. The full color illustrations reflect the vocabulary and experiences that preschoolers are exposed to every day.

Road to the Code

This developmentally sequenced 11-week program is designed to give kindergarten and first-grade students repeated opportunities to practice and enhance beginning reading and spelling abilities. Contains 44 lessons, each featuring three activities.

DK Games: Silly Sentences

Card games to learn: subject 1 verb agreement, subject 1 verb 1 object (S 1 V 1 O) sentences, humor and absurdities, speech sound articulation, questioning and answering, and present progressive verbs. Includes three color-coded decks of 40 cards each.

Speech and Language Activities for Young Learners

This literacy-based intervention program uses multisensory information to help develop articulation and phonology skills. Each chapter is based on a well-known children's book, and the activities relate to the story and reinforce story concepts. The articulation, phonological awareness, and phonological pattern activities focus on critical skills needed to become a successful speaker and reader.

Super Duper Handy Handouts

These are free informational sheets written by professionals to answer parents' and teachers' questions about speech and language development. Topics covered include signs of expressive and receptive language delays, strategies for encouraging communication, and information on pretend play and material selection.

Talking on the Go

This spiral-bound book provides parents and caregivers with ideas for stimulating speech and language skills in the following areas: vocabulary, listening and speech production, reading and writing readiness, and conversational skills. The activities are designed for children ages birth through 5 years of age.

Teaching Informational Text in K–3 Classrooms: Best Practices to Help Children Read, Write, and Learn from Nonfiction

This book provides information on selecting and using informational texts with younger children as well as resources for activities to accompany the texts. It also includes chapters on targeting comprehension, vocabulary, and writing skills.

Webber Photo Cards: Everyday Go-Togethers

This deck has card pairs that are ideal for memory-based, matching, and Go Fish games. All cards are 3 × 4 in., and the deck has content/game idea cards in six languages: English, Spanish, Japanese, Chinese, French, and German.

Webber Classifying Cards

This large, colorful card pack comes in carrying tote with seven decks, including animals, food, around the home, occupations, clothing, transportation, and numbers.

Miscellaneous

Burns, M. S., Griffin, P., & Snow, C. E. (2000). *Starting out right: A guide to promoting children's reading success.* National Academy Press.

> Clinician- and parent-friendly guide to the development of reading and spelling skills in young children. Includes specific activities to promote emergent and early literacy from infancy through mid-elementary school.

Griffith, L., & Olsen, M. A. (1992). Phonemic awareness helps beginning readers break the code. *The Reading Teacher, 45,* 516–523.

> This article contains a list of books that involve sound play for young children.

Massey, S. L. (2014). Making the case for using informational text in preschool classrooms. *Creative Education, 5*(6), 396–401.

> This journal article discusses the benefits of using informational texts as read-alouds, such as vocabulary growth and increases in language skills to support literacy development.

Reading Rockets. http://www.readingrockets.org

> This website provides literacy information pertaining to how children learn to read, difficulties in learning to read, and how to help children who are struggling to learn to read. It has many useful features, such as book finders and resources on how to engage children with different types of texts such as informational texts.

Torgesen, J. K., & Bryant, B. R. (2013). *Phonological awareness training for reading* (2nd ed.). Pro-Ed.

> Focuses on training in four areas: sound blending, sound segmenting, reading, and spelling. Skills are taught in a sequential manner through a variety of games. It includes a detailed description (script) for each activity as well as precise instructions for implementation.

Yopp, H. K. (1992). Developing phonemic awareness in young children. *The Reading Teacher, 45,* 696–703.

> This article focuses on the use of songs and melodies for training phonological awareness and provides specific suggestions.

Yopp, H. K., & Yopp, R. H. (2000). Supporting phonemic awareness in the classroom. *The Reading Teacher, 54,* 130–143.

> This article provides sample phonological awareness activities appropriate for preschool, kindergarten, and first-grade classrooms within a developmental hierarchy of difficulty.

Chapter 5

Intervention for Language in School-Age Children Through Adolescence

The initial portion of this chapter provides a description of the developmental language characteristics of two major age groups: 5- to 10-year-olds and 10- to 18-year-olds. These sections are followed by a discussion of several treatment approaches that can be appropriately used across both age ranges. Example profiles and sample activities are then presented for each age group. *The reader is encouraged to review the joint introduction to Chapters 4 and 5 for important information on the following:*

- *Definition of a language disorder*
- *Classification of language disorders*
- *Behavioral characteristics associated with language disorders*
- *Relationship between oral language and literacy*
- *Role of a speech–language pathologist (SLP) in literacy*
- *Theoretical models of intervention*
- *Treatment efficacy/evidence-based practice*

Characteristics of Students Ages 5 to 10 years

Several advancements in oral language occur during this period. Children's vocabularies increase in size and in depth of word knowledge (e.g., shades of meaning: *red* versus *crimson*; *run* versus *sprint*). Tier 2 and Tier 3 words appear with increasing frequency between kindergarten and Grade 5 (see Chapter 4, Table 4–4 for definitions and examples). Utterance length increases by an average of one word per year until about 9 years of age, when the length of oral language utterances begins to taper off. Syntactic growth is marked by the increased use of low-frequency structures (e.g., passive sentences) and an increased use of complex sentences (e.g., relative clause constructions).

Another important advance in oral language development during this period occurs in the area of *metalinguistic awareness*. Metalinguistic awareness involves explicit knowledge and the ability to manipulate the structural aspects of language independently from the meaning conveyed by the message. Many language activities require this ability to focus on language as an entity unto itself, including the phonological awareness tasks of segmenting and blending speech sounds or syllables (metaphonology); provision of formal definitions; appreciation of humor, metaphors, idioms, and other figurative language forms (metasemantics); and the ability to make grammatical judgments (metasyntax).

Of particular significance is the refinement of children's phonological awareness knowledge to the level of phonemic awareness (i.e., the ability to segment and blend *individual* speech sounds in words). It has been determined that phonemic awareness, and specifically the ability to segment words into phonemes, is the strongest predictor of early reading and writing skills (Torgesen et al., 1994; Wagner & Torgesen, 1987; Wagner et al., 1994). More recently, Murphy et al. (2016) discussed the relationship of various oral language skills and reading for preschool children with language impairments and identified phonological awareness as an early and reliable predictor of reading ability, prior to the beginning of formal reading instruction. Thus, there is a developmental relationship between oral language skills and literacy, and, further, this relationship is reciprocal. That is, phonemic awareness skills promote early reading ability, and early reading skills further the development of phonemic awareness (see Chapter 4 for additional information regarding phonological awareness and its development).

In addition to progress in oral language, children acquire basic literacy skills during the elementary school years as they begin to receive formal instruction in reading and writing. In reading, they first learn to *decode* printed words (and nonwords) by making sound–letter correspondences (i.e., use the alphabetic principle). As children gain word-recognition accuracy, their reading *fluency* improves, and they begin to read connected text with greater ease and automaticity. By middle elementary school, the focus of reading and reading instruction shifts to *reading comprehension*, or reading for meaning. Thus, third to fourth grade represents a critical transition because "learning to read" becomes "reading to learn." Table 5–1 provides definitions and stages of reading development.

Third to fourth grade is also the point at which children's writing development progresses in both *spelling* and written *composition* (writing at the text level). By middle to late elementary school, children reach the stage of conventional spelling and can correctly spell a large number of words automatically (see Chapter 4 for the developmental stages of spelling) and can spell with enough fluency to compose sentence-length text. Thus, they display advances in both the processes and products of writing. According to Hayes and Flower (1987), *writing processes* include the following:

- Planning (prewriting)—generating and organizing ideas about the topic, taking into account both the goal and target audience

- Drafting/composing—putting ideas into words and text

- Revising—reviewing and evaluating content to reorganize, consolidate, and develop new ideas

- Editing written text—polishing the flow and format of the composition

For skilled writers, these processes are overlapping and continuous until the final composition is generated. The following *writing products*, the output of writing processes, occur at the word, sentence, and text levels (Dockrell, 2014; Nelson, 2014):

- Word selection and spelling (word level)

- Grammatical complexity and morphological forms (sentence level)

- Cohesion devices that link sentences together (text level)

- Discourse type such as persuasive essay versus compare-and-contrast composition (text level)

- Capitalization and punctuation (across all levels)

Table 5–1

Definitions of Reading Processes and Stages of Reading Development

Term	Definition
Decoding	Knowledge of letter-sound correspondences (alphabetic principle) to convert print into words
Word recognition and fluency	Rapid and automatic identification of written words
Comprehension	Processes by which printed language is understood and interpreted

Stages of Development	Description
Word-Level Reading	
Logographic/Pre-alphabetic	Association of spoken words with environmental print without knowledge of letter-sound correspondences (alphabetic principle); for example, logos, brand names, street signs
Transitional	Partial knowledge of sound-letter correspondences; for example, use of initial or final letter to guess the word; sight-word vocabulary for highly familiar words
Alphabetic	Full knowledge of alphabetic principle; that is, ability to decode both familiar and unfamiliar words
Orthographic	Use of spelling patterns to recognize and pronounce commonly recurring letter patterns as units (e.g., root words, prefixes, suffixes, syllables); builds large reading vocabulary
Automatic word recognition	Proficient and fluent reading of most words by sight
Text-Level Reading	
Phase 1, 4th–6th grade	Can read familiar content (i.e., narratives); consolidates reading fluency and speed; not reading to gain new information so can concentrate on the print
Phase 2, 7th–8th grade	Reads text to learn new information (reading becomes a source of ideas); reads materials that contain one point of view to obtain facts, concepts, how to do things, rather than for nuance; begins to bring prior knowledge and experience to written text; growing importance of vocabulary/word meanings
Phase 3, 9th–12th grade	Can read multiple points of view, can read more than one set of facts, and can acquire new concepts and viewpoints from text (textbooks, reference works, mature fiction, newspapers, magazines)
Phase 4, 12th+ grade	Mature reading stage; reads for greater detail and completeness; reading becomes more qualitative, as reader constructs own knowledge using analysis, synthesis, and evaluation of information from different sources; reads at different levels to obtain desired level of detail, such as skimming versus studying text

The development of written text structures proceeds from the narrative form to various types of expository writing and persuasive essays. Narrative discourse involves story or storylike forms in which the events occur in a chronological order. Expository texts present nonchronologically sequenced events and generally convey information that is novel to the reader. Examples of different types of expository text structures are description, comparison/contrast, and cause–effect. Table 5–2 presents the differences between narrative and expository texts, and Table 5–3 lists different types of text structures and their characteristics. In addition to narrative and expository texts, there are persuasive essays. The main difference between them is that an expository essay explains and provides clarifying information, while persuasive pieces argue for a particular point of view on a debatable topic. Table 5–4 lists the main types of complex sentences.

Characteristics of Adolescents 10 to 18 years

Adolescence is the developmental period during which youngsters (a) develop a stable identity, (b) acquire independence from family, (c) develop career plans, and (d) develop moral and ethical values consistent with those of society (Erikson, 1968). There are three main stages of adolescence, and the intervention goals for each stage differ slightly. In early adolescence (10–14 years), the primary focus is on developing communication skills for academic and personal–social purposes.

Table 5–2
Narrative and Expository Text Difference

Narrative	Expository
Purpose to entertain	Purpose to inform
Familiar schema content	Unfamiliar schema content
Consistent text structure	Variable text structures
Focus on character motivations, intentions, goals	Focus on factual information and abstract ideas
Often requires taking multiple perspectives, understanding the points of view of different characters	Expected to take the perspective of the writer of the text
Can use pragmatic inferences, that is, inference from similar experiences	Must use logical-deductive inferences
Connective words not critical—primarily *and, then, so*	Connective words critical—wide variety of connectives, for example, *because, before, after, if-then, therefore*
Each text can stand alone	Expected to integrate information across texts
Can use top-down processing	Relies on bottom-up processing

Source: Adapted from "Assessing and remediating text comprehension problems," by C. E. Westby, in A. G. Kamhi & H. W. Catts (Eds.), Language and reading disabilities (3rd ed., pp. 154–223), 2012, Pearson.

Table 5–3

Expository Text Types and Characteristics

Text Type	Function	Key Words
Descriptive	Does the text tell me what something is?	None
Sequence/procedural	Does the text tell me how to do or make something?	*first . . . next . . . then; second . . . third . . . ; following this step; finally*
Cause/effect	Does the text give reasons for why something is or happens?	*because, since, then, therefore, for this reason, results, effects, consequently, so, in order, thus, then*
Problem/solution	Does the text state a problem and offer solutions to the problem?	*one problem is; a solution is*
Comparison/contrast	Does the text show how two things are the same or different?	*different, same, alike, similar, although, however, on the other hand, but, yet, still, rather than*

Source: Adapted from "Assessing and remediating text comprehension problems," by C. E. Westby, in A. G. Kamhi & H. W. Catts (Eds.), Language and reading disabilities (3rd ed., pp. 154–223), 2012, Pearson.

The goals for midadolescence (14–16 years) involve facilitation of communication skills for academic, personal-social, and vocational aims. By late adolescence (16–20 years), language intervention is concentrated on developing communication skills for personal–social and career purposes.

In the adolescent period, communication skills are refined, and higher order language abilities undergo significant development as the child's linguistic system reaches the adult form. The language demands of secondary grades also increase dramatically. For example, high school seniors are now expected to read 50 pages/week across all subject areas, and about 70% is informational text with Tier 2 and Tier 3 vocabulary.

Significant growth occurs in the metalinguistic area of nonliteral or figurative uses of language, including idioms, metaphors, proverbs, and humor. These are considered higher order language forms, because they require the ability to go beyond the conventional meaning of language for correct interpretation or use. Figurative language forms increasingly appear in both oral and written language materials beginning in middle and upper elementary school years. In fact, by eighth grade at least 20% of teacher talk and written text consist of nonliteral uses of language (Nippold, 1998; Nippold et al., 2005).

During adolescence, continued development also occurs in conversational maturity, utterance length, the comprehension/production of complex sentences and linguistic cohesion devices (see Appendix 5–A on the companion website for types of cohesion), and low-frequency syntactic structures (language forms that occur in literate texts, spoken and written, with greater frequency than in oral conversational speech, such as expanded noun phrases and expanded verb phrases). Semantic knowledge also undergoes further growth with respect to both vocabulary size and depth of word knowledge, with steep increases seen in the use of Tier 2 and Tier 3 vocabulary words. Word knowledge reflects an increased understanding of multiple meaning words (e.g., block, cold) and the literate lexicon (words that commonly occur in scholarly contexts such as textbooks, lectures, and seminars).

Table 5–4
Main Types of Complex Sentences

Types	Definition	Examples
Coordinated/ conjoined	Clauses are linked together by a coordinating conjunction. Clauses are syntactically independent.	and or but while and then or else
Embeddings	The embedded clause is subordinated to the main clause. The word "that" signals the noun phrase (NP) complement and is called a "complementizer."	The students knew that they were going on a field trip.
Complementation	Embedded clause functions in a syntactic role such as subject, object, or indirect object.	The teacher announced (that recess was cancelled).
Relative clauses	The embedded clause follows and modifies a NP. A relative pronoun is a word that introduces the relative clause (RC) (e.g., who, that, which).	The man (who came to see you) was tall.
Subject relative clauses	Relative pronoun is the subject of the RC.	The cat (that jumped onto the refrigerator) was black.
Object relatives	Relative pronoun is the object of the relative clause.	They saw the boy (whom the dog chased).
Adjectival clauses	Embeddings that modify adjective NPs.	He is ready to leave.
Adverbial clauses	Embeddings that modify adverbial noun phrases.	I had to leave while Eli was playing basketball.

Source: Adapted from "Targeting Complex Sentences in Older Children With Specific Language Impairment: Results from an Early-Phase Treatment Study," by C. H. Balthazar and C. M. Scott, 2018, *Journal of Speech, Language, and Hearing Research, 61,* 713–728.

Deepening social relationships marked by camaraderie, joking, teasing, gossiping, and slang can pose significant problems for students with language-learning impairments.

   In addition to oral language, students demonstrate advances in the written language domain, as they become mature readers and skilled writers by the end of this developmental period. Students are reading longer and more complicated texts (see Table 5–1 for stages of reading development) and can increasingly concentrate on obtaining and synthesizing new information from a variety of print materials (i.e., textbooks, essays, poems, reference sources). In both reading and writing, there is a shift in focus from content facts (simple propositions conveyed by a text, such as information about a character in a story or facts about mammals) to content schema (macrostructures that represent the organization of a text structure, such as a story, a compare–contrast essay, or an informational text). Schema knowledge provides structure that allows the reader to do the following:

- Organize sets of facts (content knowledge)

- Assimilate new text information (e.g., new facts)

- Make inferences necessary for accurate and full comprehension (e.g., predict what's coming next, understand what is not explicitly stated)

- Search for information from memory in an orderly fashion

- Improve in the reconstruction and summarization of text

Adolescents' written expression shows steady gains in the use of planning and organizational strategies; the ability to reflect on and revise/edit initial drafts for grammar, punctuation, and word choice; and the ability to meet the organizational and structural demands of different discourse genres. See Table 5–3 for different types of text structure and their characteristics.

Older students with **language learning disabilities (LLDs)** frequently demonstrate significant difficulties with both the processes and products of writing. The primary process characteristics of students with LLDs are as follows:

- Lack of planning

- Reduced use of background knowledge

- Lack of revision and editing

- Composition does not align with genre

- Reduced sense of audience (understanding audience perception)

The following are primary characteristics of the writing products of students with LLDs:

- Shorter texts

- Reduced sentence complexity (both semantic and syntactic)

- Fewer instances of complex sentences

- Fewer cohesive ties and less accurate use of cohesion

- Higher proportion of grammatical errors

- Higher proportion of punctuation errors

A final area of importance during this developmental period is **metacognitive/executive functioning**. Metacognitive abilities involve an awareness of one's own problem-solving abilities and include self-regulation behaviors that are used to guide, monitor, and evaluate the success of one's performance (Baddeley, 2007; Barkley, 1996, 1997). They include planning, attending selectively to certain aspects of a situation, shifting attention as necessary, inhibition of behavioral impulses, setting goals, and organizing/modifying one's behavior and work. Metacognition/executive functioning has been aptly described as "the brain's air traffic control system." Students show marked advances in metacognitive functioning beginning at about fourth grade, and, as a result, they gradually become more strategic learners. Metacognition is considered a higher order ability area, because these "meta" strategies must be invoked from the outset of a task and require task analysis and a great deal of planning. Metacognition also requires "mindfulness": skills that allow for intentional, adaptive, and flexible learning. Students with these higher order difficulties often have difficulty with overall organization, setting and attaining goals, planning according to the task demands, identifying errors in their own work, and initiating alternative approaches to a task (making behavioral adjustments). Knowledge of metacognitive development and deficits is necessary for SLPs because these skills and strategies are largely mediated through language, and they are not generally taught explicitly in the classroom. In traditional educational settings, students implicitly are encouraged/expected to engage in "self-talk" throughout the school day about the nature of a task/assignment, how and why they are doing it, the effectiveness of their strategies, and ways to change their behaviors and strategies.

Metacognitive intervention strategies often focus on teaching students how to learn rather than what to learn. Examples include the following:

- Explicitly teaching rules for different academic and social settings

- Teaching principles of information gathering for a range of academic subject areas

- Teaching strategies for identifying the main idea in oral and written texts

- Using context to determine meaning in academic and social situations

- Using checklists or graphic organizers to plan assignments (e.g., study guides)

- Training on how to parse morphologically complex words that occur in academic coursework

- Facilitating the use of digital technologies to access and share information for different purposes

Students with language and learning disabilities often seek postsecondary education, employment, or career opportunities. Yet, **transitioning** from secondary to postsecondary settings presents unique challenges for students with language/learning disorders and their families. Many of these individuals continue to need accommodations to function effectively in these advanced settings (Association on Higher Education and Disability [AHEAD], 2008). Qualifying for these supports requires transition documentation of a disability. Unfortunately, there is no uniformity across settings as to the type or rigor of documentation needed. For example, in some environments, the emphasis is on the "history" of disability and its functional limitations rather than a current diagnosis of the disability. In other cases, such as most 2- and 4-year academic institutions, a "recent" diagnosis is required, where "recent" is defined as not longer than the prior 3 years. SLPs, other professionals, and families need to be aware that documentation is required, that it can be burdensome, and that it takes planning and preparation. For example, if an institution, training program, or job site requires recent documentation of a diagnosis, then the SLP can plan to complete an exit evaluation accordingly. SLPs also can reinforce the importance of student and family self-advocacy to inform postsecondary settings about the student's need for support services and to follow-up as needed.

Intervention Considerations for School-Age Children and Adolescents

It is important to note that, in general, adolescents with language/learning impairments are "underserved" at the secondary level in terms of access to services by SLPs.

Intervention for school-age students revolves, in large part, around the relationship between oral language and literacy. Language therapy goals are programmed to address the demands and expectations of the educational curriculum. Therefore, service delivery is often accomplished through a variety of models, including classroom consultation and collaboration in addition to more traditional individual therapy sessions. Cirrin et al. (2010) focused on the effect of different service-delivery models (e.g., pull-out, classroom based, indirect consultation, interprofessional practice) on speech-language intervention outcomes for elementary school-age students. These authors conducted a systematic review of evidence-based studies published during the past 30 years and found that only five studies met the review criteria and addressed the effectiveness of service-delivery models. Even within this small sample, results were mixed, revealing large gaps in our knowledge of the relative effectiveness of different service delivery models. Approaches to goal selection still may include a developmental focus, depending on a student's language and learning abilities. However, strategies designed to facilitate *functional* performance are used increasingly with preteens and adolescents. Many approaches to language therapy have been designed for the wide variety of communication deficits exhibited by this population. Regardless of theoretical orientation, all intervention goals should be guided by well-designed studies that demonstrate their instructional effectiveness. See Stone et al. (2014) for a compendium of research-based practices in language instruction/intervention. Clinicians should remain sensitive to the cultural and linguistic backgrounds of each student throughout all stages of the intervention process. For intervention to be successful with the adolescent, the teen has to be a fully cooperative partner in the therapy program. The teen should be consulted regarding the selection of specific therapy objectives, and the clinician must clearly explain the rationale for each target behavior. This allows the student to take ownership of the problem, take primary responsibility for achieving the goals, and recognize that he or she is the one who will lose out if follow-through does not occur. At least two potential problems may be encountered when working with adolescents: (a) resistance to dependent relationships with adults because they are striving to achieve and demonstrate their own independence and (b) rejection of the idea of being flawed or different in any way from their peer group.

The Common Core State Standards

The Common Core State Standards (CCSS) were developed in 2010 to improve the college and career readiness of high school graduates. These national standards outline/map the hierarchy of knowledge and skills in English language arts and mathematics that students should develop within grades K–12 to be competitive in a global workforce/society. Led by state education organizations, the goals of the standards are to improve U.S. educational outcomes and provide equivalent educational opportunities for all students. The CCSS are a defined set of increasingly complex standards that are internationally benchmarked (Table 5–5 presents an example of the K–12 "staircase" of complexity for the reading–literature standard). The CCSS clearly require that the standards be taught using high-quality, research-based instruction that reflects best practices (http://www.corestandards.org/). Most states have adopted the CCSS or a modified version of the standards and are implementing them in K–12 classrooms.

SLPs have significant roles in helping students meet CCSS expectations, particularly in the English language arts (ELA) domain. The ELA standards are composed of four areas—reading, writing, speaking, and listening and language—all of which are central to the roles and responsibilities of SLP professionals for several reasons:

- Language and communication underlie all of the ELA standards.
- Language competencies are essential to successful academic, social, and career/employment outcomes.

Table 5–5
Example of Increased Complexity of CCSS Across Grade Levels for the Domain of Reading–Literature

Grade Level	Reading for Key Ideas and Details
K	With prompting and support, ask and answer questions about key details in a text.
1	Ask and answer questions about key details in a text.
2	Ask and answer such questions as *who, what, where, when, why,* and *how* to demonstrate understanding of details in a text.
3	Ask and answer questions to demonstrate understanding of a text, referring explicitly to the text as the basis for the answers.
4	Refer to details and examples in a text when explaining what the text says explicitly and when drawing inferences from the text.
5	Quote accurately from a text when explaining what the text says explicitly and when drawing inferences from the text.
6	Cite textual evidence to support analysis of what the text says explicitly as well as inferences drawn from the text.
7	Cite several pieces of textual evidence to support analysis of what the text says explicitly as well as inferences drawn from the text.
8	Cite the textual evidence that most strongly supports an analysis of what the text says explicitly as well as inferences drawn from the text.
9–10	Cite strong and thorough textual evidence to support analysis of what the text says explicitly as well as inferences drawn from the text.
11–12	Cite strong and thorough textual evidence to support analysis of what the text says explicitly as well as inferences drawn from the text, including determining where the text leaves matters uncertain.

- All students need communication skills to participate meaningfully in the classroom, to learn to read and write, and to interact with peers and adults.

- Developing subject-area knowledge (i.e., disciplinary literacy) depends on the integrity of language skills (the ability to comprehend, generate, and respond to material presented by teachers or contained in texts).

- At-risk students and students with disabilities generally do not have the requisite/foundational language and communication skills to be successful in classroom environments.

Following are examples of specific ELA standards that require language and communication skills and knowledge:

- Ask and answer questions about **unknown words** in a text.

- Describe **characters in a story** (e.g., their traits, motivations, or feelings) and explain how their actions contribute to the sequence of events.

- Determine the **meaning of words and phrases** in a text relevant to grade-level topic or subject area.

- Speak in **complete sentences** when appropriate to task and situation in order to provide requested detail or clarification.

- Follow **agreed-upon rules for discussions** and carry out assigned roles.

- Write **narratives** that recount two or more appropriately sequenced events include some details regarding what happened, use **temporal words to signal event order**, and provide some sense of closure.

- **Ask and answer questions** about information from a speaker, offering appropriate elaboration and detail.

- Write opinion pieces on topics or texts . . . and **use linking/transition words and phrases** (e.g., *because, therefore, since, for example*) to connect opinion and reasons.

- Write narratives about experiences or events **using temporal words and phrases to signal event order**.

- Demonstrate understanding of **figurative language, word relationships, and nuances in word meanings**.

- **Adapt speech to a variety of contexts and tasks**, demonstrating command of formal English when indicated or appropriate.

- Determine or clarify the meaning of **unknown and multiple-meaning words and phrases** based on grade-level reading and content, choosing flexibly from a range of strategies.

- **Use common, grade-appropriate Greek or Latin affixes and roots** as clues to the meaning of a word (e.g., audience, auditory, audible).

Many school districts are implementing CCSS within a Response to Intervention (RTI) framework, using multitiered instruction to improve student performance in the general education setting. (See Chapter 1 for a description of RTI.) Linking the CCSS with a multitiered system facilitates ongoing monitoring of student progress and prevents/reduces learning and behavior problems. It also provides a means to identify students who may be eligible for special education services.

Implementing the CCSS in an RTI framework requires "shared responsibility" among educators (Erickson, 2017; Saletta, 2018). SLPs, general education teachers, special education teachers, other professionals, and students must engage in interprofessional collaboration teaming to develop and implement instructional/intervention approaches that are coordinated, strategic, and deliberate if students in all classrooms are to achieve academic goals. Teachers and SLPs bring distinct but complementary skills sets. Working together, SLPs and teachers can give students support needed to develop and strengthen oral language and literacy skills. For example, SLPs can communicate information about areas of language to teachers (e.g., figurative language, multiple-meaning words, linguistic cohesion, complex syntax), whereas teachers know effective methods for teaching these linguistic areas to students using classroom-wide instructional activities. Following are examples of collaboration opportunities for clinicians:

- Identify initial status and progress-monitoring data to identify at-risk students.

- Develop techniques for classroom-wide implementation of standards.

- Implement team-teaching or demonstration lessons in general or special education classrooms.

- Share responsibility for providing differentiated or increasingly intense instruction for smaller groups or individual students who require additional support.

Although intended for *all* students, the CCSS do not address the needs of students with learning difficulties or students who are English-language learners. SLPs and teachers have to translate/adapt the standards-based curriculum to specific goals and objectives for Individualized Education Programs (IEPs). This includes identification and implementation of instructional strategies and scaffolds (accommodations and supports) to maximize the learning of each student. Moreover, SLPs and other educators must recognize that implementation of the CCSS does not preclude the need to teach functional skills to students with language-learning and communication difficulties.

Treatment Approaches for School-Age Children and Adolescents

There are a variety of approaches to language intervention, most of which can be implemented with students across a wide range of ages and stages of development. These approaches emphasize the provision of intervention in naturalistic contexts. This means that children/students are engaged in authentic, meaningful activities that are functionally linked to their daily or classroom activities. The basic remediation approaches described here are often used in combination and align with the expectations of the CCSS. The approaches also are appropriate for a variety of service models, including RTI (or other multitiered support systems [MTSSs]), other collaborative curriculum-based approaches, as well as small-group/individual therapy. It is important to recognize that underlying language deficits may require targeting before focusing on reading comprehension skills (Nippold, 2017).

Previewing

This is a planning strategy that is used to prepare students for upcoming lessons. For oral material, it may involve topic identification, pertinent vocabulary review, and a brief synopsis of information to be presented. In addition to these components, previews of written material may involve identification of section headings and photo captions to provide a "big picture" of the structure/content of a reading selection. The final step in previewing generally involves pausing at the end of a section to check comprehension by restating the information and ideas in the oral/written material.

Predicting

In this approach, knowledge of the subject matter is used to make predictions about content and vocabulary and to check comprehension. Different kinds of knowledge can be the focus of a prediction strategy. For example, information about the *genre* allows predictions about discourse structure. Information about the *author* can be used to make predictions about writing style, vocabulary, and content.

Think Aloud

This is a strategy for improving comprehension and monitoring of oral and written material. It focuses on both literal and inferential comprehension. Students are encouraged to engage in self-talk throughout a learning task. Clinicians orally describe their own thought processes while engaged in a difficult comprehension or problem-solving task in order to model the target behavior. For example, "I am very frustrated because I cannot understand the directions given by the teacher for my homework assignment. What can I do to help me understand it? I will use the strategy: 'Ask again and take notes.'"

K-W-L Procedure (Ogle, 1986)

This approach focuses on improving comprehension of oral or written language, using a three-column chart: K = What we KNOW; W = What we WANT to know; L = What we have LEARNED. The first two columns give clinicians information about students' present knowledge and what needs to be explicitly taught and emphasized. As a new topic/concept is introduced and previewed, students brainstorm everything they know about the topic (prior knowledge), and the clinician records this information in the K column. Then the students generate ideas about what they want to know at the completion of the lesson (W column). Following the lesson, the L column is completed as students identify what they have learned and compare this knowledge to the first two columns.

Metacognitive Stems

This strategy provides students with a structure to improve their organization skills for completion of an assignment. Clinicians teach the steps necessary to complete a task in the correct chronological sequence. As students progress through the steps, they are asked to complete phrases, such as *I'm thinking, I'm picturing, I'm noticing, I'm wondering,* and *I'm feeling.* A visual aid (e.g., poster with written thinking stems) often is provided as a reminder.

Discussion-Oriented Approach (Ebbers & Denton, 2008)

This strategy offers a forum (in classroom or smaller groups) where word meanings are talked about and explained in a conversational context. Students are provided with opportunities to share their background knowledge, ask questions, make predictions about word meanings and correct contexts for use, and validate/modify their predictions.

Social Stories (Gray, 1995)

The main focus of this approach is to improve pragmatic language skills. The clinician develops written scripts that provide explanations of appropriate communicative interaction behaviors in given social situations. These "stories" typically contain both descriptive and directive statements. Descriptive statements provide the specific words, phrases, and sentences that are appropriate in that context, whereas directive statements identify more socially appropriate alternatives to the child's current behavior. For children who cannot read, pictures and other visual supports can be used.

Computer-Driven Therapy

These approaches to language and literacy intervention utilize personal computers to present therapeutic stimuli and feedback. They are generally student paced and move sequentially through a predetermined hierarchy of difficulty levels. The clinician's primary role is to monitor and facilitate the student's learning progress rather than provide direct teaching. An example of a computer-driven program is Fast ForWord.

Instructional Strategies for Writing

In 2007 and 2014, meta-analyses of different approaches to writing instruction identified the most effective strategies (Gillespie & Graham, 2014; Graham & Perin, 2007). The reports' general findings are summarized as follows:

1. Provide exemplary models that are explicitly contrasted with weak examples.

2. Use goal setting by providing students with a goal for their writing (e.g., elements to include in a cause–effect essay), or have students choose their own goals for writing.

3. Use strategy-based approaches that are aimed at increasing the quantity and quality of students' background knowledge, knowledge of characteristics of good writing, and knowledge of different text structures.

4. Use repeated revision (e.g., "I will revise my composition three times").

5. Use the spelling editing strategy: Have students read their essays backward, because they are less likely to "fill in the gaps" and more likely to focus on the actual words.

6. Use flash drafting: Have students draft a small portion of text and revise, and then draft the next section followed by revision (this approximates the writing process of skilled writers).

7. Use graphic organizers to highlight the different elements of expository text (see Table 5–3 for details).

8. Provide extended time periods (minimum of 30 min) for student writing, with encouraging, constructive feedback provided throughout the writing activity.

9. Combine reading and writing instruction that simultaneously focuses on comprehension of text and expressing the knowledge in written form.

There are a wide variety of strategy-based approaches to writing instruction. Selected examples of effective strategies are described next.

Self-Regulated Strategy Development (SRSD; Graham & Harris, 1989; Graham et al., 2009)

This approach is used for teaching both narrative and expository texts. It focuses on both processes and products of writing and employs peer-mediated teaching as an instructional technique. It consists of six steps:

1. Develop background knowledge (brainstorm).

2. Discuss/explain the steps.

3. Model the steps (think-alouds).

4. Memorize and rehearse (through self-talk and self-evaluation to facilitate self-monitoring of own progress).

5. Support it (graduated scaffolding: students and instructor collaborate and students write with assistance).

6. Perform independently (scaffolds are faded).

SRSD employs a think (who will read this?), plan (what to say), and write (and say more) strategy to help students plan and generate a sufficient amount of text in their essays.

Genre Specific (Wong, 2000)

This five-step program focuses on teaching specific genres of expository writing, such as compare–contrast, cause–effect, and opinion essays. The program provides a rubric for each genre that includes anchors such as clarity, organization, and relevance of information. Prompt cards are used for different essay types and include introductory phrases (e.g., "This paper explains . . ."; "The cause of . . ."), explanatory phrases (e.g., "The reasons for . . ."; "As a result of . . ."), and concluding remarks (e.g., "To sum up the reasons for . . .").

Compensatory Strategies (MacArthur, 2000, 2009)

This category of approaches generally involves some form of assistive technology (AT) for struggling writers to supplement, but not replace, explicit instruction. In addition to word processing, examples of AT include voice-to-text speech-recognition software, word-prediction software, hypermedia (multimedia presentations of materials), and electronic concept map software.

Example Profiles

Following are four typical profiles of children and adolescents with language disorders. These examples have been designed to illustrate the selection of intervention targets as well as a variety of service models, therapy approaches, activities, and materials. Most are easily implemented in individual, small-group, or classroom settings.

PROFILE 1: SCHOOL AGE—5- TO 10-YEAR-OLD

Willy is an 8-year, 3-month-old male student with normal nonverbal intelligence who demonstrates a moderate broad-based language impairment. His receptive language is notable for a reduced vocabulary, difficulty understanding complex sentence constructions, and difficulty monitoring the adequacy of a speaker's message. Willy's expressive output is characterized by use of simple sentences, omission of grammatical markers, overuse of nonspecific referents, and difficulty relating information in a logical, sequential order. Willy's teacher reports that he continues to experience significant problems with basic grade-level reading materials and word problems used in mathematical instruction (i.e., addition and subtraction).

Selection of Therapy Targets. Due to the broad-based nature of Willy's language impairment, multiple components of the linguistic system will be targeted for treatment:

- In the area of semantics, categorization skills will be taught to strengthen Willy's vocabulary and concept knowledge.

- Coordinating conjunctions will be targeted to facilitate his use of syntactically more complex utterances.

- Present, past, and future verb-tense markers will be included in the therapy program, because Willy consistently omits these morphological forms in his spontaneous speech (although he evidences understanding of the time concepts).

- In the area of pragmatics, therapy will focus on increasing Willy's ability to recognize inadequate messages from other speakers and implement appropriate repair strategies.

- Instruction also will be provided in the metalinguistic area of phonemic awareness (i.e., sound blending) to facilitate the acquisition of early reading skills (i.e., decoding).

- Finally, specific vocabulary will be taught to address Willy's curriculum goals in mathematics.

Sample Activities

Semantic Categorization

1. Collect 15 picture cards depicting items in each of two semantic categories (e.g., clothes and birds) and 10 unrelated picture cards to serve as foils (e.g., book, car, horse). Provide the student with a simple definition of both target concepts. For example, a bird is an animal that has feathers, two legs, and two wings; clothes are things that you wear to cover your body, arms, and legs. Shuffle the cards and place them in a deck on the table. Instruct the student to sort the cards into two piles according to category (e.g., "Find all the birds"). As each card is sorted by the student, the clinician explains why the card belongs in either the birds or clothes category (e.g., "It's a bird because it has wings"). For unrelated foils, the clinician explains why the item should be excluded from the two primary categories (e.g., "It doesn't have feathers, and you can't wear it.").

   Note: The categorization activity can be made conceptually more sophisticated by modifying the task according to the following progression:

   a. Sort objects by function (e.g., things we eat, things we use as furniture, things we play with, things we use in a hospital).
   b. Sort objects according to semantic relationships (e.g., "What goes together?"—bat and ball, milk and cookies, hammer and nail).
   c. Sort objects by dimensions or attributes such as size, shape, color, or texture (e.g., big versus little, round versus square).
   d. Sort objects within a single category according to whether they are central or peripheral instances of the concept (e.g., robin versus emu, shirt versus scarf).

Coordinating Conjunctions

2. Develop a list of 20 sentences, each of which contains the coordinating conjunction *and*, *or*, or *but*. Print each sentence on a long strip of paper (approximately 2 × 11 in.) with the conjunction word represented by a blank line. Write each of the three conjunction words on small triangular pieces of paper. Following are example sentences:

   The waitress said, "You can order salad, rice, _____ a potato with your meal."

   Ed likes basketball, _____ he likes baseball more.

   Which one do you want: soda, hot chocolate, _____ lemonade?

   For breakfast, you can have an omelette _____ scrambled eggs.

   John _____ Billy went to the movies together.

   For lunch, Dion had a hamburger _____ french fries.

   Mary had to decide whether to go to New York by train _____ plane.

   The dentist drills _____ fills cavities in teeth.

   Rita wants to go to the movies, _____ she has no money.

   Bill wants to be a lifeguard, _____ he cannot swim that well.

   We ate all of the donuts _____ one.

   Place sentence strips face down in a pile in the center of the table. Position the conjunction triangles in a row in front of the student. Define the conjunctions by explaining when each is used:

   And is used to connect things together.

   Or is used to indicate a choice of one thing over others.

   But is used to mean "except," "with the exception of," or "on the other hand."

   Instruct the student to turn over one sentence strip. The clinician reads the sentence aloud and instructs the student to choose the triangle that best finishes the sentence and then to place it on the blank line. The clinician then reads the completed sentence aloud and instructs the student to imitate the model.

   Task difficulty can be increased by eliminating the conjunction triangles, thereby changing the multiple-choice format to a spontaneous generation task.

Verb-Tense Markers

3. Print 25 third-person singular active sentences on separate index cards. Develop three cue cards for present progressive, past, and future verb tenses in the following manner:

Yesterday	*Right Now*	*Tomorrow*
-ed	is _____ing	will

   Place the cue cards in a row on the table approximately 3 in. apart in the order illustrated. Place the deck of sentence cards on the table. Instruct the student to read each of the cue words aloud or to repeat each word following the clinician's model. Review the three verb tense forms with the student. Explain as follows:

a. When something has already occurred and is no longer happening, we attach -*ed* to the end of the action word. For example, you would say, "Yesterday, the boy order*ed* the pizza."

b. When something is happening right now, we say "is" before the action word and attach *ing* to the end of the action word. For example, you would say, "The boy *is* order*ing* the pizza."

c. When something has not yet happened but will happen in the future, we say the word "will" before the action word. For example, you would say, "Tomorrow, the boy *will* order the pizza."

Instruct the student to select the top card from the sentence deck and to inflect the sentence correctly as the clinician points to each of the cue cards. Example sentences include the following:

The girl talks on the phone.

Jose plays his guitar.

Sam walks to school.

The dog chases the cat.

Daddy paints the house.

The teacher points to the world map.

Jamie washes her hair.

Maria wishes for a puppy.

Joey kicks the football.

Mom picks apples from the trees.

Lee cheers for his team.

Monique laughs at the funny clown.

Tim practices his spelling words.

Grandma cooks dinner for the family.

The dog barks at the mailman.

As the student begins to master the past and future tense markers, the cue cards can be modified to include other lexical items that denote these concepts (e.g., *last week, when I grow up, next summer, 2 days ago*).

Recognition of Inadequate Messages

4. Prepare a list of 20 directions for completing a variety of simple tasks, and gather the necessary props. Some directions should contain ambiguous, incomplete, unintelligible, or absurd information, whereas others are clearly worded. Examples may include the following:

Direction	*Context*
Give me the red block.	There are no red blocks on the table.
Give me the pencil with the eraser.	All three pencils on the table have erasers.
Give me the #$%$#% (unintelligible).	There are three different objects on the table.
Place the pencil next to the book.	There are a book and a pencil on the table.

Put my money in the brown wallet.	There are three wallets on the table, none of which are brown.
Give me the ingredients for making pizza: dough, sauce, cheese, picture frame.	All these objects are on the table.
Cut a big hole in the white piece of paper.	There are red and white pieces of paper on the table, along with scissors and tape.
Give me three (*mumble rest of message).*	There are three paper clips, six pencils, and five pennies on the table.

Explain that the student will be asked to carry out directions using props and that some of the messages will be inadequate and require more information. This activity focuses on two strategies for obtaining this additional information: (a) asking for repetition of the direction (e.g., "Huh?" or "What did you say?") and (b) requesting clarification of the message (e.g., "Which book?" or "What color?"). Instruct the student to listen to the clinician's messages and think carefully about what is being said. After each direction is presented, instruct the student to identify whether the message was "OK" or inadequate. If the direction is identified as unclear, instruct the student to request a repair using one of the two target strategies. The clinician then revises the original message according to the type of repair requested, and the student performs the task. If the student does not recognize the need for repair, prompt with one or more of the following: "Is that clear?"; "Did I say that right?"; or "Do you get it?"

Phonemic Awareness

5. Print a list of 25 monosyllabic words with initial continuant sounds on index cards and segment each word into phonemes (see following examples). Draw a game board of a bridge that consists of 20 blank spaces, and draw a pot of gold at the end of the bridge. Place a small, wrapped "prize" on the pot of gold. Shuffle the cards and place them face down in a pile in the center of the board. Obtain a game piece that can be moved from space to space on the board and place it at the footpath to the bridge. Explain to the student that, in this game, there is a troll who lives under the bridge and who talks in a very funny way; he says all his words one sound at a time (Lundberg et al., 1980). Tell the student that he has to figure out the words and say them to move his game piece to the end of the bridge and find the hidden prize. Instruct the student to pick up the top card and give it to the clinician. The clinician plays the role of the troll and produces the segmented word, phoneme by phoneme. (Always produce the actual sound rather than the alphabet letter name.) The student blends the sounds together and "guesses" the troll's message. Following a correct guess, the clinician repeats both the segmented word and the whole word. The student is then permitted to move the game piece one space on the board. Following are some sample words:

f—or—k

s—u—n

z—oo—m

v—o—te

m—a—p

s—ou—p

v—e—s—t

n—o—se

f—u—ll

m—a—tch

Curriculum-Content Vocabulary: Math

6. Make two lists of the following words/phrases on separate poster boards and attach to the wall.

Addition Words	Subtraction Words
in all	how many more
more	how many are left
altogether	difference
sum	less
total	fewer

Write 10 to 20 simple word problems, half of which require addition and half subtraction, on 3 × 5 in. index cards. (Examples of these follow these instructions.) Obtain two containers into which the cards can be sorted. Label one container with a large plus (+) sign; label the other container with a large minus (–) sign. Provide a highlighter and game board. Explain to the student that the words on the two wall charts are clues for solving math word problems. Review each clue word on the addition chart and remind the student that these are "adding" words; then review each clue word on the subtraction chart and remind the student that these are "take away" words. Shuffle the index cards and place them face down in a pile on the table. Explain that the top card should be turned over and read aloud. Instruct the student to highlight any clue words that are recognized from the wall charts and state whether the problem requires addition or subtraction. Then have the student place the index card in the correct container. Repeat this procedure for all cards in the deck.

Example Addition Problems

a. Juan has three jelly beans and Eddie gives him three more. How many does Juan have altogether?

b. Ilana has five pencils on the desk, and Eli puts four more on the desk. What is the total number of pencils on the desk?

c. There were seven birds sitting on a fence. Five more birds joined them. How many birds are there in all?

d. Mary put six blue beads on a string. Kayla put five red beads on the string. What is the total number of beads on the string?

e. Ali drove eight blocks to Steve's house, and then both boys drove nine blocks to the store. Find the sum of the blocks they drove.

Example Subtraction Problems

a. Kate has 10 stickers and Shawna takes 4. How many are left?

b. John has five green crayons, and Daron has nine yellow crayons. How many more yellow crayons are there?

c. Marsha put 12 cards in a pile, and Kim put 7 in another pile. What is the difference between the two piles?

d. Kathy has nine books, and Stacy has six fewer books. How many books does Stacy have?

e. Jean drank 14 cups of water. Nan drank 8 cups of water. How much less water did Nan drink?

Note: This activity can be repeated using a game board with spaces color coded for plus and minus. The student rolls the dice and moves a game piece the appropriate number of spaces. If the piece lands on an "addition" space, instruct the student to remove a card from the (+) container and solve the problem. Follow the same procedure for subtraction.

PROFILE 2: SCHOOL AGE—5- TO 10-YEAR-OLD

Vivian is a 9-year, 1-month-old female student with normal nonverbal intelligence who has been diagnosed with a learning disability. She demonstrates a significant reading deficit characterized by the inability to decode written words. Weaknesses in the area of receptive language include comprehension of connected oral text, such as stories. Expressively, Vivian experiences notable difficulty with assignments that require formulating definitions for vocabulary known to be within her receptive repertoire. According to the classroom teacher, these difficulties are exacerbated by Vivian's inability to sustain focused attention. As a consequence, her academic performance across the entire fourth-grade curriculum is adversely affected.

Selection of Therapy Targets. Vivian's profile of oral language and literacy deficits warrants intervention in a variety of areas necessary to effectively learn from teacher discourse and textbook information:

- In the area of semantics, the structure and elements of formal definitions will be targeted to strengthen Vivian's network of higher order semantic knowledge.

- The framework of narrative structure will be taught to promote recall, comprehension, and production of oral and written text-level material often incorporated into fourth grade curricula.

- Finally, intervention will target the phonemic awareness skill of sound segmentation in conjunction with letter-sound correspondence training (alphabetic principle) to improve Vivian's reading decoding ability.

Sample Activities

Definitions

1. Create a Jeopardy! game, including stimulus cards, a buzzer, and play money. Use curriculum materials (e.g., textbooks, homework assignments, educational software) to develop a list of 10 to 15 familiar vocabulary words in three or four different semantic categories (see the following sample list with definitions).

Science

a. Microscope: A *microscope* is an *instrument* that makes *small objects look bigger.*

b. Solar system: A *solar system* is a *group of planets* that *revolve around a sun.*

c. Volcano: A *volcano* is a *mountain* that *explodes with lava and ash.*

Math

a. Number: A *number* is a *symbol* that *shows how many.*

b. Fraction: A *fraction* is a *number* that *compares small pieces or parts to the whole.*

c. Calculator: A *calculator* is a *machine* that *does arithmetic.*

English/Language Arts

a. Paragraph: A *paragraph* is *two or more sentences* about *a single idea.*

b. Topic sentence: A *topic sentence* is a *statement* that *gives the main idea of a paragraph.*

c. Comma: A *comma* is a *mark* that *shows a small break between parts of a sentence.*

Miscellaneous

a. Bicycle: A *bicycle* is a *vehicle* that has *two wheels.*

b. Dog: A *dog* is an *animal* that *barks.*

c. House: A *house* is a *building* that *people live in.*

For each category, print the words on the face of index cards and write increasing dollar values on the back (e.g., $100, $200, $300). Attach the cards to a wall in category columns with the dollar amounts facing out. Construct a wall chart that shows the three key elements of a formal definition, which are the word, the superordinate category name, and a relevant function/attribute of the referent, in a style that the student can understand.

Explain to the student that this activity is a Jeopardy! game in which the student will select a category and dollar level. The clinician will read the vocabulary item, and the student must sound the buzzer and respond using the formal definition structure. Correct responses receive play money in the amount listed on the back of the card; incorrect responses result in the subtraction of specified dollar amounts from the total.

Teach the student that a definition explains the meaning of a word by (a) stating the word, (b) identifying the larger category it belongs to, and (c) describing how it looks or what it does. Encourage the student to use the wall chart as a visual cue to remember all three components; for example,

Student: I'll take "living things" for $200, please.

Clinician: Spider.

Student: A *spider* is a *bug* that has *eight legs.*

Clinician: Great definition. You win $200. What category do you want next?

Note: The activity works particularly well in a small group setting.

Narrative Discourse (Oral and Written)

2. Write or identify a short story that contains at least one episode. The story should clearly illustrate the following components:

Setting: Information regarding characters and physical, social, and/or temporal environment

Problem: Occurrence that influences the character(s) to act; precipitating event

Actions: The character's overt attempt to solve the problem

Resolution: The character's success or failure in solving the problem and resultant thoughts or feelings

See the following sample story:

The Cookie Jar Incident

Once there was a stubborn young lady named Leigh-Anne who lived in New York City. Late one afternoon, she was really hungry and wanted a chocolate chip cookie. She knew that she wasn't allowed to eat sweets before dinner, but that didn't stop Leigh-Anne. She sneaked into the kitchen, stood on her tiptoes, and reached for the cookie jar. As she grabbed it, the jar fell on the floor and broke into a thousand pieces. As she heard her mother's footsteps, Leigh-Anne felt guilty about doing something she wasn't supposed to do.

Setting

Character: Leigh-Anne

Environment: New York City, late afternoon

Problem

hungry

no cookies before dinner

Actions

sneaked

stood

reached

grabbed

Resolution

jar broke

felt guilty

Obtain a large poster board and small self-stick notes. Draw a story map like the one in Figure 5–1. Explain that this map will help the student identify the main parts of a story. Using the definitions provided previously, teach the student each of the four story parts and where they belong on the map. Instruct the student to listen as the clinician reads the story aloud. Upon completion, ask the student to identify the components of each story part on the map, beginning with the setting and ending with the resolution. The clinician writes each of the student's responses on a self-stick note and has the student place it on the map in the correct box. Then jointly retell the story using the map as a visual guide. Finally, have the student write the story in his or her own words using the story map components in a "beginning–middle–end" format.

Title: _____

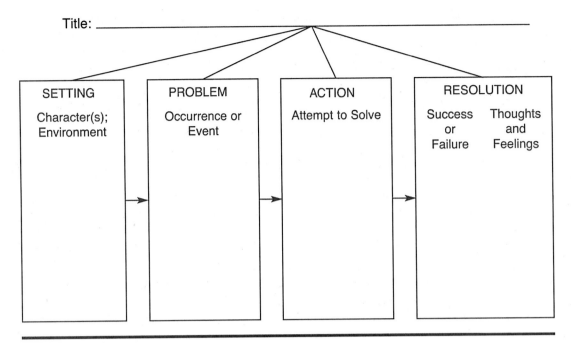

Figure 5-1
Story map. Adapted from *Stand Back," Said the Elephant, "I'm Going To Sneeze!*, by P. Thomas, 1971. Lothrop, Lee and Shepard.

Note: The difficulty level of this activity can be adjusted in a variety of ways. To branch down to an easier level, the response mode can be a multiple-choice format in which the student's task is to select the appropriate piece of story information from an array of completed self-stick notes. To branch upward, the clinician can increase the number of episodes in a given story.

Phonemic Awareness and Alphabetic Principle

3. Make a list of 30 two- and three-phoneme words that are picturable and within the student's expressive vocabulary repertoire. To incorporate exposure to the alphabetic principle, choose words with consonant-vowel (CV), VC, or CVC patterns. Avoid words that involve digraphs (e.g., h*ea*t, s*oa*p, th*ie*f) and silent vowels (e.g., gat*e*, bon*e*, sam*e*). Following is an illustrative word list:

top	cab	up	van	mop	no
cup	bus	in	fog	nut	ma
sad	sit	hi	dad	nap	me
mat	tag	go	dot	pot	us
jam	red	on	bag	pig	he

Attach the picture for each word to a "playing card." Gather six small blocks and individual alphabet letters (can be written, plastic, or cut from foam).

Tell the student that this game involves breaking words down into smaller parts. Explain that the point of the game is to figure out which words have more sounds. The cards are dealt into two equal decks. The clinician and student simultaneously turn over the top card from each deck (clinician = Deck 1; student = Deck 2). The clinician verbally segments the word from Deck 1 and lines up one block for each sound. Instruct the student to do the same for the card from Deck 2. Tell the student to identify which of the two words has more sounds. The clinician then adds the appropriate alphabet letters on top of the blocks and sounds out that word again. If the student correctly chose the word with the most sounds, the student wins both cards and sets them aside. If the choice was incorrect, the clinician wins both cards. Repeat this sequence until all cards from both decks have been played. (If the two words have the same number of sounds, each player wins one card.) The player with the most cards at the end of the game is the winner.

Note: The difficulty level of the activity can be increased or decreased according to the hierarchy in Table I-2 in the Introduction to Chapters 4 and 5.

PROFILE 3: ADOLESCENT—10- TO 18-YEAR-OLD

Pedro is a 12-year, 6-month-old male who presents with a moderate language-learning disability. He demonstrates particular difficulty with higher order language skills. Specifically, Pedro performs poorly on confrontational naming tasks and tasks that require the comprehension of figurative language forms. His oral and written narratives and expository essays omit essential information and lack a logical sequence. According to direct observation and teacher report, Pedro exhibits difficulty initiating and maintaining conversational exchanges, as evidenced by his tendency to talk about inappropriate topics and interrupt ongoing conversations. Although some minor grammatical errors were observed during timed tasks, comprehension and production of syntax and morphology were noted to be relative strengths.

Selection of Therapy Targets. Based on Pedro's overall profile, the areas to be targeted involve semantics, narrative discourse, expository writing, and conversational discourse.

- With respect to semantics, idioms were selected because they are among the earliest developing forms of figurative language.

- In addition, word finding was chosen to accommodate the increasing demand at the middle school level for accurate retrieval of specific vocabulary words in different academic subject areas.

- Narrative discourse was targeted to improve Pedro's knowledge of the organization of extended text, because text is the primary vehicle for transmitting academic knowledge.

- Expository writing instruction will focus on the processes of planning and composing for "compare-and-contrast" essays.

- The area of conversational initiation was selected to address the negative effects/perceptions that Pedro's verbal interaction style has on peers and adults in his environment.

Sample Activities

Figurative Language: Idioms

1. Select five idioms and write three different short story contexts for each. For each story, include three written alternative response choices (see the following examples). Duplicate

these materials for the student. Define an idiom for the student by explaining that idioms are expressions in which a new meaning is given to a group of words that already has a meaning. For example, the expression "over the hill" can be interpreted literally *or* as an idiom meaning that someone is old. Explain that the clinician will be reading stories containing idioms and that the student will be asked to select the most appropriate meaning from three choices. Recite the first short story aloud as the student reads along silently. Depending on the student's skill level, instruct him or her to listen to or read the choices and select the response that best fits the context of the story. After the three stories for a particular idiom have been successfully completed, ask the student to brainstorm at least one personal experience to which the specific idiom could have been applied. Examples include the following:

Kick up our heels

1) John made the football team. He was so happy and excited. He wanted to kick up his heels.

 Does this mean?   He wanted to celebrate.

 He kicked his feet in the air.

 He was upset.

2) Hannah sat in her classroom and waited for the announcement. The principal finally came on the public-address system and said: "Students, the winner of the school spelling contest is Hannah Smith. Congratulations!" Hannah felt like kicking up her heels.

 Does this mean?   She took off her shoe.

 She was thrilled.

 She was very disappointed.

3) Larry wanted to get an A in math. He was a good math student but always got Bs. The final exam was last week, and he studied harder than ever. When the mail came, Larry ran to see his report card. He opened it up, saw an A next to math, and felt like kicking up his heels.

 Does this mean?   He did not do well in math.

 He lifted his legs in the air.

 He wanted to cheer.

Shake a leg

1) Sue forgot to set her alarm for the swim meet. Her mom woke her up and said, "We have only 10 minutes to get to the pool, so shake a leg."

 Does this mean?   Sue has to hurry.

 Sue's leg is hurting.

 Sue's mom shook her leg.

2) Bobby wanted to win the bicycle race. He had trained hard for it all summer. But now he was in fourth place with just 1 mile to go. He told himself that he'd better shake a leg if he wanted to win.

Does this mean? Bobby has to slow down.

Bobby has to ride faster.

Bobby does not want to win.

3) Mom and Dad are going out to dinner for their anniversary. It's time to go, but Dad is still shaving. Mom says, "Honey, shake a leg; our reservation is in 20 minutes."

Does this mean? They will probably be early.

Dad should move his leg while shaving.

Dad should hurry up.

A fish out of water

1) Mariah was very excited about the school dance. She wanted to look really cool. She decided to wear her new faded blue jeans and her favorite flannel shirt. When she walked into the gym, all of the girls were wearing party dresses. Mariah felt like a fish out of water.

Does this mean?   Mariah doesn't like to swim.

Mariah was not wet.

Mariah felt different from everyone else.

2) Joan was going to sleep-away camp for the first time. She kissed her parents good-bye after checking in. When she walked into her cabin, all the other girls seemed to know each other. They laughed and talked like old friends. Joan felt like a fish out of water.

Does this mean?   Joan felt like she didn't fit in the group.

Joan wanted to go swimming.

Joan likes to go fishing at the lake.

3) Jason just moved to the city and was starting his senior year in high school. Jason rode his bike on the first day of school. As he entered the parking lot, he noticed that all the seniors were driving cars. Jason felt like a fish out of water.

Does this mean?   He felt like he couldn't breathe.

He felt like he didn't belong.

He felt very happy.

All thumbs

1) Jack was helping his dad build a birdhouse in the maple tree. Jack hammered the nail into the wood but kept missing it. His dad said, "Son, you're all thumbs today."

Does this mean?   Jack was clumsy.

All of Jack's fingers look like thumbs.

Jack put his thumb on the nail.

2) Kate and Nika decided to bake some chocolate chip cookies. Nika took the eggs out of the refrigerator and dropped one on the floor. Then she spilled the flour all over the table and knocked over the milk. She said to Kate, "I guess I'm all thumbs."

Does this mean?   Nika was finished with the cookies.

Nika was klutzy.

Nika's thumbs were all sticky.

3) The period bell rang and David raced to his locker to get his English book before the next class. He held his books in one hand and turned the combination, but the lock wouldn't open. He tried again and dropped all his books onto the floor. He said to himself, "I'm all thumbs."

Does this mean?   David wished that all his fingers were thumbs.

David's locker opened easily.

David was clumsy.

Word Retrieval

2. Develop a list of 20 names of objects or people. Write a synonym, category name, or other semantic cue for each word on an index card. In addition, write the initial sound (not letter) of each word on another set of index cards. Examples include the following:

Word	Semantic Cue	Phonological Cue
cook	chef	/k/
gloves	mittens	/gl/
jacket	coat	/dʒ/
comb	brush	/k/
tissues	Kleenex	/t/
van	vehicle	/v/
pencil	writing utensil	/p/
shoes	sneakers	/ʃ/
lamp	light	/l/
soda	coke	/s/
hat	cap	/h/
purse	handbag	/p/
painting	picture	/p/
carpet	rug	/k/
car	automobile	/k/
notebook	binder	/n/
jeans	clothing	/dʒ/
backpack	knapsack	/b/
sailboat	kind of boat	/s/
dollar	money	/d/

Explain that the student will be asked to guess a specific word based on two clues provided by the clinician. Further explain that the two clues represent different strategies that the student can use when trying to retrieve specific vocabulary words. Instruct the student to use the first clue to create a visual image of the object and the second clue to identify what the mystery word sounds like. For example, the clinician says, "I'm thinking of a word. It's like a 'chef' and starts with /k/." Encourage the student to refrain from responding quickly, but rather pause reflectively and think about the cues. After each item, instruct the student to produce the target word in a sentence that describes its function.

Narrative Discourse

3. Write the *main elements of a story* on separate index cards along with short definitions of each part (Stein & Glenn, 1979); for example,

Setting:	The main characters in the story (who the story is about) and where the story takes place
Problem:	The main event or problem that the main character faces
Response:	The way that the main character feels about the problem
Attempt:	What the main character actually does to try to solve the problem or achieve the goal
Outcome:	What happens at the end of the story; whether or not the character achieves the goal
Reaction:	How the main character feels about the outcome (success or failure at attaining the goal)

In addition, write one or more *question* cues for each of the main story parts on separate index cards; for example,

Setting:	Who is the story about? Where does the story take place?
Problem:	What happened to the main character? What caused the main character to act?
Response:	How does the main character feel about the problem?
Attempt:	What does the main character do to solve the problem?
Outcome:	What happens at the end of the story? Does the main character achieve the goal?
Reaction:	How does the main character feel at the end of the story?

First, review the story element definition cards with the student. Then, explain that the clinician will tell a short story aloud as the student follows the written text.

Example Story

Once upon a time, there was a 12-year-old boy named Jacob who lived in a town called Wallston. He lived about 1 mile from school and rode his bike there every day. Last week for his birthday, his parents gave him a new bike, the one he'd been asking for since June. On Wednesday morning, Jacob grabbed his backpack and headed for school. As he approached the front gate, he immediately noticed that his new bike was gone. Jacob thought to himself, "Oh no! I forgot to chain the bike last night. Somebody probably stole it. Mom will ground me for a month. I promised to take care of it." Jacob thought all day about what to do. After school, he went to the police station and spoke to one of the officers. The police officer suggested that Jacob put up signs in lots of places such as at the police station, at the post office, and in store windows. The signs should include Jacob's name, telephone number, and a description of the bike. So Jacob made the signs, put them up all over town, and walked home to wait by the telephone. At about 5:30 p.m., it rang and Jacob jumped up to answer it.

A woman named Mrs. Ramirez said, "I just saw a bike at the grocery story that matches the description on the signs." Jacob thanked the lady and ran to the market as fast as he could. Sure enough, it was his bike. His initials were on the bottom of the seat just as he had scratched them on. Jacob was so happy and relieved. As he rode home, he promised himself that he would never leave his bike unlocked again.

After the story is completed, instruct the student to answer the cue card questions either verbally or in writing. Review and discuss each answer with the student to ensure a correct response.

Then, instruct the student to use the cueing questions to construct a story of his or her own. During the initial stages of therapy, the clinician may want to provide the student with a set of choices for each part of the story to facilitate story construction. For example, the clinician might say: "Your story needs a setting. Do you want it to be about a boy named Joe or a teacher named Mr. Petry?"

Task difficulty can be increased by requiring the student to generate a spontaneous story and use the question cues as a self-monitoring strategy to check the quality of the finished product. The task also can be made more sophisticated by decreasing the number and specificity of question cues. A final set of questions might include the following:

a. Are all of the story parts included?

b. Does my story have a beginning, middle, and end?

c. Are the story parts in the correct order?

Note: This activity can be adapted to facilitate the student's production of written narratives. Mnemonic devices are effective tools for helping clients remember and sequence ideas in a logical manner (e.g., SPACE: *s*etting, *p*roblem, *a*ction, *c*onsequent *e*vent; Harris & Graham, 1996). Other acronyms can be used to revise and/or proofread written text (e.g., COPS: *c*apitalization, *o*verall appearance, *p*unctuation, *s*pelling; Schumaker et al., 1982).

Expository Writing: Descriptive Essay

4. With eyes closed, the student should brainstorm descriptive details about a favorite place. Encourage the student to identify what the place looks like and how it sounds, smells, and feels. Create a written list of the comments the student produces. Introduce the parts of a descriptive essay and explain each:

Topic/thesis statement: What the essay is about and why this topic was chosen

Content paragraphs: The particular qualities/characteristics that the student wants to focus on

Transitions: Words and phrases that provide logical connections between ideas

Conclusion: Brief summary of essay content

Conversational Initiation

5. Tell the student that today's session will focus on how to start a conversation. Explain that there are four sequential steps in initiating a conversation: (a) choosing the setting, (b) selecting the topic, (c) getting the listener's attention, and (d) introducing the topic. Design at least six scenarios, most of which are conversationally inappropriate, for each of the four steps. Explain that the clinician will read the scenarios for each step aloud. Instruct the student to show a thumbs-up or thumbs-down gesture to identify the appropriateness of each event. Example scenarios include the following:

Choosing the Setting

Your friend is on a cell phone. (thumbs down)

Your friend is sitting next to you on the bus. (thumbs up)

Two classmates are sitting in the corner and whispering to each other. (thumbs down)

You are watching a movie in a theater. (thumbs down)

A new classmate is sitting by himself in the cafeteria. (thumbs up)

You are in science class during a lecture. (thumbs down)

Selecting the Topic

Do you have any brothers or sisters? (thumbs up)

Why is your hair so short? (thumbs down)

What kind of music do you like? (thumbs up)

I heard that your parents are getting a divorce. (thumbs down)

Does your father make lots of money? (thumbs down)

You're not invited to my graduation party. (thumbs down)

Getting the Listener's Attention

Saying: "Hey, how's it going?" to the church pastor. (thumbs down)

Saying: "Good morning, Mr. Web" to the school principal. (thumbs up)

Saying: "Know what?" to a group of teachers in the hallway. (thumbs down)

Saying: "Get over here" to an upperclassman. (thumbs down)

Saying: "Excuse me" to an adult who is reading a book. (thumbs up)

Saying: "Here I am" to a group of classmates talking in the cafeteria. (thumbs down)

Introducing the Topic

Starting a conversation with, "Did you see where he went?" (thumbs down)

Starting a conversation with, "I wanted to talk to you about, you know, the assignment we . . . Remember what Ms. Jones said yesterday . . . You know what I'm talking about?" (thumbs down)

Starting a conversation with, "Everyone says that you didn't make the school play." (thumbs down)

Starting a conversation with, "I lost my doohickey, the thing I need to do the math homework problems." (thumbs down)

Starting a conversation with, "Can I talk to you about the party on Saturday night?" (thumbs up)

Starting a conversation with, "Wanna shoot hoops after school with me?" (thumbs up)

PROFILE 4: ADOLESCENT—10- TO 18-YEAR-OLD

Paul is a 17-year-old high school junior with a long-standing history of language deficits and persistent academic difficulties in the absence of overall intellectual impairment. He presents as an outgoing and friendly individual who demonstrates basic conversational competence in the areas of semantics, syntax, and morphology. Significant deficits are noted in his knowledge of higher level abstract language forms, especially multiple meaning words, metaphoric uses of language, and inferential comprehension. Recent test results indicate that Paul is reading and writing at approximately the eighth-grade level. According to classroom observation and teacher report, Paul is "disorganized" and demonstrates ineffective study habits and test-taking strategies, poor time management, and poor follow-through on class assignments. These traits are indicative of limited metacognitive functioning (i.e., the awareness of one's own problem-solving strengths and weaknesses, how to apply them, and when to use them effectively). Recently, Paul met with his guidance counselor to discuss his academic status and explore his options following graduation. He expressed a clear preference for career training over college education.

Selection of Therapy Targets. The areas to be targeted are metalinguistics, metacognition, social communication skills, inferencing, writing processes and products, and language-mediated study skills:

- In the area of metalinguistics, metaphors were selected because this figurative language form occurs frequently in the academic environment.

- Metacognitive training will focus on goal setting, self-monitoring, self-evaluation, goal outcomes, and reflection.

- Both Paul's age and current academic status indicate that he would benefit from therapy activities that focus on social-communication skills in a vocational setting.

- Inferencing was chosen as a means of improving Paul's ability to derive intended meaning from oral and written material.

- Finally, the intervention program will target language-mediated study skills to provide Paul with the requisite tools for improving his academic performance.

Sample Activities

Figurative Language: Metaphors

1. A metaphor is a nonliteral use of language in which one element (**topic**) is compared to another element (**vehicle**) on the basis of one or more common features (**ground**). Develop

a list of metaphors, and write each on an index card. Each should contain an explicitly stated topic, vehicle, and ground. Each card also should contain two alternative meanings for each metaphor. Following are examples, with the incorrect choice indicated by an asterisk (Nippold et al., 1984):

The sun was a basketball sitting in the sky.

This means that the sun

a. was orange and round.

b. was very hot.*

The giraffe was a flagpole living at the zoo.

This means the giraffe

a. was tall.

b. was on top of the flagpole.*

The skater was a top spinning on the ice.

This means the skater

a. was twirling very fast.

b. had a top next to her on the ice.*

David's nose was a grapefruit sitting on his face.

This means that David's nose

a. was big.

b. was bleeding.*

The girl's smile was a ray of sunshine on a cloudy day.

This means that the girl's smile

a. was bright.

b. was big.*

The man was a pumpkin walking down the street.

This means that the man

a. was fat.

b. was orange.*

Matt's arms were broom handles hanging at his sides.

This means that Matt's arms

a. were long and skinny.

b. were hairy.*

John's teeth were kernels of corn growing in his mouth.

This means that John's teeth

a. were yellow.

b. were chipped.*

The soldiers were cornrows going down the road.

This means that the soldiers

    a. were in straight lines.

    b. were tall.*

The runner was a jet plane flying in the sky.

    This means that the runner

    a. was fast.

    b. was getting on an airplane.*

Explain that a metaphor is a comparison between two things that are alike in some way. For example, in "The girl's hair is spaghetti," the two things that are being compared are "hair" and "spaghetti." Both are thin and long. So, this metaphor means that the girl's hair is thin and long. Explain that the student will read each metaphor aloud and, along with the clinician, identify the two things that are being compared. The student will then be presented with two choices and asked to pick the "best" meaning.

Note: Similes are easier to understand than metaphors because they have the syntactic markers *like* or *as* to signal the comparison. These markers can be used as a transition to metaphors (e.g., "The sun was [like] a basketball sitting in the sky").

Metacognition: Executive Functioning

2. Explain that this activity is designed to help the student approach problems or tasks in a systematic, organized manner. Jointly review the student's current course requirements and select a relevant assignment. For example, a civics class assignment might be a group project to develop a campaign to change some aspect of school board policy or local government ordinance. This student's group chose to petition the county council to install a stop sign at a busy intersection. As a group member, the student's responsibility is to write a persuasive letter to the appropriate government officials.

Goals and Target Behaviors	Self-Questions
a. Goal-Setting/Planning Think before acting/speaking/writing.	What do you want to do? What message do you want to send? How do you want this to come out?
b. Self-Monitoring Think about how the task is coming along. Are you devoting enough time/effort/attention?	How does your work look? Are there any problems? Do you need new or different strategies? How is your progress?
c. Self-Evaluation Rate the overall quality of the finished product and effectiveness of your performance.	Did you solve the problem(s)? Were the strategies useful? Was your work correct? Was it efficient?
d. Goal Outcome Evaluate the result of your work.	Did you achieve the goal? Was the goal realistic? Should it have been modified in some way?

e. Reflection	
Think about what the experience taught you.	Would you do things differently next time? What did you learn about your ability to solve problems?

Gather two 5 × 7 in. index cards in each of five colors for a total of 10 cards. Write goals and target behaviors from the list on one card of each color. Follow color coding and write corresponding self-questions on the remaining cards.

Introduce and discuss each of the goals and target behaviors in the order in which they were listed. Provide several examples for each component. Then have the student generate additional examples. Once the student demonstrates reliable recall of the five goals and target behaviors, begin the task by implementing the first goal (planning). Introduce the self-questions as instructional cues to facilitate achievement of the target behavior. When goal-setting is finalized, proceed to each subsequent component in the hierarchy using the self-questions to support the student's performance at each phase.

Note: The ultimate aim of this metacognitive training procedure is for the student to internalize the self-questions and use them as strategies for problem-solving across tasks.

Social Communication

3. Teach social communication skills in the context of vocational settings by using the training sequence of explanation, demonstration, and role-playing. As each activity is mastered in the therapy session, the clinician can ask school personnel to participate in simulated work environments to provide the student with practice and promote generalization of the newly learned skills. For example, the school media specialist, principal, or cafeteria staff could play the role of "employers" or "potential employers" to provide the student with opportunities to practice the skill in quasiwork environments (i.e., library, office, restaurant). Debriefing sessions can be held on a regular basis to review performance and improve the student's self-monitoring skills. Following are suggested tasks/contexts:

   Telephoning to request a job interview

   Undergoing a job interview

   Accepting a suggestion from an employer

   Accepting criticism from an employer

   Providing constructive criticism to a coworker

   Explaining a problem to a supervisor

   Complimenting a coworker

   Accepting a compliment from a coworker

Inferencing

4. Develop 20 situations that have clear logical inferences, and write each on the top portion of an index card. Explain that an inference is a conclusion reached by using information that you know to be true to make a "good guess" about what is also likely to be true. For example, Mr. Jones made several jokes in class today, so I *inferred* that he was in a good

mood. Instruct the student to read each situation and write one logical inference. After each response, discuss with the student the reason that it was a correct/incorrect inference. Examples include the following:

The principal usually makes the announcements, but today the vice principal gave them.

Tyler blushed when he saw Emily.

Tony picked up his baseball bat and walked out to the plate.

Joe hammered the nail and yelled, "Ouch!"

Ken walked into his apartment and his laptop and iPad were gone.

Chad walked by his best friend Steve without saying "Hello."

Hank rented a tuxedo for Saturday night.

Ashley is making a salad for dinner. Her eyes are stinging and tears are rolling down her cheeks.

Noah made sure to put on gloves and a hat.

Wanda put the book down after reading only half of it.

The boss walks by and gives you a pat on the back.

Alex looked at the clock and ran out of the room.

The sand burned Madison's feet.

Danny took one bite of the apple and threw it away.

Mrs. Jensen frowned as she handed Tim his math exam.

Jack smiled as he left his basketball game.

Allison took the cookies out of the oven and threw them in the trash.

Sam walked into the backyard to get some tomatoes and peas.

Mia could hear the waves from her bedroom window.

Fred searched for some change and called a tow truck driver.

Compare–Contrast Essay Structure

5. Brainstorm writing topics of great interest to the student. (The clinician can provide some examples, such as baseball and football or different types of transportation, such as a skateboard and roller blades.)

- Explain to the student that the compare–contrast essay identifies how things are alike and different. Briefly define each term (i.e., *comparison* refers to how two things are alike, whereas *contrast* refers to how they are different).

- Review/teach examples of vocabulary that signal the compare–contrast structures. Base selection of words on curricula content materials and content area learning objectives.

  Vocabulary for comparing: *similar, like, still, likewise, in the same ways, in comparison, at the same time, in the same manner.*

  Vocabulary for contrasting: *however, on the other hand, but, yet, nevertheless, conversely, rather, on the contrary, nonetheless, in contrast.*

- Make a list of salient characteristics for each of the subjects (e.g., football and baseball). Use a highlighter to indicate characteristics that are found under each subject header.

- Use the list as an aid to compose a compare-and-contrast essay in the following suggested format:

    Paragraph 1: Introduction: Begin with a sentence that will catch the reader's interest. This might be a question or a reason people find the topic interesting/important. Then, name the two subjects and say they are very similar, very different, or have many important (or interesting) similarities and differences.

    Paragraph 2: The next paragraph(s) describes features of the *first* subject. Do not mention the second subject.

    Paragraph 3: Begin this section with a transition word showing you are comparing the second subject to the first. For each comparison, use a cue word such as *like, similar to, also, unlike, on the other hand.* Be sure to include examples that clearly demonstrate that the similarities and/or differences exist. (Note: Some students may benefit from writing a paragraph about the characteristics of the second subject prior to this paragraph.)

    Final paragraph: Write a conclusion by giving a brief, general summary of the most important similarities and differences. End with a personal statement, a prediction, or another snappy clincher.

Study Skills

6. The development of language-mediated study skills is particularly critical for successful academic performance at the middle and high school levels. A compendium of important skill areas is included in Table 5–6. Training can be accomplished most effectively by using the student's actual curricular materials (e.g., lecture notes, textbook readings, homework assignments, and term projects). One effective school-based service delivery model for study skill training is the provision of a course that meets regularly and is taken for academic credit.

Helpful Hints

1. Observe/video students in a variety of daily school contexts and activities (classroom, recess, breakfast/lunch time) to gain a richer and representative sample of their verbal and non-verbal behaviors.

2. Clinicians may increase the motivation of older students by involving them in the selection of therapy targets using a forced choice format with two or three targets.

3. Whenever possible, conduct phonological awareness activities in a group setting to encourage interaction and avoid a sense of drill/rote memorization. In addition, a group setting is beneficial because it encourages interaction and participation.

4. Whenever appropriate, supplement an activity with the provision of written word or sound cues as an indirect means of facilitating word-recognition skills in students who are beginning readers.

5. Visualization is an effective strategy for some students to enhance semantic categories. For example, a student might be instructed as follows: "Close your eyes and imagine that you are in _____ (*a particular location*; e.g., classroom, supermarket). Look all around and tell me all the things you see."

Table 5–6
Language-Mediated Study Skills for Older Students and Adolescents

STUDY SKILLS

1. *Time Organization*

   Budgeting time for completion

   Establishing daily homework and study schedules

   Breaking assignments into smaller units

   Planning for deadlines

   Organizing notebook/planner

2. *Text Analysis*

   Table of contents

   Glossary

   Legends, maps, diagrams, tables

3. *Note-Taking*

   Importance of taking notes

   Different methods: mapping, outlining, abbreviating, summarizing, webbing

4. *Study Strategies*

   Active thinking method

   Scanning versus skimming versus reading

   Memory strategies: mnemonic devices, chunking, acronyms, brainstorming, visualizing

5. *Test-Taking Strategies*

   Preparation: establishing study schedule; inquiring as to type of questions that will be on test

   Review terms often used on tests: for example, prove, review, summarize, compare, contrast, criticize

   Strategies for different types of tests: fill-ins, multiple choice, matching, true/false, essay

6. *Reference Skills*

   Library and media center skills: alphabetical order, online catalogue skills, cross-referencing

   Review different types of reference sources: Internet searches, dictionary, atlas, thesaurus

CRITICAL THINKING

1. *General Thinking Behaviors*

   Observing and describing

   Developing concepts

   Hypothesizing

   Generalizing

   Predicting outcomes

   Explaining an event

   Offering alternatives

   Inferencing

continues

Table 5–6
continued

2. *Problem-Solving*

Teach steps in decision-making: define problem, break into small parts, develop options, choose option, predict outcome, critique decision made

3. *Higher-Thinking Skills*

Inductive and deductive reasoning

Solving analogies

LISTENING/READING

1. *Prelistening/Previewing*

Strategies for "getting ready" to listen/read, for example, reviewing material beforehand

2. *Listening/Reading*

Teach recognition of organizational cues and phrases, for example, *in the beginning, the first point, the key point, three main areas are, in summary*

Reading: teach identification of topic sentence, supporting sentences, details

3. *Evaluative Listening*

Teach distinction between fact and opinion in various materials: propaganda, commercials, prejudices, absurdities

ORAL AND WRITTEN EXPRESSION

1. *Organization*

Ways in which to ask questions

Strategies for organizing paragraphs

Teach forms of expository writing: description, explanation, compare–contrast

2. *Craftsmanship*

Sentence and paragraph construction: subject–verb agreement, tense agreement, topic versus supporting sentences, coherence

Editing

Proofreading: spelling, peer proofing

Source: F. Roth and E. Eyre, personal communication, July 1991.

6. A referential communication task is a good instructional mechanism for facilitating the development of a variety of pragmatic skills. It involves a speaker who is responsible for describing something (e.g., objects, shapes) so that a listener can identify the correct object or replicate the pattern. This task can be manipulated in numerous ways to focus on communicative intentions, perspective taking, and conversational discourse abilities. (See Spekman & Roth, 1984, for specific intervention suggestions.)

7. Another aspect of metalinguistic skills that can be trained is humor. One common type of humor is riddles. The appreciation of riddles requires the ability to detect ambiguity. There is a developmental progression that the clinician can keep in mind when programming targets in this area:

Phonological (6–9 years): A sound sequence can be interpreted in more than one way

    Example: Why was the doctor upset? He was out of patience (patients).

Lexical (9-12 years): A word has more than one meaning

    Example: Why didn't the skeleton cross the road? It didn't have the guts.

Syntactic (13+ years): Words in a sentence can be grouped differently

    Example: What is the difference between a running dog and a running man? The man wears trousers and the dog pants.

8. The information-giving aspect of counseling may involve educating families about the purpose and procedures of the IEP process so that they can effectively participate in decision-making for appropriate educational placements and services.

9. An important aspect of counseling with this age group often is apprising the family of the potential impact of oral language disorders on the acquisition of early reading and writing skills.

10. Story frames can facilitate a student's generation of a well-formed story. See the following examples:

    Once upon a time _____

    Suddenly _____

    Luckily _____

    In the end _____

11. With adolescents, it is important to use written materials that are relevant and age appropriate (e.g., blogs, magazines, emails, or websites on topics of interest; advertisements; bus/metro routes and schedules). Also, engage the student in relevant writing tasks, such as making shopping lists, copying recipes, writing letters of inquiry for potential jobs, preparing résumés, and practicing interviewing skills.

12. When using role-play as a technique for fostering the development of social skills, it may be useful to portray examples of both appropriate and inappropriate behaviors to highlight the differences between more and less socially acceptable behavior.

13. To facilitate peer relationships through small-group settings, it may be helpful to include a normally achieving peer who can model appropriate skills. This strategy may also buffer the effects of low acceptance and rejection that may occur in larger peer groups.

14. Inferencing can be trained in the context of paragraph-length material using a multiple-choice response format; for example,

    Hal was watching a movie on TV. It was about a man who was crossing a desert. Hal could almost feel the hot sun. Soon, Hal ran to get something he wanted very much. What do you think it was?

    a. Something to ride on

    b. Something to drink

    c. Something to play with

15. To reinforce meaning and foster generalization over time, it is preferable to use several different contexts for the same figurative language form rather than introducing several different expressions.

16. Introduce new figurative language forms in matching and multiple-choice tasks because they are easier than explanation tasks.

17. Certain types of idioms, metaphors, and so on are easier to understand than others, because their meaning is more transparent or closer to the literal meaning. For example, the idiom "keep a straight face" is more explicit than "come apart at the seams." The following examples are from Schweigert (1986, pp. 33–45):

Examples of Transparent Idioms	*Examples of Opaque Idioms*
hit the road	asleep at the switch
pain in the neck	has a green thumb
burned out	big frog in a small pond
coast is clear	piece of cake
over his head	shout from the housetops
hit the sack	build a fire under
have a ball	paddle his own canoe
on the tip of his tongue	clip his wings
up the creek without a paddle	know which side his bread is buttered on

18. Begin with predictive metaphors, because they are easier to understand than proportional metaphors. **Predictive metaphors** are based on similarity and contain only one topic and vehicle. **Proportional metaphors** contain two topics and two vehicles and express an analogical relationship, usually with one topic left unstated (e.g., The bird's nest was a piggy bank that had no coins). The analogy is *nest* is to *piggy bank* as *eggs* are to *coins* (leaving the topic of eggs to be inferred).

19. Dictionaries of English figurative language forms are commercially available. Two examples are the *Dictionary of American Slang and Colloquial Expressions* (2005; McGraw-Hill) and the *Cambridge Dictionary of American Idioms* (2003; Cambridge University Press).

20. Adolescents may demonstrate significant behavioral problems that are, in fact, related to their language impairment. Clinicians may need to provide counseling to help students function more effectively in classroom as well as clinical settings. Clinicians also may recommend that families seek services from specialized counseling professionals.

21. Instruction that addresses linguistic cohesion devices can significantly improve a student's comprehension and production of oral and written text. See Appendix 5–A on the companion website for examples of the most common types of cohesion.

Conclusion

This chapter presented basic information, protocols, and procedures for intervention for childhood language disorders at an *introductory* level. This information is intended only as a starting point in the reader's clinical education and training. For more in-depth coverage of this area, the following readings are recommended:

Nelson, N. W. (2010). *Language and literacy disorders: Infancy through adolescence.* Allyn & Bacon.

Nippold, M. A. (2016). *Later language development: School-age children, adolescents, and young adults* (4th ed.). Pro-Ed.

Owens, R. E. (2014). *Language disorders: A functional approach to assessment and intervention* (7th ed.). Allyn & Bacon.

Paul, R., Norbury, C., & Gosse, C. (2018). *Language disorders from infancy to adolescence: Listening, speaking, reading, writing, and communicating* (5th ed.). Elsevier.

Additional Resources

Crack the Books Interactive Science Books

This series of digital books is designed for use with upper elementary school-age children. Lessons are written to align with core curriculum standards and universal design parameters. The lessons can be adjusted to meet the needs of students on varying reading levels (covering first through eighth grade reading levels) without altering the content for these students. Book topics include geography, anatomy, U.S. history, and weather. The books have interactive features such as imbedded videos, pop-up definitions, voice-over options, and quizzes/tests.

Developing Language for Literacy

This resource targets strategies for using linguistic knowledge to learn basic reading skills for children ages 5 through 10. It includes a discussion of the interrelationship between language learning and the acquisition of reading skills. Topics range from the importance of prediction strategies to facilitating development of phonological awareness. It also emphasizes pragmatic activities and strategies for working with bilingual/multicultural populations. The resource can be found on the Academic Communication Associates website (https://www.acadcom.com).

Exercises for Descriptive Language Skills

For ages 4 to 10 years, this collection of activities targets skills such as sequencing story pictures and retelling stories, describing details using precise vocabulary, describing similarities and differences, creating stories and finishing incomplete stories, and giving explanations. It also includes reproducible pictures and worksheets. The resource can be found on the Academic Communication Associates website (https://www.acadcom.com).

500 Prefixes, Suffixes, and Stems Super Fun Deck

This deck presents 500 illustrated prefixes, suffixes, and stems. One side of each card presents a word part and its meaning along with two words (using the word part) and their definitions. Knowing the meaning of various word parts can greatly expand vocabulary and help to figure out the meaning of words that have never been seen or heard before. The other side is a flash card to test knowledge of the word's meaning.

Granny's Candies

This board game expands vocabulary skills with question cards from one of eight semantic areas, such as "What belongs in this group?" and "How are they alike?"

No-Glamour Grammar

Each skill is broken down into small increments of learning. The pages have few visual distractions and a consistent format so students know what to expect. Units progress in difficulty with the mastery of each grammar skill. Includes pretests and posttests for each unit to chart progress.

No-Glamour Grammar Cards
This set contains 200 cards and targets 10 grammatical concepts, including verb forms, plurals, and comparatives. The cards are designed with color pictures on the front and a list of six questions on the back.

101 Language Activities
These varied language activities promote the skills necessary to communicate effectively in the classroom. They provide motivational language and reasoning tasks using curricular topics and vocabulary.

Road to the Code
This developmentally sequenced 11-week program is designed to give kindergarten and first-grade students repeated opportunities to practice and enhance beginning reading and spelling abilities. Contains 44 lessons, each featuring three activities.

Story Magic: Developing Language Skills Using Popular Children's Stories
This book utilizes familiar children's stories, such as Jack and the Beanstalk, to increase language skills in children ages 5 to 8 years. The spiral-bound text contains simplified versions of the stories along with activities to target a variety of language skills, including vocabulary development, sequencing, and story grammar concepts. The resource can be found on the Academic Communication Associates website (https://www.acadcom.com).

Tasks of Problem Solving: Elementary (TOPS-3:E Companion)
These activities are designed for students with impairments in language and problem-solving skills. The tasks incorporate test-taking strategies, comprehension activities, and classroom decision-making skills. They also improve metacognitive skills by teaching students the vocabulary and language to describe how they are thinking.

Ten Steps to Writing Better Essays
This standards-based guide provides lessons for older students who have difficulty organizing their thoughts and materials before writing expository essays.

Webber Core Curriculum Vocabulary Card Decks
These color-coded and research-based cards will help your students learn tier-two, high-frequency vocabulary words by matching a word to its definition. The decks are divided into the following levels: PreK-K, Level One, and Level Two. They target words students need to know for success in the early grades in the areas of language arts, science, social studies, and math.

Miscellaneous

Bear, D. R., Invernizzi, M., Templeton, S, & Johnston, F. (2016). *Words their way: Word study for phonics, vocabulary, and spelling instruction* (6th ed.). Pearson.

>This clinician and teacher guide provides evidence-based activities for teaching phonological awareness, vocabulary, spelling, alphabetic principle, and reading decoding skills.

Beck, I. L., McKeown, M. G., & Kuckan, L. (2013). *Bringing words to life: Robust vocabulary instruction* (2nd ed.). Guilford Press.

This book provides practical vocabulary instruction strategies for early, intermediate, and later grades. It also identifies specific children's books with corresponding target vocabulary words.

Burns, M. S., Griffin, P., & Snow, C. E. (2000). *Starting out right: A guide to promoting children's reading success*. National Academy Press.

This is a clinician and parent-friendly guide to the development of reading and spelling skills in young children. Includes specific activities to promote emergent and early literacy from infancy through mid-elementary school.

Loh-Hagan, V., & Moss, B. (2016). *40 strategies for guiding readers through informational texts*. Guilford Press.

This book provides its readers with an understanding of informational texts as a genre as well as guidelines for selecting and assessing the complexity of informational texts. It contains subsequent sections that focus on strategies to use for skill areas such as vocabulary, comprehension, and discussion.

Marzano, R. J. (2004). *Building background knowledge for academic achievement*. Association for Supervision and Curriculum Development.

This book provides specific steps for building students' general and subject-specific background knowledge. It contains helpful vocabulary lists organized by 11 subject areas (e.g., math, science, social studies, etc.) and grade levels from kindergarten through 12th grade.

Rooney, K. J. (2010). *Strategies for learning: Empowering students for success. Grades 9–12*. Corwin.

This text presents practical strategies to help adolescent learners access curricula content across subject areas and meet the performance demands of secondary educational settings.

Roth, F. P., Worthington, C. K., & Troia, G. A. (2012). *Promoting Awareness of Speech Sounds (PASS): A phonological awareness intervention program*. Attainment.

This book focuses on training in three areas: rhyming, sound blending, and sound segmenting. Skills are taught in a sequential manner through a variety of games. It includes a detailed description (script) for each activity as well as precise instructions for implementation.

Scott, C. (2012). Learning to write. In A. Kamhi & H. Catts (Eds.), *Language and reading disabilities* (3rd ed., pp. 244–268). Pearson.

This text focuses on the differences between spoken and written language disabilities. This chapter covers writing skills and provides information on writing texts for specific genres.

Torgesen, J. K., & Bryant, B. R. (2013). *Phonological awareness training for reading* (2nd ed.). Pro-Ed.

This book and corresponding kit focus on training in four areas: sound blending, sound segmenting, reading, and spelling. Skills are taught in a sequential manner through a variety of games. It includes a detailed description (script) for each activity as well as precise instructions for implementation.

Yopp, H. K., & Yopp, R. H. (2000). Supporting phonemic awareness in the classroom. *The Reading Teacher, 54,* 130–143.

This article provides sample phonological awareness activities appropriate for preschool, kindergarten, and first-grade classrooms within a developmental hierarchy of difficulty.

Chapter 6

Intervention for Autism Spectrum Disorder (ASD)

Note: Use of person-first language (e.g., "child with autism") or identity-first language ("autistic child") is an individual choice expressed by many in the disability community (Taboas et al., 2023). Both are used in this chapter.

Overview of Autism Spectrum Disorder

Autism spectrum disorder (ASD) is a complex disorder, and its study is rapidly evolving. The original term early infantile autism was used by Kanner (1943) to describe children who showed extreme self-isolation, lack of social interaction, impaired language, and "insistence on the preservation of sameness." Asperger (1944) published an account of children with impaired communication and interaction skills whose language and intelligence were in the average to above-average range. The name for the disorder described by these researchers and others, changed to "autism" during the 1970s to 1980s. And in the 1990s, the "spectrum" terminology was added to capture the range and severity of impairment along a continuum from mild to severe. In this chapter, the authors have made a decision to include material that is widely known in the field and do not specifically endorse particular treatment strategies.

The fifth edition of the *Diagnostic and Statistical Manual of Mental Disorders* (*DSM-5*; American Psychiatric Association [APA], 2013) was released in May 2013, and it contains several *significant changes* to the definition and criteria for diagnosis of autism. First, the overall category name, "pervasive developmental disorder" (PDD) has been replaced with "autism spectrum disorder," and all of the subcategories (e.g., "Asperger's PDD-NOS") are no longer used. According to the DSM-5, this change was due primarily to the lack of evidence for discrete categories. Second, the criterion related specifically to oral language development has been removed. Now the diagnosis of ASD as a neurodevelopmental disorder is based on the demonstration of two basic symptoms prior to the age of 3 years: (a) *persistent deficits in social communication and social interaction* and (b) *restricted or repetitive patterns of behavior, interests, or activities that cause significant impairments in daily functioning*. Children who meet these criteria will be given a diagnosis of ASD with varying levels of severity: mild, moderate, or severe (Table 6–1). While language difficulties are not a core feature of ASD, a significant proportion of children with ASD experience difficulties acquiring spoken language. About 55% of children with ASD have below-average intelligence (Centers for Disease Control and Prevention [CDC], 2018). This represents a significant shift from more than a decade ago, when only one-third of children with ASD scored above the IQ cutoff for intellectual disability/impairment (Dykens & Lense, 2011). Thus, children diagnosed with moderate-to-severe ASD are likely to exhibit significant intellectual deficits. Guidelines from the American Speech-Language-Hearing Association (ASHA) state that speech-language pathologists (SLPs) play a critical role in the diagnosis of ASD, typically as part of an interdisciplinary/collaborative team (see the ASHA position statement at https://www.asha.org/practice-portal/clinical-topics/autism/#collapse_4). In addition, the *DSM-5* states that diagnoses are most valid and reliable when based on multiple sources of information, including clinician observations, caregiver history, and, when possible, self-report (APA, 2013, p. 53).

Table 6–1
Levels of Severity for Autism Spectrum Disorder

Severity Level	Social Communication	Restricted, Repetitive Behaviors
Level 3 "Requiring very substantial support"	Severe deficits in verbal and nonverbal social communication skills cause severe impairments in functioning, very limited initiation of social interactions, and minimal response to social overtures from others. For example, a person with few words of intelligible speech who rarely initiates interaction and, when he or she does, makes unusual approaches to meet needs only and responds to only very direct social approaches.	Inflexibility of behavior, extreme difficulty coping with change, or other restricted/repetitive behaviors markedly interfere with functioning in all spheres. Great distress/difficulty in changing focus or action.
Level 2 "Requiring substantial support"	Marked deficits in verbal and nonverbal social communication skills; social impairments apparent even with supports in place; limited initiation of social interactions; and reduced or abnormal responses to social overtures from others. For example, a person who speaks simple sentences, whose interaction is limited to narrow special interests, and who has markedly odd nonverbal communication.	Inflexibility of behavior, difficulty coping with change, or other restricted/repetitive behaviors appear frequently enough to be obvious to the casual observer and interfere with functioning in a variety of contexts. Distress and/or difficulty in changing focus or action.
Level 1 "Requiring support"	Without supports in place, deficits in social communication cause noticeable impairments. Difficulty initiating social interactions, and clear examples of atypical or unsuccessful responses to the social overtures of others. May appear to have decreased interest in social interactions. For example, a person who is able to speak in full sentences and engages in communication but whose to-and-fro conversation with others fails, and whose attempts to make friends are odd and typically unsuccessful.	Inflexibility of behavior causes significant interference with functioning in one or more contexts. Difficulty switching between activities. Problems of organization and planning hamper independence.

Incidence

ASD is one of the most common developmental disabilities in the United States, and is marked by gender differences, with males representing a significant majority of children diagnosed with the disorder. Over recent decades, there has been a steep increase in estimated incidence figures:

1 of every 125 children in 2004

1 of every 110 children in 2006

1 of every 88 in children in 2011/2012

1 of every 68 children in 2014 (Centers for Disease Control and Prevention [CDC], 2013, 2014)

1 of every 44 children in 2018 (Centers for Disease Control and Prevention [CDC], 2018)

Several reasons for this increased incidence have been proposed, including the following:

1. More children may have ASD (i.e., the true frequency of autism has increased).

2. There is increased awareness of the condition by health care and educational professionals as well as the general public.

3. The diagnosis may be applied more broadly than before the concept of "spectrum" was added to the definition.

4. Diagnosis is being made at increasingly early ages.

5. Better diagnostic tools are increasingly available.

Jick and Kaye (2012) examined data from three countries to clarify the reasons for the sharp increase in the diagnosis of autism in the 1990s. They compared 250 case pairs of boys with and without a diagnosis of autism in the 1980s and 1990s. Those in the nonautistic group had diagnoses of developmental delays. Several factors were compared across the two populations, including exposure to drugs, maternal rubella, preexisting medical illness of children or their mothers, vaccinations, and pregnancy history. No material differences were found, causing the authors to conclude that (a) a major cause of the steep increase in the number of boys diagnosed with autism in the 1990s is probably due to changing diagnostic practices; and (b) in the 1980s, these same children would have been diagnosed with developmental disabilities rather than autism. In summary, the factors driving the dramatic increase in incidence of diagnosis as well as the shift in the intellectual profile of children with ASD continue to be debated in this rapidly evolving communication disorder.

Etiology

The cause of autism is unknown and somewhat controversial. Most researchers agree that there is not a single etiology and multiple clinical phenotypes exist (Davidson & Ellis Weismer, 2017; Sauer et al., 2021). Overall, many researchers and clinicians believe that genetic vulnerabilities/predispositions interact with environmental risk and resilience (protective) factors to alter the development of brain structure and function, thus compromising the child's ability to learn. In addition to genetic influence, other commonly proposed contributing factors include infectious agents (e.g., maternal rubella), brain structure abnormalities (hemisphere asymmetries), physiologic brain abnormalities (e.g., deficits in coordination among neural areas), and metabolic diseases (e.g., phenylketonuria). Several well-done studies (e.g., Plotkin et al., 2009) have ruled out vaccinations (e.g., diphtheria, tetanus, and pertussis [DTaP]; measles, mumps, and rubella [MMR]) as causative factors.

In an effort to increase our understanding of the developmental mechanisms underlying the disorder, Jones et al. (2013) published an article that focused on mapping how ASD evolves from birth. Using a novel methodology, they reviewed numerous prospective studies of infants with familial history of ASD. These "high-risk" infant siblings were followed until 2 to 3 years of age, when diagnosis of ASD is usually made. A low-risk control group composed of children who have a **typically developing (TD)** older sibling and no family history of ASD was similarly followed. According to the authors, this methodology may help to identify **early markers** of ASD and facilitate prediction of clinical outcome. The studies reviewed involved several different methodologies: observation in more than one context, standardized tools, eye-tracking tasks, and neuroimaging. This design also allowed for the identification of a **broader ASD phenotype (BAP)**, which consists of a collection of subclinical traits/characteristics that are present at an elevated rate in individuals with ASD. Importantly, Jones et al. (2013) found that most of the preverbal impairments emerge during the second year of life (e.g., lower number and variety of communicative gestures, combine eye gaze with gesture to communicate). Also, social communication deficits are not always the earliest symptoms of ASD and frequently do not precede impairments in other areas (e.g., sensory, ritualistic behaviors; Elsabbagh & Johnson, 2010; Rogers, 2009; Yirmiya & Charman, 2010).

Characteristics of Children With ASD

The myriad characteristics of ASD can be divided into two major groups of "core" deficits: (a) persistent failure to develop effective social communication and (b) restricted/repetitive patterns of attention, interest, and behaviors (including fine and gross motor movement). It is important to realize that not all children with ASD will demonstrate every characteristic and not to the same degree. Behavior may vary on a daily basis.

Social Communication

Children with ASD fail to establish reciprocal social interactions with others in their environment. Rather, they tend to remain self-isolated and detached. This lack of awareness/disinterest is evidenced in their failure to anticipate arrival of parents or recognize their voices, failure to develop natural kiss and cuddle routines, and lack of social imitation (e.g., waving bye-bye). Significantly, these children do not develop joint attention, which is the ability to focus/share eye gaze with another person on the same object (Bruner, 1983). Each individual must understand that the other individual is looking at the same object and realize that there is an element of shared attention. This ability to engage in the "same line of regard" is the prerequisite for the development of referencing (e.g., pointing and other gestures). Further, children with ASD demonstrate significant difficulty with simple and more abstract forms of play. For example, when given a toy car, the child is likely to spin the wheels rather than roll the toy along the floor. In addition, pretend/symbolic play is frequently absent from the child's repertoire. Play that appears symbolic may actually be overlearned or rote behavior. These children show a lack of curiosity about the world, which is manifested, in part, as a resistance to learning new things.

Finally, emotional development is severely compromised. Children with ASD have difficulty understanding and expressing feelings and lack empathy. In 1985, Baron-Cohen et al. introduced the concept of **"theory of mind (ToM)"** or "mindblindness," which they defined as the ability to take the perspective of others, especially when that perspective is different from one's own. This includes the ability to understand that others have feelings and emotions of their own. It also includes the ability to differentiate between different emotions, label, and recognize one's own emotional states. ToM is mediated by language; it begins to develop during early childhood, at about 2 to 3 years of age. This "other awareness" is thought to affect social, emotional, communication, and language development. For example, a child might laugh when his classmate falls down at recess and scrapes his knee. The same child may not be able to select "happy" when shown pictures of "happy" and "sad" faces. Joint attention is a prerequisite skill for developing ToM; so, before any ToM strategies (e.g., perspective taking) can be meaningfully expected/introduced, a child must have first developed joint attention (Baron-Cohen et al., 1985).

Repetitive/Restricted Behaviors, Interests, and Activities

In addition to social and language impairments, children with ASD exhibit other significant deficits. Again, the reader is reminded that every child with ASD does not exhibit all of these characteristics and not to the same degree.

- Non-goal-directed behaviors (i.e., self-stimulatory behaviors such as rocking back and forth, pacing, hand waving)

- Self-injurious and aggressive behaviors (e.g., head banging, biting)

- Obsessive behaviors: Remaining fixated on a particular stimulus (e.g., learning how a vacuum cleaner works) and ignoring other stimuli (aka, overselected attention)

- Difficulty developing/following important routines (e.g., feeding/sleeping), probably as a result of inability to cope with even the smallest changes in the environment

- Hypo-/hypersensitivity to stimuli (e.g., high tolerance for pain, extreme reactions to everyday sounds, aversion to certain food or fabric textures)

- Extreme food selectivity (aka "food fetishes"): child restricts his or her intake to one or two very specific foods (e.g., Dannon strawberry yogurt; strawberry Twizzlers) and rejects all others, which can result in significant developmental and health consequences; may develop pica, ingesting or chewing on nonedible substances such as dirt, paper, wood, or plastic

- Stimulus overselectivity: Focus on isolated aspects of objects or people (e.g., fascination with sensory experiences such as lights or visual patterns)

- Difficulty integrating auditory and visual information simultaneously (e.g., hold hands over ears to reduce confusion between the senses)

- Attentional difficulties: Orienting, sustaining, and shifting attention, especially when a rapid shift of attention is required (transitions)

- Situational-specific learning (aka, "local learning"): Learning a skill in one context but not recognizing the skill in another context

Language and Speech Considerations

Although oral language development is no longer a DSM criterion for the diagnosis of ASD, it is important to understand that children with ASD exhibit significant quantitative and qualitative language impairments. The pattern of development and language use described in ASD is often strikingly different from TD children and children with other developmental disabilities. Sometimes, their language development is characterized as aberrant rather than "delayed." That is, their language development does not follow a typical developmental pattern and does not represent any stage of typical language development. Most often, these children demonstrate a failure to acquire spoken language, demonstrating significant language comprehension and production problems, even those with typical intellectual development (Kjellmer et al., 2018). For children with ASD who are verbal, their use of language is often inappropriate and out of context (e.g., failure to stay on topic during a conversation, irrelevant responses to requests/questions) and conveys a significantly lower proportion of communicative intentions than the language of nonimpaired peers and peers with other kinds of disabilities (Shumway & Wetherby, 2009). They also have difficulty understanding the nonverbal communication of others (e.g., gestures, facial expressions) and do not use meaningful gestures to communicate. A notable feature characteristic of these children's expressive language is pronoun reversal. For example, a child who is asking for juice will likely say: "You want juice" rather than the conventional "I want juice," or "He eat cookie" in response to the question: "What are you eating?" In addition, proper nouns are commonly used to refer to oneself, as in "John wants juice" rather than "I/ me want juice." These individuals often recite long passages of verbal material (entire poems, weather reports, news articles) without comprehension; this is because they have excellent "recording memory" but cannot chunk linguistic information into meaningful units.

One of the hallmark characteristics of ASD is the use of **echolalia**, which is the partial or full repetition of the speech of others (Prizant & Duchan, 1981). This linguistic behavior can be described according to when it occurs (i.e., immediate vs. delayed) or according to the function it is intended to serve (i.e., communicative vs. noncommunicative). In general, delayed echolalia is often viewed as a self-stimulatory behavior, whereas immediate echoes tend to be used when the child does not know what is expected in terms of verbalization (e.g., turn-taking filler or searching for the correct response). Although the traditional view of echolalia characterized it as an aberrant behavior that should be eliminated, Prizant (1983) found that the echoes can serve a variety of different communicative functions, such as requesting, protesting, or commenting. Some children with ASD demonstrate use of both communicative and noncommunicative echolalia. This verbal behavior is not unique to autism; children with other disabilities such as intellectual impairment, fragile X syndrome, and childhood schizophrenia may exhibit echolalia (Tager-Flusberg et al., 2005). However, compared to these other populations, a much larger proportion of children with ASD (approximately 85% of verbal communicators) produce echolalic utterances, the length of their echoed utterances are longer, and their echoes include more precise replication of the original utterance with regard to factors such as intonation, coughs, and accents (Rydell & Prizant, 1995). Table 6–2 summarizes the different aspects of echolalia.

Elimination/extinction of echolalia should not be considered an initial, appropriate, or even necessary intervention goal. Many children with ASD use echoes communicatively to request, comment, or respond to others. Echolalia may be a significant portion of the child's communicative repertoire. In some cases, it may be the primary or sole means of communication and will continue throughout the life span, particularly in stressful situations. In other cases, echolalia can be a transitional step/ phase prior to or during therapy to facilitate development of spontaneous spoken language. In general, echolalia decreases significantly as the child acquires greater receptive and expressive language skills.

In addition to communication deficits, children with ASD demonstrate speech impairment in the presence of good speech articulation skills. The main speech impairment occurs in speech prosody (melody or rhythm of speech), and this characteristic is observed even in adolescents with no discernible language impairment (Grossman et al., 2013; Rapin & Dunn, 1997).

Grossman et al. (2013) showed that high-functioning adolescents with autism performed as well as typically developing peers on receptive tasks that required them to perceptually differentiate stress patterns in speech (e.g., HOTdog versus hotDOG) as well as affective prosody (happy, sad, neutral),

Table 6–2
Examples of Different Types of Echolalia

Type	Example and Context/Intent
Immediate/ noncommunicative	Adult: Where did you go yesterday? Child: Where did you go yesterday? Adult: Wash your hands. Child: Wash your hands.
Delayed/ noncommunicative	Child: Don't throw the doll off the balcony. (Child is repeating an utterance heard 2 years previously for no apparent reason.) Child: Give this to John. Give this to John. Give this to John. Give this to John. (No referent in sight. Said intoning a melody.)
Mitigated	Adult: Why are you crying? Child: Why are you screaming? Adult: Do you want to watch *Snow White*? Child: You want to watch *Snow White*. (Meaning, "Yes, I do.")
Immediate/ communicative	Adult: Do you want a sandwich? Child: Do you want a sandwich? Yes. (Meaning that the child wants a sandwich.) Adult: Soup's on. Child: Soup's on. (Meaning that the child wants a bowl of soup.)
Delayed communicative	Child (When child is tired): It's been a long day kids, but you've done a great job. (Child is repeating a line from a Tonka Truck computer game.) Child (When child is asked to do a difficult task): And in other news . . . Child (Whenever child breaks something): Can we fix it? Yes, we can! (Child is repeating a line from *Bob the Builder*.)
Immediate/ mitigated	Adult (Pointing to a gingerbread house that was hit by a peer): It's smooshed into pieces. Child: It broke into pieces.
Delayed mitigated	Child (Whenever sees classmate crying): It's not easy being green. (Child is repeating a line from the Muppets characters.)

Note. Portions are adapted from I. Betz and E. Brady, personal communication, 2014.

but demonstrated significant differences in the production of prosody. Specifically, their production of two-syllable words was atypical, with noted exaggerated pauses between syllables, especially for second-syllable-stress items. This labored and slow enunciation pattern was in stark contrast to the briefer, more fluid productions of their typically developing peers. These abnormal prosody production patterns also have been noted by Paul et al. (2005).

Other characteristics often observed in the speech of children with ASD include the following:

- Monotone inflection at the utterance level

- Instances of singing interspersed into the child's production of connected speech

- Repetition and perseveration in individual sounds as well as some sound sequences

Emergent Literacy and Literacy

In both emergent literacy and literacy, children with ASD tend to show strengths in form and weakness in meaning (Boyle et al., 2019; Westerveld & Paynter, 2021). Some children demonstrate *hyperlexia*: an advanced ability to recognize the written word in the presence of delayed or deviant language development (Mehegan & Dreifuss, 1972; Westerveld et al., 2017). Hyperlexia also has been characterized as a compulsive preoccupation with the written word.

At the emergent literacy stage, children can name letters, but do not understand what people read and write (Chen & Kou, 2017; Lanter et al., 2012; Lindgren et al., 2009). At the literacy stage, the same pattern is seen. Decoding and spelling are strengths for children with ASD, whereas reading comprehension is quite challenging. Specifically, children with high-functioning ASD perform as well as or even better than typically developing peers (matched for age and IQ) on word-reading and spelling tasks, whereas their reading comprehension is very poor. Moreover, children who demonstrate accurate reading comprehension at the word level often experience severe difficulties at the passage level for both reading accuracy and comprehension (Arciuli et al., 2013).

Medications

About 70% of children with autism are prescribed psychoactive medications to ameliorate disruptive behaviors, which range from impulsivity to self-injury to overt aggression to mood disorders. SLPs need to understand the potential side effects of medication and be able to differentiate these effects from the actual symptoms of ASD. Side effects are not well understood. Efficacy data for most classes of drugs are increasing, but they are still somewhat limited (Goel et al., 2018). Classes of drugs that are commonly used in the ASD population include the following:

- *Antipsychotics:* Risperdal, Haldol

- *Stimulants:* Ritalin, Cylert

- *Nonstimulants:* Stratera

- *Secretin and serotonin reuptake inhibitors (SSRIs):* Prozac, Paxil

- *Antiseizure medication:* Ativan, Keppra

- *Complementary and alternative medicine (CAM) interventions:* Insufficient evidence about effectiveness or adverse effects

Outcomes

Language skills and IQ are the strongest predictors of a child's outcome (Gotham et al., 2012; Pellicano, 2013; Witwer & Lecavalier, 2008). Specifically, a good outcome is best predicted by attainment of meaningful communication and demonstration of normal nonverbal IQ by 5 years of age.

In addition to overall prognosis and outcome, researchers have traced the development of specific skill areas in small samples of individuals with ASD over time and examined how change in one area affects another. One area of focus is metacognition/executive functioning with children/adolescents in the average or high-functioning range of intelligence between 4 and 19 years old (Bennett et al., 2013; Pellicano, 2012). Metacognitive/executive functioning abilities involve an awareness of one's own problem-solving abilities and include self-regulation behaviors that are used to guide, monitor, and evaluate the success of one's performance (Baddeley, 2007; Barkley, 1996, 1997). Findings suggest a positive link between executive functioning, ToM development, and language development. Overall, children/adolescents with the strongest executive functioning skills (planning, carrying out complex tasks) demonstrated the strongest ToM (taking the perspective of another). These findings suggest that intervention focused on executive functioning and ToM may yield overall developmental benefits, including advances in language and communication. Because these studies involved small sample sizes, the results must be viewed as promising, but preliminary. Autism is a lifelong developmental disorder, but most of the research studies are cross-sectional (e.g., Kalk et al., 2010). A few longitudinal studies followed large samples of children with ASD over two decades and provide insight into the trajectories for ASD from early identification through adolescence and into adulthood. The findings of Lord and her colleagues (2012) are representative. These authors followed 300 children from age 2 years to 21 years and found three distinct subgroups:

- About 10% of children showed dramatic improvement by middle adolescence (i.e., live independently, self-supporting, professional careers, marry).

- Another 10% worsened over time.

- Eighty percent continue to demonstrate significant deficits over time with regard to core symptoms/severity.

These subgroups remained surprisingly stable over time, with little variability within or across the groups.

In summary, most children with ASD continue to demonstrate significant deficits throughout life and may not be able to live independently. But even those with the mildest symptoms have residual deficits in the social domain (viewed as "eccentric"), exhibiting highly stereotypic interactions (e.g., scripts), difficulty in turn taking and reciprocal conversations, poor coordination of eye contact and speech, and unusual speech patterns. These limitations may affect their ability to adjust to new social demands in academic, vocational, and community settings. When working with adolescents, SLPs may need to include transitional objectives and functional outcomes to prepare these individuals for employment in highly structured jobs such as computer programming, sorting/assembling materials, or stocking shelves.

Treatment Efficacy/Evidence-Based Practice

The unprecedented increase in the prevalence of ASD in the U.S. population has fueled a strong demand for information on evidence-based practices with this group of individuals. Given the wide range of intervention approaches that have been developed over the past 60 years (e.g., behavioral, dietary, educational, etc.), combing through the existing ASD treatment literature can be daunting for the practicing clinician. Fortunately, there have been several systematic reviews of intervention practices published since 2015 (Will et al., 2018). The National Standards Project (NSP) published an update of their systematic review in 2015 (https://tinyurl.com/yc28x98a). This study identified 14 intervention approaches deemed to have adequate evidence presented in the literature. In addition, the National Clearinghouse on Autism Evidence and Practice (NCAEP, 2017; https://tinyurl.com/5n93vee4) also conducted a systematic review of current interventions for autism and identified 27 approaches deemed to demonstrate solid evidence in the literature. Although the two reviews differed somewhat in their methodology and criteria for determining "established approaches," four approaches were identified by both entities as effective: cognitive-behavioral therapy, naturalistic intervention, parent training, and peer training—these will be described in detail under the subsequent header of "Treatment Approaches." It should be noted that all four of these intervention strategies are highly compatible with a social model of disability.

Treatment for Autism

Theoretical Models

Three primary theoretical orientations underlie the treatment of autism: functional/ behavioral; developmental; and social/neurodiversity affirming models:

- *Functional/behavioral* (Lovaas et al., 1973): This framework places primary emphasis on improving a child's effectiveness as a communicator. Intervention does not follow any developmental sequence and is not limited to verbal speech. Target behaviors are selected based on environmental/social factors such as instructional/family priorities, in addition to the individual's disability.

- *Developmental* (Tager-Flusberg et al., 2009): This framework focuses on spoken language skills and moves away from terminology related to "functional speech and language." It uses benchmark criteria based on typical language development as a rubric for language intervention programming. The hierarchy progresses from meaningful gestures/vocalizations, to single words, to phrases/sentences, and culminates with complex language forms.

- *Social/neurodiversity affirming* (DeThorne & Gerlach-Houck, 2023; DeThorne & Searsmith, 2021; Schuck et al., 2021): This framework focuses on enhancing a child's daily function in society by providing supports, accommodations, and modifications that address physical, environmental, and sensory barriers experienced by the child. It also targets people's attitudes that may assume that disabled individuals cannot do certain things.

These three philosophical orientations are not mutually exclusive and are frequently combined to varying degrees (i.e., hybrid). In general, selection of a model is heavily influenced by the client's cognitive profile. Developmental approaches are usually appropriate for children with mild or no cognitive impairment, whereas functional approaches may be appropriate for children whose cognitive abilities are severely compromised and approaches based on a social model of disability can be incorporated into intervention programs for all autistic clients. These theoretical models can be implemented in different settings or contexts (e.g., location, communicative partner, activity).

The degree to which programming is child directed or clinician directed may vary across settings over time. Before specific treatment approaches are presented, the particular pattern of language, communication, and social development demonstrated by these children necessitates discussion of important programming considerations:

- *Universal design principles for learning (UDL):* All instruction and intervention should align with UDL, in terms of providing the child/adolescent with multiple means of access to the curriculum, multiple means of expressing knowledge, and multiple opportunities for meaningful practice of the newly learned skills to sustain motivation for learning.

- *Early intervention (EI):* The environment has the greatest influence on brain structure and function during the first few years of life. Thus, maturation coupled with early, appropriate stimulation capitalizes on neural plasticity. Another benefit of EI often is minimization of the emergence of the maladaptive behaviors and behavioral difficulties that are frequently part of the developmental course of ASD (Boyd et al., 2010). A systematic review conducted by Landa (2018) indicates that young children with ASD benefit from EI and supports combining parent-mediated and clinician-implemented intervention to maximize gains.

- *Comprehensive and intensive intervention:* Because of the pervasiveness of ASD, it is recommended that intervention programming address multiple areas of deficits, across all of a child's daily settings and activities, with an intensity of 25 to 40 hr/week (National Autism Project, National Autism Center, 2009). This comprehensive approach should be implemented over extended periods of time, because ASD is a life span disorder (Boyd et al., 2010).

- *Structure versus flexibility:* Children with ASD function best in environments that are predictable—where rules and expectations are clear and consistent. However, excessive reliance on structure has the potential to become a hindrance and even an obstacle to learning new skills and adapting to changes in daily routines. These children need some degree of flexibility to learn new skills. SLPs are encouraged to use small, incremental changes/transitions (e.g., new materials; new location in room; order of activities) and to let students know of these changes in advance.

- *Generalization:* Children with ASD learn in situation-specific ways and thus do not generalize spontaneously to other contexts. Target behaviors need to be explicitly taught across all daily environments and activities, including home, school, day care, and community settings. A pull-out model may create an artificial context that does not provide the child with consistent connections to real life contexts (e.g., Wetherby & Prizant, 2000).

- *Behavior and emotions:* Individuals with ASD often emulate the emotions of their communication partner. If a question, direction, or request is given in a directive, strident, or loud manner, distress is a likely result, and this negativity can escalate rapidly. Clinicians are encouraged to use a positive, soft, and even tone when interacting with their clients, even when the intended message is disapproving.

- *Visual supports:* Many individuals with autism spontaneously convert spoken/verbal messages into sequences of visual images; that is, they are visual thinkers (Grandin, 2010). These children benefit from strategies that utilize their strength in visual processing, such as picture schedules, behavior graphing, and so on. Visual supports also help children transition from one activity/context to another.

- *Interdisciplinary/collaborative team:* The nature of ASD necessitates an integrated approach to intervention in which there is coordinated and cooperative involvement of the SLP, classroom teacher, parents/families, and other professionals (Lewis et al., 2018). The team also may include the following:
  - Occupational therapist for teaching fine motor and self-care skills and sensory integration.
  - Nutritionist for addressing feeding problems and nutrient intake (Sharp et al., 2013).
  - Social worker to help families access available resources, self-help, and support groups. Moreover, a family-based strategy recognizes the impact that this impairment has on the entire family dynamic. It also emphasizes that "improvements" must be measured in terms of family adjustment as well as child progress (Woods & Brown, 2011).
  - Physician for managing seizures and psychiatric comorbidities—most common are anxiety disorders and depression.
  - Psychologist/psychiatrist for addressing management of behaviors such as self-injury and severe tantrums.
  - Psychopharmacologist to prescribe medications, especially if problematic behaviors are severe, chronic, and unresponsive to behavioral interventions (Self et al., 2010).

Treatment Approaches

This section presents information on a variety of intervention models and techniques for ASD. The reader is encouraged to develop a large repertoire of treatment strategies to maximize the effectiveness of treatment programming for each child. This chapter does not discuss comprehensive treatment models that address the broad range of deficit areas exhibited by children with ASD, such as Learning Experiences and Alternative Program for Preschoolers and Their Parents (LEAP; Strain & Hoyson, 2000), More Than Words (Carter et al., 2011), Preschool Autism Communication Trial (PACT; Green et al., 2010), and the Early Start Denver Model (Dawson et al., 2010; Rogers et al., 2000). For additional information on these and other comprehensive models, refer to Odom, Boyd, et al., (2010).

It is important for student clinicians to consider the "spectrum" aspect of an ASD diagnosis. For nonverbal or minimally verbal children (MVC), the focus is often on preverbal communication skills, such as eye gaze gestures. With MVC children, an alternative or augmentative system of communication (AAC) is frequently adopted (Kasari, 2014). It may be used as a step toward useful speech, or it may serve as a child's main form of communication. AAC is used to supplement, enhance, or replace spoken language. It has many forms, including no tech (e.g., signs, gestures) and low tech (e.g., pictures, photographs). In 2018, Brignell et al. presented a comprehensive review of treatment approaches for the MVC population. In contrast to MVC, children at the higher end of the verbal spectrum require interventions that focus on functional use of structural language (e.g., phrase/sentence construction, word meaning). Group social skills approaches are commonly used for these children and focus on components such as behavioral modeling of a specific cognitive, social, or communication role-play practice during sessions and receiving individualized feedback (Wolstencroft et al., 2018).

Some of the approaches discussed in the next section clearly align with a particular theoretical model, whereas others cross philosophical or conceptual categories and can be adapted for use within more than one theoretical orientation. It is important to remember that age of onset of treatment, treatment intensity, and spectrum level are more important than use of a specific treatment program or model (Warren et al., 2011). Hsieh et al. (2018) suggest that the four approaches most commonly utilized by SLPs in the United States include social skill training, AAC, Picture Exchange Communication, and social stories.

The first four approaches were identified by both the NSP and NCAEP systematic reviews as solidly "evidence-based." However, given the complex and sometimes controversial nature of intervention in ASD, clinicians are strongly encouraged to become acquainted with the breadth of practices available and the extent to which they are supported in the current literature. When combined with the SLP's clinical judgment and the needs/values of the child/family with ASD, this will ensure that intervention is individualized for each client and programmed and implemented in the most efficacious manner possible.

Cognitive behavioral therapy (CBT) was originally developed for adults with depression (Beck et al., 1979) and aims to teach patients to identify their own thoughts, expectations, and attitudes in order to change false and negative beliefs. This intervention has been adapted for use with autism and is most appropriate for older children and adolescents with a level 1 ASD profile with strong cognitive skills (Scarpa et al., 2013). The purpose of CBT is to help clients identify and change maladaptive "thinking patterns," which can then positively influence emotional reactions and decrease problem behaviors. It promotes the ability to tolerate emotions/problematic events and mitigate anxiety by choosing new ways to behave. This intervention approach is relatively short-term and highly directive which requires substantive CBT training for the clinician. Major focus is placed on developing self-awareness, self-control, and constructive strategies to repair emotions (all of which are difficult for autistic individuals). Ultimately, the autistic individual is guided to communicate and manage emotions for successful interpersonal interactions within the daily environment.

Naturalistic Teaching Strategies

Naturalistic teaching strategies (NTS) are primarily child directed and refer to a variety of techniques that are naturally occurring in familiar contexts, including the home, school, and community (Gengoux et al., 2021; Tiede & Walton, 2019). This approach uses activities and materials that the child is likely to encounter on a daily basis to improve language, communication, and social skills.

The following steps can guide the intervention:

- Observe the child to find out what motivates him or her, and then structure teaching interactions around those interests.

- Use materials your child is likely to encounter on a daily basis such as books, stuffed animals, or cars that are available at home and at school.

- Provide consequences that are naturally found in the environment and have a direct relationship to the activity being conducted. For example, food might be a natural and direct reinforcer at lunch and getting toys "powered on" might be a natural and direct reinforcer during playtime.

- Provide loosely structured teaching sessions that vary based on the child's interests for that day. For example, if therapy is focusing on specific morpho-syntactic structures (e.g., past tense, plurals), the clinician will need to be flexible in choosing materials that are of maximal interest to the child on a given day.

Different names have been given in the literature to the intervention strategies included in the naturalistic intervention category. These include: focused stimulation, incidental teaching, milieu teaching, embedded teaching, responsive education, and prelinguistic milieu.

Parent Training Intervention

Parents and caregivers play a significant role in treatment programs for their ASD children. Sometimes parents receive direct instruction on how to implement various communication strategies. They also may serve as the child's therapist and provide direct instruction in a natural environment (Kaiser et al., 2022; Liao et al., 2022). In addition, parent training can take many other forms including the following:

- Group training with other parents/caregivers

- Support groups with educational elements

- Written training materials for expanding communication/language skills

Examples of skill targets for parents to learn may include the following:

- Consistent focus on joint attention

- Establishing and enhancing the child's imitation skills

- Repetition and expansion of grammatical language structures during daily activities

- Anticipatory waiting to increase the frequency of communication initiations

Peer-Based Interventions

Some children on the spectrum frequently try to interact with peers, but may do so in unexpected or socially inappropriate ways (Odom, 2019). Peer-training strategies facilitate skill growth for children with ASD by teaching typical peers on how to initiate and respond during social interactions with an autistic child. These programs can be used in home (don't overlook siblings), school, and community settings (Park et al., 2022). Factors to consider when designing a peer-training intervention include the following:

- The age and skill level of the children (with and without ASD) should be similar. Choose peers who are socially skilled, compliant, regularly available, willing to participate, and able to imitate the target communication behaviors modeled by the clinician.

- The activities included in the session should address the interests and preferences of the peers as well as the client to ensure high motivation.

- Teach the peers how do the following: get the attention of the child with ASD, facilitate sharing of toys/games/devices, provide help and affection, model appropriate play skills, and help organize play activities.

- After training, have the peers interact with the autistic child in a structured setting during a familiar activity. This strategy will allow the peers to practice their new skills in a comfortable environment prior to expectation for independent implementation.

- The group instructor should use prompts and feedback to facilitate interactions between the children.

- Intervention should be conducted in multiple settings and with multiple peers to increase the frequency and consistency of implementation across settings.

Different names of peer training programs may appear in the literature and include Project LEAP, peer networks, circle of friends, buddy skills package, integrated play groups, peer initiation training, and peer-mediated social interaction training.

 Note: The following approaches were not identified as "established" in the overlap between the systematic reviews conducted by NSP 2015 and NCAEP 2017. An asterisk indicates approaches that met criteria as "evidence-based" by one of the reviews, but not both.

Applied Behavior Analysis

Applied behavior analysis (ABA) represents a class of interventions that apply behavioral science principles to address behavior problems and learning in children with autism and other developmental disorders. All ABA approaches are based on Skinner's (1957) behavioral principles of operant conditioning: a stimulus, or antecedent event, is presented to elicit a target response, which is immediately followed by a consequent event (reward or punishment) to increase desired behaviors or decrease unwanted behaviors. The proper implementation of ABA requires objective observation and analysis of behavior. ABA has several forms, some of which focus on the reduction of disruptive behaviors (e.g., self-injury, aggression, repetitive, ritualistic mannerisms), whereas others are aimed at increasing adaptive behaviors, communication, and spoken language. All ABA approaches break complex tasks, actions, and behaviors into smaller, sequential parts for easier access by the child. Most ABA approaches are intensive, consisting of 30 to 40 hr of one-to-one therapy per week. Emphasis also is placed on the role of parents as primary intervention agents.

     Discrete trial training (DTT), a form of ABA therapy developed by Lovaas et al. (1973), is based on the learning principle that if a behavior is rewarded, it is more likely to be repeated. Although ABA is sometimes referred to as the "Lovaas method," this version, DTT, is one specific type of ABA. The clinician presents a stimulus (e.g., question or request to stand up), along with the correct response. Following each correct response, the child is rewarded with consequent events such as praise, food, or other incentives. Incorrect responses are ignored. This immediate schedule of reinforcement for correct behaviors is used to clearly establish the expected behavior and provide immediate feedback to the child about the accuracy of his or her response.

     Pivotal response teaching (PRT) is an ABA approach developed in the 1970s by Koegel and Koegel that uses naturalistic procedures that focus primarily on two "pivotal" areas: motivation to learn and initiation of activities. As such, PRT is specifically designed to increase a child's motivation to participate in learning new skills. Target behaviors are selected based on each child's developmental level and may include social skills (e.g., turn taking), adaptive behaviors (dressing, feeding), and language-learning skills. The intent of PRT is to increase and generalize skills in language, play, and social interaction in a child-directed format.

     Reciprocal imitation therapy (RIT) is a variation of PRT developed by Ingersoll and Lalonde (2010) for teaching play skills. Within the context of a play environment, it is specifically aimed at teaching spontaneous, reciprocal imitation skills to young children with autism. The clinician imitates actions and/or vocalizations of the child in an obvious manner, and then the child is rewarded for any subsequent attempted imitative behavior. Assistance is provided through prompting, modeling, and physical guidance.

DIR/Floortime (Developmental, Individual Difference, Relationship-Based) (Greenspan, 1990)

DIR is a framework developed by Greenspan (1990) that identifies six developmental milestones for healthy emotional and intellectual growth: (a) attending, (b) relating, (c) purposeful communication,

(d) problem-solving interactions, (e) using ideas creatively, and (f) using ideas logically. This model emphasizes identification of each child's individual differences in the way he or she processes sounds, sights, sensations, and movements. It also focuses on how parents, caregivers, therapists, and educators can tailor their interactions/relationships with the child to provide maximal opportunities to achieve the described milestones. Floortime is the technique for implementing this model of intervention for children with ASD. Adults in the child's environment are encouraged to "get down on the floor" and engage in the following set of steps 6 to 10 times per day for 20-min periods:

1. Pay attention to the child's individual behaviors.

2. Locate an "entry point" into the child's system by imitating/joining in his or her behavior (e.g., jumping, rubbing a spot on the table).

3. Engage the child this way for a few minutes and then introduce variations on the theme for both of you to embrace.

4. Gradually lead the child into mastering the milestones identified previously to create the experience of a "shared world" between the child and adult.

Functional Communication Training (FCT) *(Durand, 1990; Franzone, 2009)*

FCT is aimed at replacing a child's disruptive behaviors with more appropriate and effective communication behaviors or skills. FCT is a highly systematic and structured program that utilizes the basic principles of operant conditioning (antecedent event response–consequent event). The clinician first identifies the function of the interfering behavior (e.g., biting classmates to get a wanted toy) and then teaches a more conventional replacement behavior (e.g., pointing) that serves the same communicative purpose as the interfering behavior. The replacement behavior should allow the child to obtain his or her goal just as easily, or more easily, than the disruptive behavior. The replacement behavior can be nonverbal (e.g., pointing, sign, informal gestures) or verbal (e.g., "Please"; "I want the truck"; "Want"). The clinician structures each session to elicit several instances of the interfering behavior to provide the child with numerous opportunities to practice using the replacement behavior.

Picture Exchange Communication System

The **Picture Exchange Communication System** (PECS), developed by Bondy and Frost (1994), is a structured AAC system that promotes symbolic communication in nonverbal children with autism (or children with limited speech), encouraging spontaneous initiations. Its overall goal is to help children begin to discover/understand the power of communication. It uses a combination of incidental teaching and behavioral methods to foster meaningful communication interactions. It starts with a basic goal: to develop the concept of how to use a picture/object (symbol) to obtain a desired item or action. It progresses through six phases, beginning with simple requests and moving to single words, phrases, comments, and answering questions. At all steps of the program, children make choices/decisions that allow them to have more control over their world through the use of communication. In a typical early session, the clinician places an item (object or picture) on the table for which the child has previously shown desire. When the child reaches (makes a physical request) for the item, the SLP places it in the child's hand and helps the child to "exchange" the item (symbol) for the desired object. The immediacy of the exchange demonstrates the social interactive nature of communication in a highly concrete and functional way. This is important because children with autism often are not reinforced by typical social rewards associated with the act of communication, such as eye contact, a smile, or praise. Some children using PECS later develop speech, others may move to a more sophisticated AAC system, and still others continue to use PECS as their major form of communication both at home and at school.

Relationship Development Intervention (RDI) *(Gutstein & Sheely, 2002)*

This approach is a home-centered treatment program for young children with ASD and is a parent-implemented method. Developed by Gutstein in the 1990s, it is based on his theoretical construct of "dynamic intelligence," which Gutstein defines as the ability to think flexibly. Flexible thinking includes the ability to take the perspective of others, adapt to changes in the environment, and integrate information from a variety of sources (e.g., auditory, visual, tactile). The main premise is that individuals with autism can participate in authentic social and emotional relationships if they are exposed to them in a gradual, systematic way. The goal of RDI intervention is the gradual development of a child's reciprocal social communication that underlies the ability to form emotional bonds and interpersonal connections/relationships. Parents receive formal training in behavioral methods to slowly and systematically change/shape the interaction patterns between themselves and their children in everyday activities and settings. RDI has several core objectives to foster flexible thinking, such as emotional referencing (the ability to learn from the emotional and subjective experiences of others), social coordination (the ability to control one's behavior to successfully participate in social relationships), declarative language (the ability to use verbal and nonverbal communication to express curiosity, invite interactions, share perceptions and feelings, and coordinate with others), and relational information processing (the ability to solve problems that lack clear-cut solutions).

In a typical session, parents or other caregivers use an ordered set of developmentally sensitive objectives based on routine daily activities. For example, in the early stages of training, spoken language may be limited to encourage eye contact, joint attention, and other forms of nonverbal communication. The objectives gradually expand as the child's abilities increase.

Social Communication, Emotional Regulation, and Transactional Support (SCERTS)

The SCERTS program (Wetherby & Prizant, 2000) focuses on the core deficits of children with ASD and emphasizes communication, social relatedness, and sensory domains using a family-centered model (Prizant et al., 2003). Intervention occurs in an integrated manner because, according to the program's authors, the difficulties presented by children with ASD do not occur in isolation, and therefore must be treated as a whole. For example, mealtime is a daily activity that involves skills from each of these areas. Intervention planning is individualized according to the strengths, natural motivations, and needs of each child and the priorities of the family. Family involvement, support, and education are deemed essential to enhance a child's development and progress. The following are the main elements of the SCERTS model:

- *Communication and language:* A social-pragmatic approach to language therapy is used that focuses on the functional use of preverbal and verbal communication skills in natural and semistructured interactions. Nonspeech communication systems such as the Picture Exchange Communication System (PECS) and picture symbols often are incorporated to facilitate communication initiation and responsiveness. Both ABA and developmentally based strategies are used.

- *Social relatedness and social-emotional reciprocity:* Greenspan's DIR/Floor Time approach is the approach of choice to treat deficits in these areas because of its emphasis on developmental progressions in naturalistic contexts. (See later section on DIR for further information.)

- *Sensory processing:* Sensory integration therapy and environmental modifications, adaptations, and supports are integral parts of SCERTS, because many children with autism have motor planning problems and difficulties with daily living skills (e.g., feeding, dressing).

Social Stories *(Gray, 1994, 1998; Gray & Garand, 1993)*

The **social stories** approach is designed for higher functioning children and adolescents with autism (i.e., children whose cognitive status ranges from mild intellectual disabilities to above-average intellectual function). For each child, "scripts/stories" are written that provide explanations of appropriate behaviors in social situations with which the individual is having difficulty. The scripts are tailored to the client's level of language comprehension.

Most stories contain three sequential statements: descriptive statements, perspective statements, and directive statements. Descriptive statements are intended to help a child understand a particular situation and provide words, phrases, or sentences for a situation that the child cannot generate on his or her own. Perspective statements facilitate the child's ability to verbally identify the feelings, wants, and motivations of other people. Directive statements provide specific social cues that tell the children what they could do in a situation that would be more socially appropriate than their current responses. For children who cannot read, visual scripts and visual modeling serve as the social stories. Social stories also foster executive functioning skills, particularly in the areas of planning and self-monitoring. Role-playing and repeated reading are common strategies used to teach social stories, along with traditional techniques of prompting, modeling, imitating, and other types of cues. Typical examples of social story topics include joining a game, praising others for accomplishments, waiting your turn in an activity, raising your hand in class, or monitoring one's own production of inappropriate/disruptive vocalizations.

Treatment and Education of Autistic and Communication-Related Handicapped Children (TEACCH) *(Mesibov & Shea, 2010; Schopler & Reichler, 1971)*

The **TEACCH** approach was originally developed in 1971 as a home-based approach. It has evolved to include a classroom-based focus, and the current version is described here. TEACCH can be used with children at a wide range of ages and can incorporate **assistive technology (AT) or AAC** for children who are nonverbal. The structured classroom-based approach to teaching is based on the premise that children with autism are predominantly visual learners. Structured teaching involves four components:

1. Organize the physical environment to maximize learning and to minimize distractions.

2. Use visual teaching to capitalize on the child's relative strength in visual/spatial information processing (e.g., photographs, schedule boards, written words).

3. Individualize goals and activities to engage the child's attention (e.g., use stimuli related to the child's favorite superhero when teaching turn taking).

4. Facilitate meaningful child-initiated communication (e.g., provide opportunities for the child to make choices versus prompted responses).

Video Modeling *(Charlop et al., 2018)*

This is an instructional technique that uses a video format to teach a variety of social and communication behaviors to children with autism (Bellini & Akullian, 2007). Target behaviors are scripted and videotaped by the clinician (referred to as an *other-as-model method*). The child watches repeated videotaped presentations of adults or peers engaging in exchanges using appropriate communicative behaviors. **Video modeling** can be used to teach basic communication skills (e.g., establishing joint attention during play) and more complex communication behaviors (e.g., increasing utterance length during conversational exchanges; Charlop et al., 2018). It also can be effective for improving a variety of emotional, behavioral, and daily living skills in children with ASD. For older and more advanced children, a "self-as-model" procedure can be used where the client acts as his or her own model. The clinician then edits the video so that only desired behaviors are shown.

Example Profiles

PROFILE 1: MILD IMPAIRMENT—12-YEAR-OLD

Thomas is a 12-year-old boy who was diagnosed with level 1 autism (mild) in second grade. He is enrolled in a seventh-grade general education program, and his academic skills range between average and superior. He tends to answer questions from teachers and others tangentially and in excessive detail. He exhibits difficulty with the rules for initiating conversation and responding appropriately to topics introduced by others. In addition, the teacher and the family report that he consistently interrupts others despite frequent reminders to wait his conversational turn. In general, he does not seem to understand nonverbal cues such as the facial expressions and body language of others. Since childhood, Thomas has had difficulty establishing friendships and has just recently begun to express an awareness of his exclusion from peer groups.

Selection of Therapy Targets and Suggested Intervention Strategies. Based on Thomas's profile, barrier reduction, pragmatic language, and executive function are three main areas selected for intervention. A potential goal for neurodiversity-affirming intervention is to educate Thomas' peers on effective ways to initiate and maintain conversations with him. A potential pragmatic goal is to improve his ability to recognize and interpret nonverbal communication behaviors. For executive function, a primary goal is to improve Thomas's ability to monitor and inhibit/decrease his persistent conversational interruption behaviors. Although several intervention strategies are applicable in this scenario, peer training, social stories, and video modeling may be particularly appropriate.

PROFILE 2: SEVERE IMPAIRMENT—3-YEAR-OLD

Dominic is a 3½-year-old male child who received a diagnosis of level 3 autism (severe) at 2½ years old. He is enrolled in a full-day special education preschool program where he continues to receive services. Dominic displays many classic characteristics of ASD, including the following:

- Extreme social isolation
- Self-stimulatory behaviors and unprovoked aggression toward others

- Frequent echolalia, which may be a combination of communicative and noncommunicative echoes
- Hypersensitivity to tactile stimuli (e.g., hugging, food textures)
- Severe impairment in receptive and expressive language with moderate intellectual impairment
- Excellent rote memory skills
- Somewhat intact visual/spatial skills

Overall, Dominic does not appear to be interested in communicating with others in his environment.

Selection of Therapy Targets and Suggested Intervention Strategies. Based on Dominic's profile, the following are suggested as main targets of intervention:

- Establishing a larger repertoire of functional communication behaviors
- Increasing the frequency of social interactions in the home environment
- Decreasing unwanted and aggressive behaviors

Several intervention approaches may be appropriate in this case. A parent training program may be effective in promoting more frequent social/interpersonal interactions in the home environment (perhaps using PECS symbols). The functional communication therapy (FCT) strategy may be useful in expanding Dominic's repertoire of functional communication behaviors. The combination of these two approaches may yield a reduction in disruptive behaviors.

PROFILE 3: AT-RISK—18-MONTH-OLD

Lilly is an 18-month-old girl with normal hearing who is at risk for ASD based on the results of a recent evaluation. Lilly was referred for the evaluation by her parents, who are concerned that their daughter's development is very different from that of their other children (Larry, age 4 years; Toby, age 6 years). Lilly has a positive family history of ASD; her maternal aunt and uncle were diagnosed with autism during childhood. Based on both parental report and clinical evaluation, Lilly shows inconsistent eye contact with parents, siblings, and other familiar persons. She demonstrates a social smile and joint attention but is difficult to engage in social games such as peek-a-boo or in imitative vocal play, both of which require turn taking. Lilly shows excessive interest in a restricted set of objects and activities, such as her talking monkey and running in and out of a toy house. During the evaluation, some functional play was observed. For example, she kissed a baby doll and when given a toy car, she rolled it on the floor. Her true level of language comprehension was difficult to determine, although below age expectations, as her on-task attention was fleeting and highly distractible. Expressively, Lilly communicated mainly by vocalizations paired with gestures, about half of which the clinician was able to identify as meaningful. Isolated instances of single words (e.g., "no" and "cookie") were noted.

Selection of Therapy Targets and Suggested Intervention Strategies. Based on Lilly's current profile, she would benefit from family-based language stimulation activities implemented in the home environment. The following are recommended as major areas of focus:

- Turn taking

- Increasing ability to follow simple directions

- Expanding repertoire of speech sounds and single words relevant to her daily environment

A naturalistic intervention approach seems most appropriate based on Lilly's age and current communication skills. Materials, activities, and reinforcers found in her daily environment should be emphasized. Reciprocal imitation therapy, Floortime, and SCERTS also may be useful because these strategies advocate for engaging in child-directed play (imitating what the child does) and shaping that interaction into more functional communication behaviors. Lilly's language development and social communication status should be monitored closely, and a reevaluation should be scheduled in 6 months unless specific parental concerns arise.

Helpful Hints

1. From a neurodiversity affirming perspective, it is important that young children are enrolled in early intervention programs that value neurodiversity, rather than programs that prioritize changing the child's behavior to fit neurotypical norms.

2. Include parents and families as full participants on the interdisciplinary team from the beginning of the therapeutic process. Parents, especially keen observers, can provide basic information about their child's preferred and nonpreferred tasks, activities, toys, foods, and so forth. Clinicians also are encouraged to help parents identify and prioritize the behaviors of their child that are most disruptive to the family dynamic at home.

3. Avoid using indirect forms of communication, such as indirect requests (e.g., "That cake sure looks good"); because individuals with ASD have difficulty reading social cues, direct forms of communication generally are more effective (e.g., "Give me some cake, please").

4. Because individuals with ASD learn in situation-specific ways, we cannot expect them to generalize a skill learned in one situation to another context, or even in the same context at a different time of day. Each context may represent a separate behavioral objective.

5. Older students with high-functioning ASD may benefit from joining networking groups where they can share ideas, voice frustrations, and get suggestions from others who have had similar experiences. Alternatively, local groups can be sought that provide opportunities for social interaction and group social activities.

6. High-functioning individuals with ASD may be misdiagnosed as learning disabled (LD) because they share many of the same presenting behaviors. But, inappropriate diagnosis most often results in inappropriate instruction/intervention strategies, especially programming that does not have a central focus on social communication and interaction.

7. Counsel families, teachers, and others who interact with the child on a regular basis that the communication style of individuals with ASD is frequently "too direct," making others uncomfortable. This directness, however, is a sign that these individuals cannot read the social cues of others or the environment.

8. The clinician and family are encouraged to use visual schedules to build predictability into the daily routines of both children and adolescents.

9. Books are helpful to expose children to emotions and feelings in a nonthreatening way. Titles are available across the age/developmental range. Examples include *Taking a Bath with the Dog and Other Things That Make Me Happy* (Scott Menchin), *When Sophie Gets Angry—Really, Really Angry* (Molly Bang), *I'm Mad* (Elizabeth Cray), and *The Way I Feel* (Janice Cain).

10. Many individuals with high-functioning ASD pursue postsecondary education. Clinicians can provide guidance, resources, and encouragement regarding colleges and universities that serve this population or have programs to support their needs.

11. When working with individuals from culturally and linguistically diverse backgrounds, the perceptions/beliefs of family members regarding appropriate social communication are of critical importance.

12. Often as children's intentional communication improves, a decrease may be noted in unwanted/undesirable behaviors. With the significant growth in technology, clinicians are encouraged to explore the availability of computer programs or "apps" that might be useful for children with ASD, particularly with regard to easy portability into the home environment.

Conclusion

This chapter has presented basic information and considerations for ASD issues in intervention at an *introductory* level. This information is intended only as a starting point in the reader's clinical education and training. For in-depth coverage of this area, the following readings are recommended:

Buron, K. D., & Wolfberg, P. (Eds.). (2014). *Learners on the autism spectrum: Preparing highly qualified educators and related practitioners* (2nd ed.). AAPC Publishing.

Murray-Slutsky, C., & Paris, B. A. (2014). *Autism interventions: Exploring the spectrum of autism* (2nd ed.). Hammill Institute on Disabilities.

Prelock, P., & McCauley, R. (Eds.). (2021). *Treatment of autism spectrum disorders: Evidence-based intervention strategies for communication and social interactions (CLI)* (2nd. ed.). Brookes.

Volkmar, F., Rogers, S., Paul, R., & Pelphrey, K. (Eds.). (2014). *Handbook of autism and pervasive developmental disorders* (4th ed.). Wiley.

Additional Resources

Note: There is a wide variety of resources available for addressing autism spectrum disorders. The following list represents a limited number of these resources, with no intended focus on any particular approach to intervention.

Social Communication Disorders in Children: Speech-Language Pathologists Can Help [ASHA Brochure]

This comprehensive brochure is aimed at parents and families who have concerns about the social communication development of their child. It offers suggestions for promoting social interactions and a list of age-appropriate social communication skills for infants through adolescents.

Speech-Language Pathologists and Your Child With Autism [ASHA Brochure]

Parents are the target audience for this brochure, which describes how SLPs can help children diagnosed with ASD to develop social and communication skills. It also provides a checklist of strategies that parents can use in daily interactions with their child.

Autism and PDD Adolescent Social Skills Lessons

This title refers to a series of workbooks, with each workbook targeting a specific skill. These workbooks can be used with individuals in middle school through adulthood, with topics that include social interaction, behavior management, health and hygiene, and vocational skills. Lessons are supported by pictures to facilitate practice of the targeted skills. These lessons aim to provide individuals with the nonverbal and verbal language skills to navigate social situations encountered in daily life.

Autism and PDD Answering Questions

This set of two workbooks is divided by level/difficulty of questions targeted. These workbooks contain visual supports to help individuals on the autism spectrum to process and use more abstract forms of language. Workbook Level 1 is intended for children ages 3 to 5 years and workbook Level 2 is intended for children ages 5 to 9 years. Various question forms are targeted, including "what" questions, "why" questions, and questions targeting problem-solving skills. For more targeted practice on a specific question type (e.g., "why" questions), the *Autism and PPD More Picture Stories and Language Activities* has a series of workbooks that each target a specific question type.

Autism and PDD Early Intervention

This is a series of workbooks that target prelinguistic skills in children ages 1 to 3 years. Topics covered include joint attention, eating routines, dressing routines, and play skills. The lessons focus on the characters of a boy, a girl, and a bear. The lessons and stories target early vocabulary/concepts and support these skills with colorful visuals and sign language images.

Autism and PDD Picture Stories and Language Activities Social Skills

This is a set of five workbooks that cover social skills in a variety of settings (e.g., home, school, community). The lessons are designed to follow a consistent format to facilitate learning and provide a secure, predictable session. These workbooks use the characters of Matt and Molly to engage children in lessons that depict hypothetical events.

Autism and PDD Things I Can Say and Do

This is a series of workbooks that target social skills that pertain to specific contexts or scenarios. The lessons provide individuals with language skills/phrases to use in context-specific communicative exchanges. Organizational tools/worksheets are provided to individualize lessons to each client. Topics/concepts covered include body parts/clothing, feelings and actions, holidays, weather, seasons, and months.

The Autism Spectrum Disorders IEP Companion

This book provides information on some of the common issues related to communication and behavioral skills that arise in the school setting. It gives advice for treatment planning and considerations during the IEP process, including sensory needs, transitions, and classroom and instructional accommodations. Chapters are divided into skill areas (i.e., social pragmatics, communication) and provide examples of goals and objectives.

The Basic Reading Comprehension Kit for Hyperlexia and Autism
For children ages 5 to 12 years, this kit aims to bridge the gap between a child's ability to decode and comprehend what he or she has read. In particular, it provides strategies for visual imaging skills and sequencing skills in order to support the visual learning style of children with ASD.

Practical Theory of Mind Games
For children 4 to 12 years of age, these lessons target inferencing skills pertaining to social situations. This resource is divided into three sections based on the underlying principles of theory of mind (ToM) deficits, stories and games to teach lessons on inference skills, and discussions of the emotional differences between individuals. This resource includes a CD-ROM to access and print the lessons.

Autism Navigator
Autism Navigator is a web-based instructional program developed by the Florida State University Autism Institute to increase the capacity of primary care, early intervention, and other service providers, as well as families, to better serve young children with or at risk for ASD.

The Source for Intervention in Autism Spectrum Disorders
This resource provides information on issues pertaining to ASD, such as related disorders, theory of mind, and learning styles. This information is then used to develop goals and strategies for intervention as well as activities to use with this population. This book provides advice for working with individuals from the toddler years through adulthood and targets expressive/receptive language, literacy skills, behavioral skills, and functional life skills.

Autism and PDD Photo Cards: Wh- Questions
This is a set of 240 photographs to engage students in question-asking/answering interactions. The photos depict scenes and have targets to elicit a question and/or to respond to a question. Picture tasks cover a variety of question types (e.g., "where" questions, "who" questions). Cues and prompts are provided to help with question formulation. This resource can be used with individuals ages 4 to 12 years.

Educating Students With Autism: A Quick Start Manual
This book is meant for educators as well as related service providers, such as SLPs. It contains chapters on topics such as different treatment approaches, strategies for providing structure to daily life, and communication skills to target. It also provides resources for further information on autism as well as the types of support organizations and programs that are available.

Early Start for Young Children With Autism/PDD: Practical Interventions
This is a workbook with information for working with children ages 2 to 5 years. It covers topics such as establishing routines, targeting behavioral issues, implementing visual schedules and calendars, and incorporating play into intervention. The workbook also contains forms that pertain to the lessons and topics covered.

What Do You Say . . . What Do You Do . . . At School?
This board game can be used for children in grades kindergarten through 8 and targets social skills that pertain to the school setting. Skills targeted include reasoning, making inferences, and con-

versational skills. The questions require students to act out situations and verbally problem solve these situations rather than to select an answer from a field of answers. There is a separate game for targeting social skills in the community setting.

"Say and Do" Workbook Series

These workbooks can be used with children in grades kindergarten through 4. The lessons present a social scene and then discuss appropriate versus inappropriate responses/actions for these situations. The scenes depict a variety of situations that a child might encounter, including stores, school, and phone conversations. The titles in the series are as follows: social scenes for home, school, and community; early social scenes for school; and social scenes for daily living skills and feelings.

Simply Social 7 at School

For children in grades 2 through 12, this workbook provides scripted scenarios in order to help children on the autism spectrum to develop social language skills. The workbook targets skills such as conversational skills, turn taking, using and understanding facial expressions, and understanding figurative language. The workbook also includes a social skills checklist to help identify and target each child's pragmatic language needs.

Positive Pragmatic Game Boards

These game boards consist of a set of five double-sided boards, for a total of 10 board games. Each game targets a specific pragmatic language skill. The skills targeted include topic maintenance, making requests, identifying and expressing feelings, and giving information on a specified topic.

Social Skills Quick Take Along

This small, laminated booklet contains 600 questions covering 15 areas within the topic of social language skills. Question sections target areas such as formulating apologies in response to a given situation as well as formulating appropriate utterances in response to given social situations. Its smaller format (5 × 3 in.) is designed for on-the-go use.

Social Thinking (Michelle Garcia Winner)

Social Thinking offers a variety of products and programs for targeting pragmatic language skills. One program, called SuperFlex, consists of a series of comic books with characters that represent various pragmatic behaviors, such as reacting appropriately to situations and perspective-taking skills. The books, including *You are a Social Detective!*, help students to learn about different characters' traits as well as develop strategies for working on social language skills in relation to these difficulties. Another product is a workbook (*A 5 Could Make Me Lose Control!*) that can be used to develop 5-point rating scales to help individuals identify sources of anxiety or frustration as well as strategies to mediate these feelings.

Chapter 7

Intervention for Adult Aphasia With Introduction to Traumatic Brain Injury

The majority of this chapter covers adult aphasia, which is a language-based disorder. In addition, an overview of traumatic brain injury (TBI) is provided. Dementia and right-hemisphere dysfunction are beyond the scope of this chapter. Selected references are provided at the end of this chapter for readers interested in these topics.

Aphasia

Aphasia is a language disorder due to brain damage that results in impairment in the comprehension and/or formulation of language and can affect both the spoken and written modalities. The major cause of aphasia is stroke due to hemorrhage or blockage of blood flow to the brain. Strokes are also referred to as cerebrovascular accidents (CVAs). Other etiologies include tumors, head trauma, and certain disease processes, such as encephalitis. According to the National Institute on Deafness and Other Communication Disorders (NIDCD), in the United States, there are 180,000 new aphasia cases a year, and 1 of every 272 Americans are affected with aphasia. Approximately one-third of the cases are attributed to cerebrovascular accidents. The most common type is global aphasia. There is an equal incidence of aphasia caused by CVA between men and women. However, the incidence is age dependent. Those younger than 65 years old have a 15% chance of being affected compared to those older than 85 years old, who have a 43% chance of developing the condition. Overall, 25% to 40% of stroke survivors develop aphasia due to damage to the language-processing regions of the brain.

Aphasia is associated with damage to the dominant hemisphere for language in the brain, which is the left hemisphere in most individuals. It frequently is accompanied by motor and sensory deficits. As the left hemisphere controls the contralateral (or opposite) side of the body, these motor and sensory impairments are most often right-sided in individuals with aphasia. Common motor impairments are **hemiplegia** or **hemiparesis**, paralysis or weakness on one side of the body, respectively. **Hemianopsia** is a visual field deficit in which an individual cannot see to the right or left of midline in one or both eyes. (Other pertinent medical terms are located in the Glossary in Appendix C on the companion website.)

Classification of Aphasia Syndromes

Historically, there has been an enormous amount of effort devoted to the classification of aphasic types and syndromes. This work has resulted in the development of several different approaches to classification, including site of lesion taxonomies (e.g., Goodglass et al., 2001; Kertesz, 1979), linguistic structure paradigms (Jakobson, 1964), and modality-oriented systems that address behavioral symptoms of language impairment (e.g., Schuell et al., 1964). A detailed discussion of the similarities and differences among the various aphasia taxonomies is beyond the scope of this chapter.

(See Chapey [2008] for comprehensive reviews of classification issues and approaches.) From a treatment-oriented perspective, we find it clinically useful to adopt the Boston group's (Goodglass et al., 2001; Raymer & Rothi, 2017) approach to classification, which includes two main categories of aphasia: nonfluent and fluent. This classification system is based on quality of output and involves both oral and written modalities. Within each category, the degree of severity may range from mild to profound.

The profile of **nonfluent aphasias** is one of poor output with relatively spared comprehension. It generally is characterized by reduced vocabulary; agrammatism; and impairments of articulation, rate, and prosody (rhythm, stress, and intonation)—resulting in labored and effortful production.

Fluent aphasia consists of impairment in language comprehension with maintenance of normal melodic speech contour. The main characteristics are word-retrieval difficulties, paraphasias (phonemic and semantic), neologisms, perseveration, and the maintenance of normal melodic speech contour.

Definitions of key terms related to language deficits in aphasia are presented in Table 7–1. The major categories of fluent and nonfluent aphasia can be further divided into selected subtypes, as

Table 7–1
Terminology Related to Language Deficits in Aphasia

Term	Definition
Agrammatism	Syntactic deficit characterized by omission of function words and grammatical inflections. Semantic aspects of language remain intact. Speech output consists primarily of content words. Example: When asked to describe a picture of a picnic with someone sleeping in a hammock, the client responds, "Food … man bed … he sleep."
Word-retrieval problems	Difficulty accessing a word from one's mental vocabulary. Severe naming difficulty is termed **anomia**. Example: When asked to name a hammock in a picture, the client responds, "It's to sleep in … under trees … you know, with a rope."
Paraphasia	Errors in speech output characterized by the production of unintended sounds, syllables, or words. The two main types are phonemic and semantic. **Phonemic paraphasias** (also known as literal paraphasias) consist of *extraneous* or *transposed* sounds and syllables or *substitution* of one correctly articulated phoneme for another. Example: When asked to name a hammock in a picture, the client may respond with one of the following: "hammerock," "hackamm," "pammock," respectively. **Semantic paraphasias** involve unintended substitution of one word for another, usually within the same semantic category. Example: When asked to name a hammock, the client responds, "It's a bed."
Neologism	Invented word that has no true meaning but adheres to the phonological rules of a given language. These errors tend to occur primarily with nouns and verbs rather than function words. Example: When asked to name a hammock in a picture, the client responds, "That's a blick."
Perseveration	Inappropriate continuation of a response after the presentation of a new stimulus. Example: After successfully naming a hammock in a picture, the client continues to respond "hammock" when shown the next three pictures of a chair, key, and glove.

shown in Table 7–2. Note: Odd language use is not restricted to adults with communication disorders. The following instances are examples from a typical adult that have been observed by or reported to the authors (F. Roth, personal communication, October 15, 2014). Some of the examples are spontaneous comments, while others are portions of conversations:

- In the context of techs working on fixing a website, "They have to create a new aneurysm" (intended meaning = algorithm).

- "Killing two eggs with one stone."

- Speaker A: "I don't like this soup because it is immoral."

  Speaker B: "How can any soup be immoral?"

  Speaker A: "I should have said Swanson. Immoral is a famous chef." (intended meaning of Immoral = Emeril).

- "I've been running around like a chicken without a hat . . . no wait . . . that's not right. I've been running around like a chicken without an egg."

Table 7–2
Classification of Aphasia Syndromes

Syndrome Type	Characteristics
Nonfluent Aphasias	
Broca's	Agrammatism; effortful articulation of phrase-length utterances; impaired prosody and intonation; concomitant apraxia of speech; good comprehension; lesion in the posterior inferior frontal lobe, as well as central and inferior parietal regions
Transcortical motor	Little to no initiation of spontaneous speech; output similar to Broca's but excellent imitation (even of long utterances); relatively intact comprehension; lesion in the medial-frontal cortex, involving the supplementary motor area
Global	Severe deficits in all areas of language comprehension and production; output may be limited to stereotypic utterances; lesion encompasses both pre- and postrolandic speech zones
Fluent Aphasias	
Wernicke's	Fluent but often meaningless speech (jargon); impaired comprehension; good articulation, intonation, and prosody; lesion in the posterior portion of the first temporal gyrus of the left hemisphere
Conduction	Relatively fluent speech; frequent phonemic paraphasias; marked difficulty with imitation; good language comprehension; lesion in the arcuate fasciculus, deep supramarginal gyrus, or superior temporal gyrus
Anomic	Significant word-finding difficulties in the presence of otherwise fluent and grammatical speech; good comprehension; lesion in the angular gyrus region

Source: Adapted from *Introduction to Communication Disorders* (3rd ed.), by M. N. Hegde, 2001, Austin, TX: Pro-Ed.

- "Wow, you live close away."

- Speaker A: "He's not the brightest bulb in the . . . What's that saying?"

  Speaker B: "You mean 'drawer'?"

  Speaker A: "No, that's silly."

Treatment Efficacy/Evidence-Based Practice

As part of the natural recovery process, the brain regains some of its speech, language, and motor functions after an injury. The greatest amount of this **spontaneous recovery** occurs during the first two to three months. However, changes may continue to be noted for a period of up to 1 year after onset. Following the period of spontaneous recovery, individuals may demonstrate varying degrees of gradual improvement, in some cases months or years after the initial brain injury. Several factors influence the degree of spontaneous early recovery and ultimate prognosis (Basso, 2018; Yamajai & Maeshima, 2021). These include the size, location, and etiology of the lesion; type and severity of the initial aphasia (particularly verbal comprehension); age at onset; and overall health of the client (Kertesz, 1979; Kertesz & McCabe, 1977; Kiran & Thompson, 2019; Pedersen et al., 2004). The most predictive indicator of long-term recovery is initial aphasia severity, along with lesion site and size (Plowman et al., 2011). In general, lesions located in the temporoparietal region are associated with a poorer prognosis. Studies also indicate that hemorrhagic strokes have a more remarkable recovery pattern than those due to blockage of cerebral blood flow (i.e., embolism or thrombosis). As a rule, prognosis is more favorable for younger clients and for those without additional medical problems. During spontaneous recovery, the initial aphasia syndrome may evolve into a different (usually milder) classification type.

Historically, there has been controversy over the efficacy of aphasia therapy. Some studies have suggested that any objective improvement seen in a client's status is attributable to the brain's spontaneous recovery rather than a result of treatment effects (e.g., Sarno et al., 1970). Others contend that aphasia treatment results in measurable gains in communicative functioning through both traditional and group treatment models (e.g., Elman & Bernstein-Ellis, 1999; Wertz et al., 1981). Evidence indicates that speech and language treatment is effective in improving discourse (Dipper et al., 2021) as well as receptive and expressive language skills in individuals with stroke-induced aphasia (Brady et al., 2012; Teasell, 2018; Zheng, Lynch, & Taylor, 2016). In part, this controversy is a result of methodological problems associated with obtaining matched subject samples and the ethical dilemma of withholding treatment from individuals assigned to control-group conditions.

To confound the issue further, disagreement also exists regarding the optimal time to initiate therapy. The main source of contention is whether to initiate therapy immediately or wait until the spontaneous recovery process has run its course. The available data do not adequately solve the problem of separating spontaneous recovery changes from treatment effects. Several studies have reported that delaying initiation of treatment had no significant negative impact on client progress (Sarno & Levita, 1971; Sarno et al., 1970; Wertz et al., 1986). However, most clinicians advocate early intervention based on the premise that treatment may serve to accelerate the natural process of spontaneous recovery.

Holland et al. (1996) and Robey (1998) conducted major systematic reviews of aphasia treatment efficacy and concluded that aphasia therapy is efficacious in that treated clients make significantly more improvement than untreated clients. More recent literature reviews on treatment efficacy have been reported by Brady et al. (2022), Doogan et al. (2018), and Stahl et al. (2018). Overall findings include positive evidence for the following:

Age: Individuals under the age of 65 years tend to make greater gains in therapy

Intensity: An overall total of 20 to 50 intervention hours resulted in more positive outcomes

Duration: Continuation of intervention beyond a 4-week period may contribute substantially to improved recovery

Maintenance: Longer term gains in therapy were noted for individuals with diagnoses in the milder range of aphasia and with no accompanying deficits in executive functioning.

Some researchers argue that early intervention targeting linguistic tasks (e.g., semantics, phonology) benefits individuals with aphasia more than deferring treatment (Nouwens et al., 2013). Moreover, it is posited that the focus on linguistic tasks rather than functional communication tasks increases blood flow to linguistic regions of the brain, thus supporting communicative gains in these areas early on in the recovery process (Nouwens et al., 2013). The systematic review of semantic feature therapy by Efstratiadou et al. (2018) concluded that semantic feature analysis is effective intervention, particularly with moderate or mild fluent aphasia.

In addition to the question of when to commence treatment, research also has been conducted to investigate the optimal duration for treatment. In a meta-analysis of research studies on treatment gains with chronic aphasia, several studies yielded evidence supporting the continuation of treatment beyond the early intervention phases for gains in communication skills as well as executive function skills (Korner-Bitensky, 2013). Further support for ongoing intervention was found in a 2011 study of individuals with chronic aphasia in Italy. Researchers found evidence that if therapy is intensive enough, gains can be noted even in cases of chronic aphasia (Basso & Macis, 2011). Raymer et al. (2008) also reviewed literature that found greater gains from continued treatment of aphasia versus dismissal from treatment. It was purported that treatment often is discontinued too early and/or is not intensive enough with cases of chronic aphasia (Basso & Macis, 2011). As individuals with chronic aphasia will have long-term deficits, the authors stressed the role of caregivers in providing language stimulation and daily practice for maintenance of therapeutic gains (Basso & Macis, 2011).

In summary, evidence indicates that speech-language treatment is effective in improving communication and receptive/expressive language skills in individuals with stroke-induced aphasia.

Treatment for Aphasia

The overall goal of aphasia therapy is to improve a client's communication skills to the highest degree possible within the constraints of the neurological damage. The majority of individuals with aphasia will experience at least some residual language deficits throughout their lifetimes. For this reason, clinicians must decide when to shift the focus of treatment from a "cure" to a "care" orientation. The goal of treatment changes from recovery of premorbid language skills to establishing compensatory/maintenance strategies for functional language skills (Teasell et al., 2016). To devise an appropriate and effective intervention program, the clinician must have thorough knowledge of prognostic variables as well as familiarity with the most predictable patterns of recovery that are associated with the different aphasia subtypes (Ellis & Urban, 2016). For example, one common recovery pattern is for a global aphasia to evolve into a chronic Broca's aphasia. Few well-designed studies evaluate aphasia therapy in terms of optimal frequency, duration, or the relative value of different methods. This is especially true in the area of fluent aphasia (Brady et al., 2016). Therefore, SLPs should design intervention programs in accordance with individual clients' presenting clinical profiles as well as premorbid status factors such as intellectual level, education, and reading ability. In addition, cultural and linguistic differences should be considered across instructional and interpersonal aspects of therapy. Very few individuals with aphasia are completely unable to comprehend auditory information, and, conversely, few have perfectly preserved auditory comprehension skills. The goal of the SLP is to recognize both spared areas of function in clients with severe aphasia and subtle areas of weakness in clients with mild aphasia.

Neuroplasticity

Another factor to consider when planning intervention is neuroplasticity, the brain's ability to restructure its neural networks in response to internal and external stimuli. Neuroplasticity is associated with learning in the intact brain and thus relearning in cases of brain damage (Kleim & Jones, 2008). Neural rewiring can manifest itself in several different ways. For example, neural regions adjacent to the lesion may adopt some of the functions attributed to the affected area. In addition, right-hemisphere sites that parallel the affected left-hemisphere areas may start performing functions once attributed to the lesioned area (Kiran et al., 2019; Torres et al., 2013; Wilson & Schneck, 2020). Focusing on brains with damaged tissue, Kleim and Jones (2008) provide a summary of the research on neuroplasticity by outlining 10 principles that can be used to inform treatment plans in relation to speech-language therapy.

One component of neuroplasticity that is currently being debated involves the severity of the brain damage. Although limited, there are some studies that provide evidence for neuroplasticity occurring even in cases of severely damaged tissue. In a study examining brain-stimulation techniques, two patients with substantial lesions corresponding to global aphasia showed behavioral changes from intervention (Galletta et al., 2016). In addition, Johansson's (2011) literature review of melodic intonation therapy (MIT) that shows gains made by patients with severe nonfluent aphasia were a result of MIT intervention.

Neuroplasticity Principle	Relation to Speech-Language Therapy
1. Use it or lose it	Because damage to neural connections has occurred, intervention tasks should target these damaged connections to stimulate that area of the brain to promote the restructuring of these areas as well as to prevent further degradation.
2. Use it to improve it	This principle purports that neuroplasticity can be induced through activities that target damaged neural regions and that this practice can improve a person's ability with the targeted skill.
3. Specificity matters	Specificity refers both to the neural region where change is expected and to the task being trained. Because it is a damaged brain, the process of learning is different from typical learning. Thus, neural changes are often limited and noted strictly in relation to the targeted task rather than being widespread in nature, impacting associated tasks/neural regions.
4. Repetition matters	Repetition of a targeted skill is important to both establishing the behavioral change and neural remodeling as well as to helping to maintain the change.

Neuroplasticity Principle	Relation to Speech-Language Therapy
5. Intensity matters	It is important to note that it is possible for intervention to be too intense and thus negatively impact the client's progress, especially early on in the process. However, this principle provides evidence that the greater the intensity (e.g., the number of trials), the greater the long-term effect of the intervention. Treatment schedules can be altered during the recovery process, starting off slowly in the acute phase and increasing in intensity as the patient enters the chronic phase (Raymer et al., 2008).
6. Time matters	Because neural remodeling occurs spontaneously after damage to the brain, consideration must be given for when to commence treatment. Indeed, evidence from animal studies has demonstrated that early intervention can have a negative impact if too intense (Raymer et al., 2008). However, intervention can be viewed as augmenting and directing the neural restructuring already under way. Although not conclusive, early intervention seems to be effective, especially in preventing further loss of skills.
7. Salience matters	The relevance of the activities and targeted skills to the client's daily life is an important factor in promoting therapeutic gains; without motivation, the client is likely to be less engaged in therapy and the neural response will not be as great.
8. Age matters	Because atrophy naturally occurs in typically aging brains, the age at which a person experiences brain damage may have implications for the level of decline that he or she is already experiencing. However, other factors, such as mental and physical status preinsult, are important to consider when setting goals, projecting progress, and identifying treatment outcomes.
9. Transference matters	This principle refers to rewiring that is noted in one neural region as a result of targeted plasticity in a related region. Planning intervention to target more complex stimuli can also result in transference within a given linguistic skill area. For example, targeting complex stimuli (e.g., atypical items in a categorization task, such as penguin and ostrich for the bird category) facilitates learning of less complex stimuli within the same category (e.g., robin, eagle; Raymer et al., 2008). In addition to changes transferring from one neural region to another, an individual's abilities (e.g., cognitive status) preinsult can transfer and influence the progression of recovery.
10. Interference matters	There are several ways in which intervention and/or the individual's actions may induce plasticity that does not have a positive effect on the individual's recovery. For example, an individual may develop compensatory strategies that are not as sophisticated or efficient as the original skill. Further, attempts to rewire one skill may interfere with the neural networks underlying a different skill.

Sources: Adapted from "Principles of Experience-Dependent Neural Plasticity: Implications for Rehabilitation After Brain Damage," by J. A. Kleim and T. A. Jones, 2008, *Journal of Speech, Language, and Hearing Research*, 51(1), S225–S239; "Translational Research in Aphasia: From Neuroscience to Neurorehabilitation," by A. M. Raymer et al., 2008, *Journal of Speech, Language, and Hearing Research*, 51, 259–275.

Theoretical Orientations to Aphasia Treatment

There are two main theoretical orientations to aphasia treatment:

1. **Restorative/linguistic:** This model of intervention is based on the assumption that an aphasic individual's linguistic knowledge has been disrupted, and these skills can be strengthened or restored through direct instruction (Murray & Clark, 2006). The main emphasis of this approach is intensive and repeated participation in therapy activities to improve compromised linguistic functions (e.g., syntax, word finding, and phonology). It encompasses both comprehension and production of oral and written language targets. Restorative therapy techniques are frequently referred to using the terms *neuropsychological* or *neurolinguistic* (Chapey, 2008).

2. **Substitutive/compensatory:** This approach is based on the premise that language function has been lost in individuals with aphasia. However, the focus of therapy is on establishing functional communication. The procedures are designed to encourage use of whatever modalities are available to the individual to convey messages successfully to listeners (Davis, 2007; Davis & Wilcox, 1981; Simmons-Mackie, 2001, 2008). These may include speaking, gesturing, signing, writing, facial expressions, drawing, and so on. The focus of this "consequence-oriented" model is on the tasks and responsibilities of everyday living and resuming a role in society (Holland, 2008). The selection of functional therapy goals can be guided by the communicative behaviors identified in the Functional Assessment of Communication Skills developed by the American Speech-Language-Hearing Association (Frattali et al., 2003). This framework specifies 43 communicative behaviors that are grouped according to four domains: (a) social communication; (b) basic needs; (c) reading, writing, and number concepts; and (d) daily planning. Therapy goals also can be selected based on the functional endpoints of aphasia treatment suggested by Holland (1995), which are outlined in Table 7–3. The unit of analysis in this treatment paradigm is always the communicative effectiveness within the dyad (speaker + listener) rather than the client as an individual.

In summary, the restorative/linguistic model targets specific impairments in the linguistic system, whereas the substitutive/compensatory model focuses on the successful exchange of communicative messages rather than the form of those messages. Clinicians are encouraged to use whatever combination of these approaches is best suited to individual clients. In addition, a promising new direction in aphasia treatment is the use of pharmacotherapy. This approach uses drug treatment to restore equilibrium to disrupted neurotransmitter systems, which in turn should facilitate linguistic/cognitive recovery (Cahana-Amitay et al., 2013; Murray & Clark, 2006; Steele, 2009). This approach is generally used in conjunction with other forms of aphasia intervention.

Guidelines for Programming and Implementing Therapy

Therapy may focus on improving a client's abilities in listening, speaking, reading, and writing. In the restorative/linguistic model, intervention is programmed according to hierarchies of difficulty (refer to Chapter 1 for detailed information on basic therapy programming). The hierarchies are based on neurolinguistic research that has explored how adults with and without aphasia comprehend and produce language (e.g., Berndt et al., 1997; Goodglass & Wingfield, 1998; Hillis & Newhart, 2008; Mitchum & Berndt, 2008). Following is a sample hierarchy for the selection and sequencing

Table 7–3
Long-Term Functional Goals for Aphasia Therapy

---

1. Communicate to obtain assistance in emergency situations.
   Example: Call 911.

2. Express feelings.
   Example: Make attitudes and emotions known.

3. Convey basic needs.
   Example: Communicate hunger, thirst, fatigue.

4. Follow simple directions.
   Example: Set alarm clock.

5. Engage in social relationships or situations.
   Example: Enjoy social interactions to the degree commensurate with preaphasia status.

6. Declare autonomy and independence through action, thought, or opinion.
   Example: Indicate disagreement or difference of opinion.

7. Resume activities that were pleasurable prior to onset of aphasia.
   Example: Enjoy hobbies or grandchildren.

8. Take on some routine responsibility.
   Example: Put out trash, water plants.

9. Keep up with news events.
   Example: Read headlines, watch TV news.

10. Function as an individual independent of the aphasic impairment at least for brief time periods.
    Example: Attend a concert or sports event.

Source: Adapted from *Current Realities of Aphasia Rehabilitation: Time Constraints, Documentation Demands, and Functional Outcomes*, by A. Holland, 1995, paper presented at Mid-America Rehabilitation Hospital, Overland Park, KS.

of therapy targets in the area of verbal expression. This general therapeutic progression also can be applied to each of the other language modalities (listening, reading, and writing).

1. Intervention may begin at the nonverbal level by establishing pointing responses.

2. Single-word tasks that target word retrieval can then be introduced in the form of responsive or confrontation naming. In **responsive naming**, a clinician provides a verbal descriptive phrase to elicit a target label (e.g., "The object that we use to sweep the floor is called a _____"). A **confrontation naming** task is more difficult because it requires the client to name a visual stimulus (e.g., picture or object) without any contextual support.

3. Phrase-length responses can then be targeted through sentence completion activities that require the client to fill in a word or phrase that accurately completes a sentence stem.

4. Finally, sentence-level formulation may be required, in which a client might be asked to describe pictures or the function of objects or respond to direct questions posed by the clinician.

This hierarchy of difficulty focuses on utterance length as the critical factor. However, aphasia therapy entails much more than simply increasing the length of a target response. Several factors can be manipulated while maintaining the same response length. For example, a clinician may decrease the amount of support provided in the form of modeling, cues, and prompts to encourage a client to become a more independent communicator. In addition, therapy can be designed to elicit responses at more sophisticated levels of linguistic complexity (e.g., maintaining a phrase-length response while moving from literal language forms to figurative forms such as idioms, metaphors, and humor). At the single-word level, more complex language forms such as antonyms and synonyms can be elicited through the use of word association tasks. Further, the latency between clinician stimulus and client response also can be manipulated. Once the accuracy of a target behavior has been established, task difficulty can be boosted by increasing the speed of the expected response without altering either the length or linguistic complexity of the utterance. In contrast, preliminary data from single-subject research on individuals with agrammatic aphasia suggest that generalization of sentence production is facilitated when the direction of therapy progresses from more complex to less complex syntactic structures (Thompson et al., 2003).

Another important component of intervention programming for aphasia is the use of **group therapy** as well as individual sessions (Elman, 2007). An ideal model allows a client to learn new communication behaviors in individual sessions and provides group settings for opportunities to practice and expand these skills in an interactional situation. Group settings also provide a milieu in which clients can socialize and identify with peers who have problems similar to their own. In addition to therapy groups, intervention for aphasia often includes group sessions for family training and counseling. Family members can facilitate the aphasic individual's everyday communication performance by learning and implementing the techniques used by the clinician in therapy sessions. Family counseling is an essential aspect of aphasia therapy. Families may require guidance about how to talk to the affected family member. Specific suggestions are provided in Appendix 7–A on the companion website. Of all communication disorders, aphasia is the one that causes the most severe adjustment problems for families because of its sudden and abrupt onset. Virtually overnight, a family member experiences dramatic changes in health and personality as well as in the ability to communicate.

Finally, one common technique used with clients who present with word-retrieval deficits is **self-cueing**. These are strategies that can be used by a client to trigger the verbal production of a specific word and include the following:

- Automatic sequences (e.g., days of the week)

- Paired verbal associates (e.g., bread and _____ [*butter*])

- Sentence completion (e.g., We use a broom to sweep the _____ [*floor*])

- Idiomatic expressions (e.g., Look before you _____ [*leap*])

- Alternative words (e.g., synonyms and antonyms)

- Rhyming words (e.g., sounds like *fall*)

- Phonemic cues (e.g., initial sound/syllable of target word)

- Writing the initial letter, syllable, or entire word

- Subordinate category cues (e.g., Pizza and hot dogs are types of _____ [*food*])

- Air tracing (i.e., writing a word in the air with one's finger)

- Gesture or pantomime cues (e.g., pretending to drink from a cup)

- Object or action attributes (e.g., asking questions such as "Which one is sharp?" and "Which one is slow?" about two or more pictures)

Consider three approaches when planning intervention for aphasia: therapist controlled, therapist led, and patient focused (Leach et al., 2010). The main factor that differentiates these approaches is the amount of contribution from the clinician versus the individual with aphasia and his or her family members. Leach et al. (2010) advocate for a patient-focused approach when possible, because this approach has been found to have a positive impact on the client's motivation and achievement of goals. A patient-focused approach also provides insight into the types of skills that are priorities for intervention. Survey results of 50 poststroke individuals with aphasia revealed a variety of highly desired intervention goals, including the ability to communicate needs and opinions, an increase in autonomy, the ability to return to social and work activities, and the ability to participate in volunteer work and to help others (Worrall et al., 2011). Patient education is stressed as an important component of intervention, especially in terms of setting realistic goals and understanding the rationale for therapeutic activities (Leach et al., 2010).

Specific Intervention Procedures

Numerous procedures have been used in the rehabilitation of individuals with aphasia. This section briefly describes several of the most common programs identified in the clinical research literature.

Constraint-Induced Language Therapy
(Pulvermuller et al., 2001; Pulvermuller et al., 2005)

Note: Some studies refer to this approach as constraint-induced aphasia therapy (CIAT).

Constraint-induced language therapy (CILT) is a promising intervention strategy that is currently undergoing substantial clinical study. CILT is specifically beneficial for individuals with stroke-induced aphasia, although results are considered preliminary (Mozeiko et al., 2018; Pierce et al., 2019; Zhang et al., 2017). It is a restorative/linguistic approach and is built on three main principles:

1. Massed practice (intensive therapy over a relatively short period of consecutive days, such as 30 hr of practice over a 2-week period)

2. Shaping by successive approximation (presenting tasks in small steps of gradually increasing linguistic difficulty within natural communication contexts)

3. Constraint (restriction of the client's use of any compensatory/nonverbal communication strategies)

Although CILT requires intensive intervention, there is evidence that its emphasis on verbal communication is of equal importance in attaining communicative gains (Raymer et al., 2008; Wang et al., 2020). In addition, studies indicate that family involvement in this therapeutic intervention is especially important for generalization of linguistic gains; thus, family and caregivers are encouraged to monitor and to remind individuals to use verbal means for communication throughout daily communicative exchanges (Johansson, 2011).

In contrast, Rose (2013) presented evidence that gestures and other modalities should not be constrained in therapy and daily communication. This opposing view is based on several properties of gestures within the context of language and communication:

- Gestures are not viewed as an arbitrary component of communication; rather, gestures are posited to contribute to language production through means such as helping an individual to retrieve words and thus to maintain fluency.

- Neurological representations of language are not discrete from motor and sensory domains in the brain; thus, the neurological overlap can be targeted to promote gains in each system.

- Studies have found that people with aphasia tend to utilize gestures more frequently in their communicative interactions than people who do not have aphasia.

- Avoidance or targeted nonuse of a skill can have a negative impact on this skill; thus, it may be more difficult for an individual with aphasia to utilize gestures or other modalities in the future if they have gone extended periods avoiding these skills.

Stimulation Facilitation *(Schuell et al., 1964)*

Stimulation facilitation is not a specific procedure but rather a general approach to aphasia treatment that incorporates the basic principles of competent intervention (Coelho et al., 2008). Specific characteristics of this approach, as advocated by Schuell et al., are as follows: (a) the focus of therapy is intensive auditory stimulation to elicit language; (b) a client's incorrect responses are met with increased stimulation rather than corrective feedback; (c) the highest possible number of responses should be elicited in each session; (d) target behaviors are elicited through continual repetition of the clinician's stimulus rather than via direct instruction; and (e) therapy tasks are focused mainly on the semantic and syntactic components of the linguistic system.

Melodic Intonation Therapy *(Albert et al., 1973)*

Melodic intonation therapy (MIT) is a restorative/linguistic technique that utilizes "intoning" to facilitate verbal expression in clients who demonstrate severely restricted verbal output and relatively good speech comprehension. This approach uses variations in pitch, tempo/rhythm, and stress to recruit participation of the right hemisphere to improve verbal production in clients with damage to the language-dominant left hemisphere (García-Casares et al., 2022; Haro-Martínez et al., 2021; Marchina et al., 2023; Slavin & Fabus, 2018). The MIT program consists of a 15-step hierarchy (Helm-Estabrooks & Albert, 2004; Helm-Estabrooks & Holland, 1998; Sparks, 2001; Sparks & Holland, 1976), which is presented in a condensed form as follows:

1. Client taps out rhythm while listening to clinician's hummed and intoned utterance.

2. Client and clinician intone utterance in unison.

3. Clinician fades out of unison production.

4. Client independently imitates clinician's model of intoned utterance.

5. Client's response is no longer intoned but produced in unison with exaggerated inflection and then gradually shaped to approximate more normal speech prosody.

6. Clinician fades out of unison production.

7. Client independently imitates clinician's model of spoken utterance.

8. Client fades imitative response and spontaneously produces the spoken utterance in response to clinician questions.

MIT generally begins with utterances consisting of two and three-syllable words and short, commonly used phrases. Longer and more complex utterances are gradually introduced at later stages in the program. Each step in the program has specific scoring procedures. At all levels of stimulus difficulty, it is recommended that the utterance should be produced slowly and with continuous voicing.

The most suitable candidates for MIT are aphasic individuals who demonstrate the following characteristics:

- Unilateral stroke in the left frontal lobe (Broca's area), often extending to the parietal region

- Severely limited verbal output with poor speech articulation

- Extremely poor speech imitation skills

- Relatively spared comprehension of verbal input

- Emotionally stable with good attention span

MIT is not the only therapeutic approach based on shared neurologic pathways for speech and singing. Magee et al. (2017) and Tomaino (2012) discuss several other therapeutic strategies that can be used along with MIT to help individuals with nonfluent aphasia:

- *Familiar songs:* The practice of singing a familiar song can be used to transfer gains made in singing rhythm to speech rhythm. Clinicians also can use familiar lyrics as a cloze task, singing the first part of the lyric and pausing for the patient to fill in the end of the lyric. In addition to familiar lyrics, a familiar melody can be paired with common social phrases (e.g., How are you?) to assist patients with the fluent production of the phrases.

- *Breathing exercises:* The use of controlled exhalations can help patients to produce speech sounds and simple syllables. This strategy uses any breathing pattern that is intact and accessible to patients, such as yawning or sighing, to facilitate speech productions.

- *Oral-motor exercises:* The provision of exaggerated models of the oral-motor movements needed to produce lyrics and/or targeted phrases, with the patient imitating the movements while repeating the phrases.

Gesture and Naming Therapy (Caute et al., 2013; Marshall et al., 2012; Rose et al., 2017)

Two modalities are discretely targeted during intervention with this treatment approach: gesture and verbal modalities. If deemed necessary, the written modality can be used in place of the verbal modality based on individual ability. Treatment follows the same hierarchy for both modalities, with equal time given to each during a therapy session:

1. Recognition-level tasks are used in the initial phase of therapy, with individuals associating gestures and/or words with corresponding pictures.

2. Production-level tasks initially require the individual with aphasia to produce gestures/ words corresponding to a picture presented by the therapist.

3. Higher level production tasks require the individual with aphasia to produce targets that are not known by the clinician and that the clinician must then identify from a field of (a) nonrelated targets and then (b) related targets.

Gestural Program: *Visual Action Therapy* (Helm-Estabrooks & Albert, 2004)

Visual action therapy (VAT) is a substitutive/compensatory approach to aphasia intervention that enhances an individual's functional communication skills through the use of representational gestures rather than speech. This nonvocal strategy, designed for severely impaired or globally aphasic individuals, focuses on the production of messages at the single-gesture level. VAT is a hierarchically structured three-level program that utilizes objects, realistic line drawings of the objects, and action pictures depicting a figure appropriately manipulating the objects. Ultimately, the client progresses from matching pictures and objects to the spontaneous use of symbolic hand/arm or mouth/face gestures to communicate simple messages. Currently, there are three VAT program variations: (a) **proximal limb** (focuses on gestures composed of gross movements of the shoulder, arms, and fingers; e.g., sawing), (b) **distal limb** (focuses on gestures composed of finer movements of the hand and fingers; e.g., turning a screwdriver), and (c) **bucco-facial** (focuses on gestures composed of movements of the mouth and face; e.g., whistling). All three VAT variations follow the same basic training sequence, summarized as follows:

1. Client matches and then points to objects and pictures in seven-way discrimination tasks.

2. Client is taught to demonstrate appropriate use of each object through clinician modeling and shaping until spontaneous performance is achieved.

3. Clinician points to a specific action picture and client is required to pick up the corresponding object from an array of seven and demonstrate its use.

4. Client locates or points to a specific object from an array of seven in response to pantomime gestures produced by the clinician.

5. Client is required to produce an appropriate pantomime gesture when shown each of the seven objects.

6. Client is shown two randomly selected objects, which are then hidden; one object is then returned to view and the client is encouraged to self-initiate the correct gesture for the one that remains hidden.

In subsequent levels of this technique, the use of real objects is discontinued. Pantomime gestures and action pictures are utilized as stimuli. Appropriate candidates for VAT demonstrate the following characteristics:

Limb VAT (Proximal/Distal)	Bucco-Facial VAT
Unilateral damage to left hemisphere, especially anterior language areas	Unilateral damage to left hemisphere, especially primary language zones
Global aphasia, severe impairments, relatively intact verbal comprehension modalities, moderate to severe limb apraxia	Severely impaired verbal output in spoken and written language
Alert and cooperative with good attention span	Alert and cooperative with good attention span

Promoting Aphasics' Communicative Effectiveness
(Davis, 1993; Davis & Wilcox, 1981)

Promoting aphasics' communicative effectiveness (PACE) is another example of a substitutive/ compensatory approach to aphasia intervention. Therapy is conducted in the context of naturalistic conversation between the clinician and client. The goal is to improve a client's ability to convey intended messages using whatever means of communication available to the individual. In 1981, Davis and Wilcox identified four principles that underlie the implementation of PACE:

1. The clinician and client are to be egalitarian communication partners and take an equal number of turns as speaker and listener. The purpose is to create an interaction pattern that adheres to the turn-taking rules of everyday conversation. It also provides a built-in, natural mechanism for the clinician to model a range of appropriate communication styles that the client can incorporate into subsequent messages.

2. The messages that are communicated must contain new information rather than information that is already known to both communication partners. This requirement encourages the speaker to reformulate or revise messages that initially meet with listener confusion.

3. Messages can be exchanged using any vocal or nonvocal modality or combinations of modalities.

4. The clinician provides feedback regarding the communicative effectiveness of messages conveyed by the client; errors in linguistic form of messages are not addressed.

Implementation of these four principles is accomplished through a picture description task in which the clinician and client take turns acting as the sender of a message. The designated sender chooses one picture from a face-down pile (being careful to keep it from the listener's view) and describes it using any available communication modalities. Unlike most intervention programming, PACE requires that the clinician be unaware of the specific stimulus items selected by the client from the pile. The aim of this task is for the speaker to successfully transmit the intended information to the listener.

PACE is a flexible treatment technique that has been used with individuals with various types and degrees of aphasia. These include both fluent aphasic and nonfluent aphasic adults. According to Davis and Wilcox (1981), the pragmatic orientation of PACE makes it a suitable component of any aphasia treatment program regardless of the severity of linguistic impairment.

Script Training *(Cherney, Halper, et al., 2008; Holland & Ramage, 2004; Youmans et al., 2005)*

This approach is based on the instance theory of automatization, which states that automaticity occurs through the retrieval and practice of skills as a complete set rather than through targeted practice of each component within the set (Youmans et al., 2005). Script training merges components of functional therapy and linguistic therapy: it targets functional phrases with an emphasis on massed practice, a condition that is not naturally a part of functional communication. The ultimate goal of script training therapy is to increase the automaticity of speech productions, even if the automaticity is limited to a set of scripts/contexts (i.e., scripted islands of fluent speech; Youmans et al., 2005). Thus, it has implications for individuals with aphasia who have difficulty with word retrieval and/or fluent speech. Therapy typically consists of the following steps:

1. The client selects several contexts for scripts and then identifies the desired concepts/vocabulary of the script for the clinician. Scripts can be conversational in style or monologue based if the individual desires to practice telling a story.

2. Script training typically commences at the receptive level, with individuals listening to the targeted phrases modeled for them. Training can be conducted face to face in therapy sessions or through the use of computer software, with an SLP monitoring progress at specified time intervals.

3. Script production starts at the phrase level; intensive targeting of each phrase continues until it is mastered, and the individual then moves on to the next phrase, until the entire script is mastered. Cues, such as choral reading, are provided as needed throughout the training process.

4. Once mastered, the entire script is then practiced with communicative partners. These practice conversations can be varied to enable individuals with aphasia to further practice conversational skills. Variations include practicing with different conversational partners and partners using different prosodic inflections during exchanges.

Response Elaboration Training *(Kearns, 1985; Wambaugh & Martinez, 2000; Wambaugh et al., 2013)*

The main goal of response elaboration training (RET) is for clients to regain flexible and creative use of language. Some individuals with aphasia may communicate primarily with nouns and/or at the single-word or short-phrase level. RET utilizes a loosely structured treatment protocol to help patients increase the variety of words and phrases used in communicative exchanges. Client responses are judged in a more flexible manner; the clinician evaluates the amount and type of information being conveyed in a response rather than trying to elicit a specific response or grammatical form. Each stimulus presented during a therapy session is worked on using the following steps:

- The clinician presents the client with a picture and gives the instruction to talk about the picture.

- After the client responds, the clinician gives a response that either expands on what the client said or provides a verbal model for the client. The model may be a repetition of the client's response or an example of another possible response.

- The clinician asks a wh- question pertaining to the picture and/or the client's response to elicit another comment from the client.

- After the client responds, the clinician models a response that includes information from the client's response as well as previous discussion of the picture.

- The client is asked to repeat the modeled elaboration from the previous step.

- The clinician repeats the model one final time for reinforcement.

Life Participation Approach to Aphasia (Elman & Bernstein-Ellis, 1999; Lyon, 1998; Simmons-Mackie et al., 2016)

This approach broadens the functional/compensatory orientation to aphasia intervention. The overriding philosophy of the life participation approach to aphasia is to maximize the client's reengagement in life and base all therapeutic decision-making on the life concerns identified by clients and their families (Chiou & Yu, 2018; Haley et al., 2019). Therapeutic goals are designed explicitly to help clients translate newly learned skills to everyday life experiences. The main emphases of this intervention model include the following:

- All individuals with aphasia are entitled to receive services as needed at all stages of recovery.

- Both personal/intrinsic and environmental/extrinsic factors should be incorporated into therapeutic programming. These range on a continuum from obstructive to facilitative and should be identified on a case-by-case basis.

- Success is measured by documented changes in life areas defined as important by clients and their families.

Noninvasive Electrical Brain Stimulation Techniques (Barwood & Murdoch, 2013; Chrysikou & Hamilton, 2011; Martin et al., 2009)

The use of magnetic impulses to stimulate targeted areas of the brain is being explored for its therapeutic applications to treating damaged areas of the brain, thus with potential implications for speech, language, and swallowing disorders. This approach is considered noninvasive because it involves the application of electrical currents to the brain through an intact skull. Studies using a type of electrical stimulation called rTMS (repetitive transcranial magnetic stimulation) have provided evidence of neuroplasticity through behavioral changes in patients' abilities to complete naming tasks (Bucur & Papagno 2019; Harvey & Hamilton, 2022; Kielar et al., 2022). Barwood et al. (2012) used rTMS to suppress neural activation in a region of the right hemisphere, promoting more activation to the associated linguistic area in the left hemisphere. This treatment protocol was found to improve both accuracy as well as response times during naming tasks up to 8 months posttreatment (Barwood et al., 2012).

Another noninvasive brain-stimulation technique, transcranial direct-current stimulation, also has been found to have a positive effect on lexical retrieval skills (Torres et al., 2013). Because most of the current research has focused on cases of nonfluent, chronic aphasia and naming tasks, further information is needed about the relationship between brain stimulation and language gains (Yang, 2017). Current evidence for poststroke aphasia treatment includes discussion on whether this technique should be viewed as an alternative or an augmentative approach to traditional language therapy, whether certain neural areas or lesion severities are more responsive to stimulation than others, and whether the gains made through brain stimulation are transient or permanent in nature.

Pharmacotherapy (Berthier et al., 2011)

The use of medications to treat language deficits in aphasia is an area currently being explored in the literature. One study examined the use of several different medicines with individuals with mild to moderate severities of aphasia. The study found support for two different medicinal agents (i.e., dopaminergic and cholinergic agents) with regard to gains in expressive language skills, specifically naming skills and overall fluency (Tanaka et al., 2006). Neurotransmitters, such as dopamine, are often targeted in pharmacotherapy for aphasia treatment based on the theory that increasing neural activity in targeted brain areas via neurotransmitters will increase neural recovery in these regions (Berthier & Davila 2015; Berthier, 2021). Yang (2017) presents a comprehensive summary on pharmacotherapy and aphasia. Common findings among the research studies reviewed included the following:

- Greater gains in language skills were seen when pharmacotherapy was used in conjunction with speech and language therapy.

- Individuals with chronic aphasia still benefited from pharmacotherapy.

- Individuals with mild to moderate aphasia were the best candidates, as individuals with severe aphasia typically did not benefit from pharmacotherapy.

- Language gains were reported in a variety of linguistic skill areas depending on the drug therapy used, including fluency, comprehension, and functional communication skills.

Example Profiles

Following are three profiles representative of the communication problems exhibited by individuals with different types of aphasia (Wernicke's, Broca's, and global). These examples have been designed to illustrate the selection of intervention targets as well as specific therapy activities and materials. Most of the chosen activities can be implemented in either individual or group therapy settings.

PROFILE 1: FLUENT APHASIA—39-YEAR-OLD

Mr. Chang is a 39-year-old right-handed male who presented with a severe-profound fluent aphasia (Wernicke's) after sustaining a left parietal CVA 9 months ago. His initial status was characterized by intelligible verbal output and frequent semantic and phonemic paraphasias. No evidence of dysarthria or apraxia of speech was observed. It was noted that the content of Mr. Chang's output was often unrelated to the topic at hand. He demonstrated severe word-retrieval difficulties and significant auditory comprehension deficits, including an inability to answer yes/no questions. Mr. Chang did not demonstrate the ability to point to objects, pictures, or body parts named, nor did he follow any single- or multiple-step commands. His automatic writing of the alphabet was incomplete, although Mr. Chang accurately wrote his name and the numbers 1 to 20. Reading comprehension was poor, but he did demonstrate the ability to match written word stimuli to objects and pictures.

Mr. Chang received speech-language intervention services for several months poststroke. His current communication status is characterized by occasional semantic and phonemic paraphasias and moderate word-finding deficits. His auditory comprehension skills have improved; Mr. Chang correctly answers simple questions, identifies objects named by others, and inconsistently follows simple single-stage commands, such as, "Put the pencil next to the book." Writing is Mr. Chang's strongest communication modality as evidenced by his ability to write paragraph-length passages with minimal difficulty. Reading comprehension skills are also relatively strong in the areas of word recognition and sentence comprehension.

Mr. Chang's verbal description of the "cookie theft" picture from the Boston Diagnostic Aphasia Examination (Goodglass et al., 2001) is as follows:

> All right well there's a rolly dolly, whatever it is. And the dirl and be and the willy it fall and the fell and he fall down into the drom. And well the waver, water it's all out off for the end. And the mon, mother doing the dibs all the way and she's for the wauby be.

Selection of Therapy Targets. The areas to be targeted are word retrieval and auditory comprehension. These were selected for two main reasons. First, word retrieval and comprehension are Mr. Chang's most impaired language skills and continue to have the greatest negative impact on his ability to communicate effectively in everyday situations. Second, these areas have shown improvement with therapeutic intervention in the past, suggesting the potential for continued growth.

Sample Activities

(All three activities are based on a substitutive/compensatory approach.)

1. Assemble a pile of 20 pictures of common objects and place them face down on a table. Based on the PACE approach, explain that the clinician and client will take turns selecting pictures from the pile and describing them without showing them. Instruct the client to use any means of communication to convey the contents of each selected picture (e.g., oral naming, oral description of physical appearance of the object, pantomime the function of the object, draw the object, write the name of the object). Emphasize that the purpose of this activity is to successfully communicate the intended message rather than to retrieve a specific label. When a strategy is ineffective and results in listener confusion, encourage the client to reformulate the message using another communication mode. The clinician should use his or her turn as speaker to model various communication strategies. The client's communication effectiveness is measured by the clinician's ability to accurately identify the object pictured.

2. Identify a topic that is meaningful or of interest to the client (e.g., favorite hobby, job, family) and collect 25 identical pairs of picture cards that relate to this theme. Based on pretreatment baseline data, select two self-cueing strategies that will be taught to facilitate the client's retrieval of each verbal label (e.g., air tracing and sentence completion). Demonstrate each technique several times, and ask the client to imitate these strategies. Shuffle the deck and deal seven cards to each player. Explain that the object of the activity is to make pairs for all the cards in a player's hand by asking the other player(s), "Do you have a _____?" Instruct the client to use one or both of the self-cueing strategies for every request. The clinician continues to model the tracing and sentence completion procedures during his or her turn.

3. Collect five common objects (e.g., pencil, book, cup, spoon, comb). With these objects in mind, develop a list of 20 single-stage commands that contain three linguistic units (e.g., "Put the *spoon* in the *cup*"; *Give me the book* and the *pencil*"). Place the objects on the table and explain that the client will be given short instructions involving the manipulation of the objects. Instruct the client to write down the first letter of each important word in the direction as a strategy to facilitate comprehension of the verbal command. If the client demonstrates significant difficulty, the clinician can implement the following modifications: (a) reduce speech rate during presentation of stimulus commands, (b) increase redundancy by stating each direction twice before the client responds, and (c) increase the acceptable latency period between the clinician's stimulus presentation and the initiation of the client's response. These strategies will provide the client with needed extra processing time and can be faded gradually as performance improves.

PROFILE 2: NONFLUENT APHASIA—63-YEAR-OLD

Mr. Sanders is a 63-year-old right-handed male who presented with a moderate-to-severe nonfluent aphasia (Broca's) after suffering a left frontal intercranial hemorrhage 2 months ago. Currently, Mr. Sanders's verbal output is characterized by one- and two-word utterances in which the subject noun phrase and verb phrase are often separated by distinctive pauses. His output consists mainly of content words, with the frequent omission of grammatical markers. Significant word-retrieval difficulties are not noted. The ability to imitate verbal utterances is poor even at the single-word level. Mr. Sanders's output is pragmatically appropriate and reflects relatively intact comprehension of verbal material. He demonstrates the ability to identify many objects and pictures when named by the clinician and follows one- and two-step commands with minimal difficulty. Articulation is awkward and labored, with phoneme distortion errors most prevalent. However, it was noted that Mr. Sanders consistently articulated his last name correctly. Minimal use of stress and intonation patterns results in a notable lack of speech melody. Writing skills are consistent with oral output with regard to both vocabulary and syntax; reading comprehension skills are mildly impaired.

Mr. Sanders's verbal description of the "cookie theft" picture from the Boston Diagnostic Aphasia Examination (Goodglass et al., 2001) is as follows:

uh … mother … uh … she talking to the … uh … the … uh … I don't know … two cup … cookie in jar … fall down … wash … and stool … uh … tipping … boy … uh … get hurt

Selection of Therapy Targets. The areas to be targeted are utterance length and syntactic complexity as well as speech prosody. Because the content and use components of Mr. Sanders's linguistic system are relatively intact, utterance length and complexity were chosen to improve the form component of his verbal repertoire. Speech prosody was targeted because it is an essential component of intelligibility. Improved function in this area will facilitate listeners' ability to predict the content of Mr. Sanders's messages despite his articulatory deficits.

Sample Activities

(Activities 1, 2, and 4 are restorative techniques; activity 3 is based on the substitutive/compensatory approach.)

1. For MIT, Step 1, arrange seating to ensure that the client can readily see the clinician's mouth. Select stimulus items for this step of MIT with the following considerations in mind: (a) the stimuli must be meaningful and useful to the individual client, (b) stimuli in this early stage of the program should include a heavy concentration of sounds that are easy to visualize (i.e., bilabials), (c) short, simple phrases should be used (e.g., imperatives such as "Stand up," "Open the door"), and (d) an extensive list of high-probability items is necessary so that any given stimulus utterance is not presented too often. Following is a sample list of stimulus items for Mr. Sanders at this MIT level:

watch TV	salt and pepper
take a nap	good morning
bowl of soup	peach pie
make the bed	cup of coffee
read the paper	start the car

   Graphically, plot the intonation patterns for each stimulus item before the session begins. (See the following example.)

   Set criteria for an acceptable response. The clinician takes the client's hand and hums the plotted intonation pattern for a stimulus while tapping the client's hand on the table once for each syllable. Next, the clinician intones (rather than hums) the same prosody pattern using words and continues to tap the client's hand once for each syllable. Avoid a staccato rhythm, because continuous voicing facilitates verbal production. After a brief pause, repeat the intoned utterance with client hand tapping. Signal the client to join the clinician in unison repetition of the intoned phrase with assisted hand tapping. If the client's response is acceptable, carry this phrase through to Step 3, in which the clinician fades the verbal model partway through the phrase so that the client must finish the utterance alone. The clinician continues to tap the rhythm with the client's hand. If the response is not adequate, pause for several seconds, choose the next item from the stimulus list, and repeat the steps outlined previously. (For detailed information regarding the implementation of MIT, refer to Helm Estabrooks & Albert [2004] and Sparks [2001].)

2. Devise a list of 25 sentence pairs for a cloze task to train production of the regular plural form of nouns. Examples include the following:

   This is one book. These are two (*books*).

   He saw one cookie. He saw two (*cookies*).

   She washed a dish. She washed all the (*dishes*).

   I see the dog. I see lots of (*dogs*).

   The plant has one flower. This plant has many (*flowers*).

   Gather two pictures that depict common objects for each sentence pair. One should contain a single exemplar of the object and the other multiple exemplars of the same object. Explain to the client that this activity focuses on the production of the plural of nouns. Place the first pair of pictures on the table and demonstrate the activity by pointing to the singleton picture when saying the first sentence and pointing to the multiple picture while producing the second sentence with the correct plural noun form included. For the remaining sentence pairs, the clinician leaves the second sentence unfinished and instructs the client to complete the sentence fragment by supplying the plural noun form.

3. Create a conversational script like the following one, according to the guidelines listed in Appendix 7–B on the companion website.

 a. I can't watch the Orioles anymore.

 b. This time they lost to Chicago.

 c. And Chicago beat them by 10 runs.

 d. They need to get a new coach.

Instruct the client to read the script aloud one sentence at a time. When the client encounters difficulties verbalizing the scripted information, suggest self-cueing strategies to facilitate production of the utterance. Examples include chunking utterances into shorter units, gesturing to convey meaning, and using techniques to trigger word retrieval. Next, video record the client reading the script to a familiar listener who is unacquainted with its content. Coach the listener to concentrate on obtaining the gist of the message rather than focusing on specific words and details. The clinician, client, and familiar listener should evaluate the recording according to the following parameters:

 a. How successful was the scripted interaction?

 b. What did the speaker/listener find most helpful?

 c. What did the speaker/listener find least helpful?

 d. What else could have been done by the client, listener, or clinician to facilitate the interaction?

Continue this cycle of coaching and evaluation with increasingly unfamiliar listeners.

4. Develop a list of 20 two-syllable word pairs that have dual intonation patterns. For these pairs, differential stress significantly affects meaning. Stress on the first syllable (indicated in boldface) signals that the word functions as a noun, whereas stress on the second syllable indicates that the word is being used as a verb. Examples include the following:

present/pre**sent**	**con**tract/con**tract**
defect/de**fect**	**re**cord/re**cord**
permit/per**mit**	**con**test/con**test**
convict/con**vict**	**re**fuse/re**fuse**
produce/pro**duce**	**ob**ject/ob**ject**
rebel/re**bel**	**con**vert/con**vert**
contrast/con**trast**	**des**ert/de**sert**
discharge/dis**charge**	**pro**ject/pro**ject**
protest/pro**test**	**sub**ject/sub**ject**
survey/sur**vey**	**ad**dress/ad**dress**

Write each pair on a separate index card and underline or boldface the stressed syllable for each word. Develop a pair of questions or fill-in-the-blank statements for each word that are designed to elicit both noun and verb intonation patterns. For example, queries for the first pair might be: "What do you buy for somebody's birthday?" and "In honor of [insert famous name here]'s great accomplishments, I now _____ him with this award." Instruct the client to choose one index card from the pile and practice both stress patterns in unison with the clinician. The clinician then presents the stimulus question/statement for the noun form and asks the client to look at the index card and spontaneously produce the target word with the appropriate stress pattern. Present the second question/statement to elicit the verb stress pattern indicated on the index card. Repeat this procedure for the remaining word pairs. Task difficulty can be increased by eliciting noun and verb forms in random order.

PROFILE 3: GLOBAL APHASIA—71-YEAR-OLD

Mrs. Marshall is a 71-year-old right-handed female who presents with a global aphasia and a right hemiplegia and limb apraxia subsequent to a thrombosis of the middle cerebral artery that resulted in extensive damage to the pre- and postrolandic areas 6 months ago. Her communicative status has not changed substantially since that time.

Currently, Mrs. Marshall demonstrates significant impairment in both language comprehension and language production in all modalities. She exhibits understanding of some simple yes/no questions—such as, "Is your name Polly?"—and identifies body parts named by the clinician with approximately 50% accuracy. Mrs. Marshall does not appear to comprehend even simple one-step verbal commands. She relies heavily on nonverbal means to communicate, including facial expressions and head nods to indicate yes/no responses and a pointing gesture. Her speech output is limited to stereotypic utterances and neologisms that consist of both real and nonsense words. These are produced with differential stress and intonation and seem to express several communicative intentions. Reading comprehension is extremely poor even at the familiar single-word level. Writing skills are slightly better in that Mrs. Marshall can copy written words with occasional errors but does not exhibit the ability to generate legible written words spontaneously. Overall, she appears alert, attentive, and somewhat frustrated by her inability to communicate.

Mrs. Marshall's verbal description of the "cookie theft" picture from the Boston Diagnostic Aphasia Examination (Goodglass et al., 2001) is as follows:

I can't. I don't think that . . . What is this? . . . I just don't have that. Oh yeah, right here. That's all.

Selection of Therapy Targets. Based on the severity of Mrs. Marshall's deficits, the areas to be targeted are auditory comprehension and functional communication skills. Auditory comprehension was chosen to establish a core receptive vocabulary that is meaningful within the context of her daily activities. Mrs. Marshall's verbal expression appears so limited that even after 6 months she does not represent a good candidate for intervention. Therefore, the substitutive/compensatory approaches of PACE and Amer-Ind will be implemented to facilitate the effectiveness of her relatively stronger nonverbal communication skills. VAT was not considered an appropriate strategy for two reasons. First, the prescribed repertoire of gestural meanings was not deemed to be functional for Mrs. Marshall. Second, this approach requires the ability to perform a seven-way object and picture discrimination task as an initial level of training, which is clearly beyond her auditory comprehension abilities.

Sample Activities

(All three activities are based on a substitutive/compensatory approach.)

1. Consult the client's family members and friends to identify vocabulary items that are most important to Mrs. Marshall. Items may include names of significant others, pets, favorite foods, terms for hobbies and other leisure interests (e.g., knitting, art, TV, and so on), frequently visited locations, and money terms. Select 20 of these items and gather large color pictures of each one (photographs are highly desirable). Complete the following three steps. Step 1: Place each picture card one at a time face up on a table. Name each picture and then point to it to provide a model for the client. Step 2: Present each picture again, name it, and physically assist the client to point to the picture. Step 3: Place two pictures face up on the table, name one, and signal the client to identify the target item by pointing. If the client experiences significant difficulty with the two-way discrimination task in Step 3, reduce the field to a single picture while still requiring a spontaneous pointing response.

2. Gather 25 colored photographs or easily recognizable pictures that depict activities or objects of daily living that are relevant for Mrs. Marshall. These may include brushing teeth, bathing, eating, sleeping, dressing, drinking, church, dentures, toilet, and doctor. Place the stack of pictures face down on the table. Based on the PACE approach, select one picture from the pile and model several different strategies for communicating the contents of the picture to the client (e.g., oral naming, description of activity/object characteristics, pantomiming action or object function, drawing, and rudimentary written cues). Repeat this modeling as necessary. Client and clinician take turns selecting pictures from the stack. The clinician should use his or her turn as speaker to emphasize that the purpose of this activity is to successfully communicate the intended meaning by whatever means possible rather than to elicit a particular lexical item. Encourage the client to reformulate a message using another communication strategy if the initial attempt is not successful. The client's ability to effectively convey messages is measured by the clinician's success in guessing the identity of the stimulus picture. It is important to recognize that the client's turn as listener requires an identification response. In the event that the client cannot provide an oral label for the picture described by the clinician, an alternative response mode should be made available. This can be accomplished in the following manner: (a) provide a duplicate set of the 25 pictures; (b) display an array of three pictures, including the target and two foils; and (c) instruct the client to indicate the correct stimulus through pointing.

3. Identify three different communication situations that Mrs. Marshall encounters on a daily or weekly basis (e.g., neighbor visits, doctor appointments, and hair-cutting appointments). From the concept illustration section in Skelly (1979), select five concrete and relevant Amer-Ind signals for each situation, such as the following:

Neighbor	*Doctor*	*Hairdresser*
hello/goodbye	pain	cut
sit	tired	okay
drink	medicine	comb
eat	nurse	thanks
walk	puzzled	money

(*Note:* Mrs. Marshall's hemiplegia necessitates that the signals chosen can be executed with the left hand.)

Choose one scenario and gather objects and/or pictures that represent the signals to be trained. For the "neighbor" scenario, these might include a chair, a cup, a pretzel, a picture of people entering/leaving a room, and a picture of two women taking a walk. Demonstrate each signal with the corresponding object or picture several times. For example, the concept of "walk" is represented by the following signal: the left arm is extended in front of the body with the elbow at shoulder level; the palm of the hand is down and index/middle fingers are extended pointing down, while the hand slowly advances to the right; the extended fingers alternate moving forward, conveying the action of legs walking. Consult Skelly (1979) for explanations and visual illustrations of other Amer-Ind signals.

Place three of the referents on the table, model one of the signals, and encourage the client to identify the appropriate referent. Repeat this procedure until the client reliably recognizes the five target signals.

Place an object/picture on the table, model the corresponding gesture, and require the client to imitate it. If the client demonstrates difficulty with this task, provide physical assistance to shape the response. Once successful and unassisted imitation has been established for a given scenario, gradually fade the clinician's model and elicit more spontaneous and functional productions of the signals through clinician questions or role-playing.

Helpful Hints

1. Keep in mind that there is a basic hierarchy of picture difficulty. One can increase the complexity of a picture description task by progressing from object pictures to action pictures to pictures denoting location and then to a series of pictures describing a logical sequence of events.

2. Remember that individuals with aphasia (particularly those of advanced age) often present with concomitant physical or emotional problems that may affect their ability to communicate. Poor performance on therapy tasks may not be attributable to the aphasia per se but to any of several other factors, including hearing impairment, poor visual acuity or visual field deficits, medication imbalances or side effects, depression, and so on.

3. As a general rule, clients with auditory comprehension deficits benefit from substantial repetition and redundancy of verbal input.

4. Clinicians should consistently use a slower speech rate when interacting with clients with aphasia. Rate of speech may have a significant impact on these individuals' ability to process verbal information.

5. Individuals with global aphasia may benefit from the provision of a *communication book/ augmentative device* that contains pictures of familiar objects, people, and events from their daily environment. For additional information, refer to Brock (2016) and Russo et al. (2017).

6. In the early stages of intervention, clinicians may have to rely heavily on yes/no questions to provide clients with a mechanism for expressing strong feelings of frustration, anxiety, or confusion.

7. Software technology for aphasia intervention is increasingly available from many sources. Clinicians are encouraged to seek out programs with demonstrated efficacy or outcome data (Lavoie et al., 2017; Lavoie et al., 2019; Repetto et al., 2021).

8. Family participation in therapy should be maximized. Clinicians are encouraged to actively engage family members and caregivers in therapy to promote the practice of therapy targets throughout the client's daily activities.

9. Tracking progress in aphasia therapy can be made more efficient/effective if the SLP develops working definitions of what will constitute minimal → moderate → maximal cueing for a given client prior to the start of intervention.

Conclusion

This section has presented basic information, protocols, and procedures for aphasia intervention at an *introductory* level. This material is intended only as a starting point in the reader's clinical education and training. For more in-depth coverage of this area as well as for information on other cognitive-communication disorders, the following readings are recommended.

Aphasia

Barnes, M., Dobkin, B., & Bogousslavsky, J. (Eds.). (2005). *Recovery after stroke*. Cambridge University Press.

Blumstein, S. E. (2022). *When words betray us: Language, the brain, and aphasia*. Springer Publishing.

Brookshire, R. H. (2014). *Introduction to neurogenic communication disorders* (8th ed.). C.V. Mosby.

Chapey, R. (2008). *Language intervention strategies in aphasia and related neurogenic communication disorders* (5th ed.). Lippincott Williams & Wilkins.

Elman, R. J. (2006). *Group treatment of neurogenic communication disorders: The expert clinician's approach*. Plural Publishing.

Helm-Estabrooks, N., & Holland, A. (1998). *Approaches to the treatment of aphasia*. Singular Publishing.

Tanner, D. C. (2008). *The family guide to surviving stroke and communication disorders. A primer for health care professionals* (2nd ed.). Jones & Bartlett.

Winstein, C. J., Stein, J., Arena, R., Bates, B., Cherney, L. R., Cramer, S. C.,... Zorowitz, R. D. (2016). Guidelines for adult stroke rehabilitation and recovery: A guideline for healthcare professionals from the American Heart Association/American Stroke Association. *Stroke, 47*, e98–e169.

Right-Hemisphere Dysfunction

Beeman, M. J., & Chiarello, C. (Eds.) (2013). *Right hemisphere language comprehension: Perspectives from cognitive neuroscience*. Psychology Press.

Myers, P. S. (2008). Communication disorders associated with right hemisphere damage. In R. Chapey (Ed.), *Language intervention strategies in aphasia and related neurogenic communication disorders* (5th ed., pp. 809–828). Lippincott Williams & Wilkins.

Tompkins, C.A. (2012). Rehabilitation for cognitive-communication disorders in right hemisphere brain damage. *Archives of Physical Medicine and Rehabilitation, 93*(1), S61–S69.

Dementia

Bayles, K. A., & Tomoeda, C. K. (2013). *Cognitive-communication disorders of dementia: Definition, diagnosis, and treatment.* Plural Publishing.

Bourgeois, M. S., & Hickey, E. M. (2009). *Dementia: From diagnosis to management—A functional approach.* Psychology Press.

Krishnamoorthy, E. S., Prince, M. J., & Cummings, J. L. (Eds.). (2010). *Dementia: A global approach.* Cambridge University Press.

Murray, L. L., & Peak, E. J. (2016). Behavioral/nonpharmacological approaches to addressing cognitive-linguistic symptoms in individuals with dementia. *Perspectives of the ASHA Special Interest Group, 1*(15), 12–25.

Weiner, M. F., & Lipton, A. M. (2009). *Textbook of Alzheimer disease and other dementias.* American Psychiatric Publishing.

Additional Resources

Aphasia

Cognitive Reorganization: A Stimulus Handbook, Third Edition

Includes more than 4,200 stimuli plus activities for functional applications to help meet the diverse needs of clients who cannot use functional language skills in any organized, sequential, or pragmatic way. Responses may be written, verbal, or graphic.

Functional Memory Manual

This workbook provides strategies for increasing memory recall for individuals with mild to severe memory deficits. It contains chapters on topics such as attention, visual recall, and auditory recall.

Focus on Function: Gaining Essential Communication, Second Edition

Targets independent living skills for adolescents and adults by having them practice a variety of daily tasks. Includes reproducible evaluation forms, task cards, picture cards, manipulatives, and practical activities that emphasize everyday verbal, phone, reading, writing, and numerical skills.

Following Directions Series Software

Computer software that includes eight activities to help clients learn to follow one level, sequential, and two-level commands using spatial relations concepts and directional terms. The program uses Laureate's Optimized Intervention technology to tailor programs to a student's individual needs. Also includes 10 activities to improve clients' ability to follow directions and develop right/left discrimination concepts through activities such as simple left- and right-hand matching, practice crossing midline, and moving objects to left and right using hands in mirrored and nonmirrored positions.

Language Activity Resource Kit (LARK), Second Edition

A portable kit with objects (two of each), illustrated cards, color photographs, word and phrase cards, and line drawings of the objects in use. Designed especially for the itinerant SLP treating adults with aphasia and/or TBI. Optional LARK workbook with reproducible worksheets can be purchased.

Speechmark Aphasia Resource Book: Practical Ways to Help People With Aphasia

This book is meant to target overall communication skills. The activities included target areas such as answering questions, visual memory, categorization, colors, verbs, and gestures. A DVD is also included.

Problem-Solving Photo Scenes

A set of 75, 5× 7 in. color photographs that depict functional home and community scenes. Each picture contains five question prompts to target recall, problem-solving, and reasoning skills.

Results for Adults: Aphasia Book 1

This workbook is a collection of individual pictures and scenes. Prompts are provided to target auditory comprehension skills, such as picture identification and answering yes/no questions, and verbal expression skills, such as sentence completion tasks and naming. The book contains two levels of difficulty.

My House, My Town, and My School Software

These talking instructional computer software programs were designed to help clients understand and express the language they encounter during daily routines. Each program has four different activities designed to increase understanding of object names and their functions or descriptions: Discover Names, Identify Names, Discover Functions, and Identify Functions. In My House, the scenes represent typical rooms in a house: a bedroom, bathroom, dining room, kitchen, living room, and utility room. In My Town, a doctor's office, dentist's office, restaurant, park, city neighborhood, and suburban neighborhood are included.

Lingraphica App

Lingraphica is a company devoted to providing resources to individuals with aphasia. Some of the apps focus on facilitating communication, such as SmallTalk Conversational Phrases and SmallTalk Daily Activities. Other apps provide practice for therapy targets for both expressive and receptive language tasks. The TalkPath Speaking app contains naming and speech repetition exercises for memory and word retrieval skills. Receptively, the TalkPath Listening app provides practice answering yes/no and wh- questions as well as identifying associations through matching object pairs.

Workbook for Aphasia

This workbook is for adults with mild-to-moderate language and cognitive deficits. Target areas include word usage, development of syntax, use of factual information, and concrete and abstract reasoning.

Speech Therapy Aphasia Rehabilitation (STAR) Workbooks

A set of two workbooks that target expressive and receptive language skills. The first workbook contains color photographs and exercises to target skills such as naming, using descriptive language, reading, writing, and answering wh- questions. The second workbook includes receptive language activities focusing on following directions, comprehension, and calculation. The exercises can be sent home with clients for additional practice.

Tactus Therapy Solutions

A collection of apps that are divided into categories by communication disorder. With regard to aphasia, there are apps to target skills such as conversational skills, category knowledge, and answering questions. Other features include difficulty that adjusts based on performance, exercise scores that can be shared with SLPs, availability in other languages, and practice modes that provide supports.

Traumatic Brain Injury (Coauthored by Emily DeAngelis)

Traumatic brain injury (TBI) results from an external insult to the brain from causes such as vehicular accidents, gunshot wounds, falls, sports-related injuries, and explosions. It is estimated that 2.87 million cases of TBI occur annually in the United States. Of these cases, most are mild in severity and due to falls (Centers for Disease Control and Prevention [CDC], 2019b). Resulting damage and deficits vary based on the type and severity of the insult. There are two main classifications of TBI: closed head injury and penetrating head injury. A **closed head injury (CHI)** results in damage to a widespread area of the brain. The force of the insult or blow is significant and can cause tearing of cell structures. Additionally, the blow or jolt can cause the brain to move back and forth in the skull (coup and contrecoup motions), resulting in multiple points of damage (Coelho et al., 2013). In a **penetrating head injury (PHI)**, damage tends to be concentrated in a specific neurologic region(s) (Coelho et al., 2013).

In mild TBI (mTBI), there are brief changes in consciousness and memory. In more severe cases, memory loss and periods of unconsciousness are more pronounced. Post-traumatic amnesia (PTA) refers to the state of confusion that occurs as the individual regains consciousness and awareness (Ponsford, Janzen, et al., 2014). Although uncommon, aphasia may result from TBI depending on the extent of damage with a CHI or the location of damage with a PHI (Coelho et al., 2013; Ylvisaker et al., 2008). A multitude of symptoms may accompany TBI, including headaches, blurry vision, dizziness, sleeping problems, irritability, anxiety, and depression. TBI can also cause epilepsy and increase the risk of conditions that become more prevalent with age such as Alzheimer's disease or Parkinson's disease. These comorbidities are important for SLPs to consider when developing and implementing treatment plans because they may affect a client's motivation, perseverance, and self-monitoring abilities. Of most concern for SLPs are core deficits in one or more of the following domains: communication, executive functioning, attention/memory, and behavior. These four domains are highly intertwined and often integrated in treatment plans.

Communication

Due to the nature of the underlying injury, communication impairments resulting from TBI present differently than other communication disorders. The term cognitive communication impairment serves to note this distinction and the role that cognition plays in the communication profile of an individual with TBI (MacDonald, 2017; Togher et al., 2014). Cognitive communication impairments typically occur at the discourse and **macrostructure** levels of language (Coelho et al., 2013). The **macrostructure** level involves higher level linguistic skills such as cohesion devices for conversation, stories, and personal accounts (Peach, 2013). The local or microstructure level involves lexical/word choice and syntactic organization at the sentence level and is generally more intact. These higher-level language impairments are due to the impact of deficits in cognitive skills such as attention, working memory, and information processing (Togher et al., 2014).

In addition to discourse difficulties, other aspects of language may be impaired. Comprehension often becomes difficult, especially with increased linguistic complexity and utterance length or when abstract topics are discussed (MacDonald & Wiseman-Hakes, 2010). Reading and writing difficulties can occur due to challenges with attention, organization, and information processing (MacDonald, 2017; Togher et al., 2014). Speech production also may be affected due to physical damage to the oral mechanism or due to dysarthria resulting from the neurologic insult (Cherney et al., 2010).

Executive Functioning

The communication difficulties of individuals with TBI are often accompanied by deficits in **executive functioning (EF)**—a term that encompasses the cognitive processes necessary for goal-directed behaviors (Coelho et al., 2013; Tate et al., 2014; Ylvisaker et al., 2008). For example, individuals with TBI experience difficulties identifying and sequencing the steps needed to reach logical solutions (i.e., problem-solving). Self-awareness is another frequent problem and may include difficulty in monitoring and appraising one's thoughts and behaviors. EF difficulties may also include reduced ability to regulate and express emotions (i.e., poor coping with disappointment or anger). This reduced self-awareness and lack of emotional regulation can contribute to problematic social uses of language. Individuals with TBI are often judged by society to demonstrate less-than-adequate social skills in many areas of daily function. These pragmatic challenges include difficulties in taking the listener's perspective into account, formulating socially appropriate messages, and making accurate inferences about other people's feelings. See Dahlberg et al. (2006) for further information on the social language aspects associated with TBI.

Attention and Memory

Attention is a complex cognitive component encompassing several processes (e.g., orientation, engagement, object recognition) as well as types (e.g., sustained, divided; Ponsford, Bayley, et al., 2014). An individual may experience difficulty with various levels of attention, including arousal, selection, and processing speed (Whyte et al., 2010). With regard to communication skills, difficulty with attention may manifest as distractibility in noisy environments, lack of sustained concentration, and reduced speed of speech processing. Thus, aspects of daily life such as workplace and academic performance can be negatively affected by attention skills.

Memory is another aspect of cognition with many components that affect communication skills:

- Working memory: The system for temporarily storing and controlling the information required to carry out complicated cognitive tasks such as reasoning and comprehension.

- Short-term memory: A component of memory that can store limited amounts of information for short durations.

- Long-term memory: A component of memory with the capacity for storing greater amounts of information for longer or indefinite periods of time.

(See Cowan [2008] for further explanation of memory components.)

Impairments to processes such as encoding, storage, and retrieval often make it difficult for persons with TBI to learn and/or retrieve information (Velikonja et al., 2014). Deficits in the area of working memory can cause an individual to struggle with maintaining thoughts across conversational exchanges. Depending on the severity of the memory deficits, individuals may have difficulty with a variety of activities of daily living and other preinjury responsibilities. These individuals may benefit from environmental modifications (e.g., placing labels and reminders around the house) and the use of assistive devices to help them regain some of their functional skills.

Behavior

Patients with brain injuries, especially injuries in or near the frontal lobe, often demonstrate deficits in behavioral control (Ylvisaker et al., 2007). These behavioral disorders may manifest themselves externally as aggression, irritability, reduced inhibitions with anger, and inappropriate verbal outputs, or internally as depression, social withdrawal, feelings of awkwardness in social situations, and rigidity (Ylvisaker et al., 2007). Behavioral disturbances also may be related to frustrations that arise from impairments secondary to TBI. Thus, behavioral issues may persist despite improvements in communication or cognitive skills.

Treatment Efficacy/Evidence-Based Practice

Due to the variety of deficits within the TBI population, treatment efficacy studies cover a range of approaches. For organizational purposes, three main categories are addressed. One focus examines discourse-based and social-communication approaches for treating TBI (Lê et al., 2022; Steel et al., 2021). Interventions such as cognitive pragmatic treatment and discourse processing treatment fall within this category and have been found to yield positive results. In particular, Lê et al. (2022) concluded that five elements of therapy play a major role in treatment gains:

- feedback

- social contexts (simulated or actual)

- functional practice

- metalinguistic and/or metacognitive strategies

- hierarchical training

Another category of treatment approaches focuses on communication partner training (Behn et al., 2021; Wiseman-Hakes et al., 2020). Studies within this domain also note the importance of social contexts when designing and implementing therapy. The third category deals with technology-based interventions, either through telehealth services or virtual reality applications (Aulisio et al., 2020; Avramović et al., 2023; Betts et al., 2018; Maggio et al., 2019). While the evidence for virtual reality treatment is more limited, studies investigating telehealth services have found them to be similarly effective to face-to-face service delivery.

Additionally, studies found evidence to support the use of the following strategies and intervention approaches (Königs et al., 2018; Hallock et al., 2016; MacDonald & Wiseman-Hakes, 2010; Radomski et al., 2016; Teasell et al., 2018; Ylvisaker et al., 2007):

- Incorporation of metacognitive strategies (e.g., self-monitoring skills)

- Individualization of goals based on daily routines (e.g., relevance, social validity)

- Initiation of therapy early in the recovery process with dosage intensity ranging from low to high, according to individual client needs

- Implementation of cognitive remediation strategies including dual-task training, executive function training, and attention process training

- Development of self-regulation techniques

- Participation in simulated or real-life scenarios rather than drill-based activities

- Usage of positive behavioral intervention approaches

Intervention research on military members with mTBI has increased steadily, as researchers and rehabilitation specialists seek to identify treatment strategies and programs that represent best/preferred practices (Belanger et al., 2009; Helmick, 2010). One treatment approach that appears to be successful with veterans is telehealth services (therapy services that are delivered remotely; Riegler et al., 2017). Overall, several challenges remain with regard to the development of treatment plans for combat-related mTBI and include limited evidence regarding the effectiveness of cognitive rehabilitation for mTBI; the existence of multiple comorbidities (e.g., physical injuries to other parts of the body, post-traumatic stress, acoustic trauma, sensory impairments, depression); and patient compliance with rehabilitation recommendations while deployed or in post-deployment settings (Belanger et al., 2009; Lew et al., 2009; Tanielian & Jaycox, 2008; Vanderploeg et al., 2009). See ASHA's *Clinician's Guide to Cognitive Rehabilitation in Mild Traumatic Brain Injury: Application for Military Service Members and Veterans* for further information on intervention with this population.

Treatment for Traumatic Brain Injury

SLPs treat individuals with TBI in a variety of settings throughout the rehabilitation process, including intensive care units, acute/subacute rehabilitation hospital settings, and outpatient services (Ylvisaker et al., 2008). The ultimate aim of intervention for TBI is to increase an individual's independence with activities of daily living, which includes social interactions and return to work (RTW) activities (Douglas et al., 2016). A related field is vocational rehabilitation (VR) or services that assist an individual in finding and maintaining employment (Meulenbroek et al., 2022). Both of these facets, RTW and VR, provide SLPs with opportunities for interprofessional collaboration.

Another main goal of TBI rehabilitation is to increase self-awareness and psychosocial skills (e.g., coping, anxiety, mood, self-esteem, and self-concept). Treatment approaches may change over the course of the recovery process to match a patient's progress and remaining difficulties. For example, the SLP may be consulted during the time that the patient is in a coma, with the focus on providing care education to the family and monitoring the patient's sensory responses. Treatment in the acute care setting also may include reestablishing underlying cognitive skills such as attention.

Key Elements of Effective Treatments

It is important for SLPs to select approaches that address an individual's primary presenting deficit(s) in the areas of communication, executive functioning, attention, memory, and behavior. Individual sessions are beneficial in the initial stages of therapy to establish therapy targets (e.g., initiating augmentative communication systems, conversational topic maintenance skills) in a structured setting. Subsequently, group treatment sessions provide clients with opportunities to practice those targeted skills within a larger setting. Group therapy also facilitates social support networks during the rehabilitation process (Patterson et al., 2016).

Various rehabilitation approaches are reported in the literature. These generally focus on improving executive function skills (Gilmore et al., 2019; O'Neil-Pirozzi, 2011). An additional focus of rehabilitation protocols includes social interaction skills (Braden et al., 2010; Hawley & Newman, 2010). Regardless of the specific approach used, there are several key elements that comprise effective programming (Teasell et al., 2018):

- Rehabilitation is person centered and matched to individual needs, strengths, and capacities.

- Treatment addresses cognitive, social, emotional, and functional aspects of communication simultaneously rather than sequentially.

- Intervention encompasses both micro- and macro-level deficits. Although it is important to remediate cognitive deficits, focus is simultaneously placed on the client's real-world circumstances.

- A coordinated interdisciplinary team approach is important for effective treatment, especially for individuals with moderate to severe injuries.

- Intervention for TBI incorporates a strong focus on the role of the family in communicative interactions.

- Programming identifies realistic communication goals for the patient and family.

- Optimizing/maximizing skills is the primary aim rather than restoring preinjury levels of function.

Helpful Hints

1. Organizations such as the Brain Trauma Foundation and the Brain Injury Association of America provide educational information and other resources for individuals with TBI and their caregivers. In addition to providing information, BrainLine has several resources, such as a question-and-answer page, that present information from the perspective of the individual with TBI.

2. Apps are available (e.g., mTBI pocket guide) that provide education and resources on treatment strategies for TBI. In addition, personal digital assistants may be used as part of the rehabilitation process (Thomas, Alves, et al., 2017).

3. Augmentative and alternative communication (AAC) devices can be incorporated into therapy to support expressive language skills. In cases of severe impairment, SLPs may identify AAC strategies as a primary mode of communication.

4. Individuals with TBI also may suffer from hearing loss. Recommendations for patients with hearing loss (e.g., reduce background noise when possible, face the communicative partner) may be beneficial in facilitating communication skills for individuals with TBI.

5. Certain medications for symptoms related to TBI (e.g., pain medications) can have an adverse impact on cognitive and communication skills.

6. External memory aids (e.g., calendars, planners) assist individuals in recalling information as well as in maintaining connections to current events.

7. Telehealth services, such as video conferencing, promote collaboration among team members throughout the rehabilitation process. SLPs can utilize this technology to assist clients in their transition back into their communities.

Conclusion

This section has presented basic information, protocols, and procedures for TBI at an *introductory* level. This material is intended only as a starting point in the reader's clinical education and training. For more in-depth coverage of these areas, the following readings are recommended:

Academy of Neurologic Communication Disorders and Sciences. (2019). *Evidence based clinical research*. https://www.ancds.org/evidence-based-practice

Evidence-Based Review of Moderate-to-Severe Acquired Brain Injury. (2019). *About ERABI.* https://erabi.ca/about-erabi/

Mattingly, E., & Roth, C. R. (2022). Traumatic brain injury in older adults: Epidemiology, etiology, rehabilitation, and outcomes. *Perspectives of the ASHA Special Interest Groups, 7*(4), 1166–1181.

McDonald, S., Togher, L., & Code, C. (Eds.). (2013). *Social and communication disorders following traumatic brain injury* (2nd ed.). Psychology Press.

Ostergen, J. A. (2017). *Cognitive rehabilitation therapy for traumatic brain injury: A guide for speech-language pathologists.* Plural Publishing.

Silver, J. M., McAllister, T. W., & Arciniegas, D. B. (Eds.). (2018). *Textbook of traumatic brain injury.* American Psychiatric Pub.

Working Group to Develop a Clinician's Guide to Cognitive Rehabilitation in mTBI. (2016). *Clinician's guide to cognitive rehabilitation in mild traumatic brain injury: Application for military service members and veterans.* American Speech-Language-Hearing Association. https://tinyurl.com/2p87frz6

Additional Resources

Traumatic Brain Injury

CARDS Cognition, Attention, and Recall Drill Set
Set of playing cards with different games and activities that are designed to target specific cognitive skills. There are individual card sets for memory and for attention.

Results for Adults: Cognition
A workbook with lessons that target the following cognitive skills: memory, problem solving, reasoning, and planning. Designed for individuals 15 years of age and older.

Workbook of Activities for Language and Cognition (WALC)
A series of workbooks that provide lessons to target deficits in language and cognition. Each workbook has its own focus, with activities designed to provide practice in specific language and cognitive skills. Several workbooks are described in greater detail in the following sections.

WALC 2 Cognitive Rehab
This workbook is also available in Spanish. It contains 300 pages of exercises targeting the following cognitive skills: attention (e.g., word search, crossword puzzles); memory (e.g., word retrieval tasks); sequential thought (e.g., ordering steps of activities of daily living); and reasoning (e.g., identifying opposites, completing analogies).

WALC 5 Neuro Rehab
This workbook contains lessons organized by cognitive skill as well as ideas for extending these activities for further practice. Topics include orientation, memory, organization, verbal problem-solving, abstract reasoning, and writing. The activities are designed to be functional to promote carryover beyond the therapy setting.

WALC 10 Memory

This workbook helps clients to identify memory strategies that best work for them and then provides practice using these memory strategies in various contexts.

WALC 11 Language for Home Activities

This workbook contains functional lessons to help increase client functioning in their homes and daily lives. The emphasis on home and daily living is meant to increase client participation and motivation to participate in rehabilitation.

Chapter 8

Intervention for Motor-Speech Disorders
The Dysarthrias, Apraxia of Speech, and Dysphagia

Dysarthria is a speech impairment that involves an impaired ability to execute the motor movements necessary for speech production. Apraxia is also a speech-motor impairment but involves a deficit in the planning and sequencing of movement. The term **dysphagia** refers to difficulty at any stage of the swallowing process. Discussion of this topic is included in this chapter because it is a frequent co-occurring impairment with speech-motor disorders such as dysarthria and **apraxia**. These deficits may occur alone or coexist in the same individual. There is a lack of consensus concerning many issues related to each of these disorders, including basic terminology. To minimize confusion, the technical vocabulary used in this chapter was selected for its common usage and clarity.

Treatment for Motor-Speech Disorders

The optimal goal of therapy for motor-speech disorders is to improve intelligibility within the limits of a client's neurological impairment. Articulation and prosody interact to exert a powerful influence on speech intelligibility. For this reason, therapy designed to improve intelligibility focuses primarily on the modification of these two parameters. Intervention tasks in this paradigm are programmed to progress along a continuum of difficulty from simple automatic responses (e.g., counting from 1 to 10) to more volitional and complex behaviors (e.g., responding to a question such as, "What did you do last evening?"). Each client's unique characteristics will determine the most appropriate starting point along this continuum. In general, it is recommended that treatment be initiated as soon as possible to discourage a client's tendency to develop undesirable compensatory speech behaviors (e.g., pharyngeal fricatives).

The concept of drill is fundamental to any therapy program that seeks to directly modify motor-speech behaviors in any of the communication subsystems (respiration, resonance, phonation, articulation, prosody). Because speech is a complex motor skill, intense repetitive practice is more successful in changing this behavior than a therapy approach that relies on cognitive learning (e.g., explanation, modeling). Drill activities are most effective when a single presentation of a stimulus is followed by multiple productions of the target response by the client. Re-presenting the stimulus to elicit each production breaks the cycle of the motor-learning chain (Darley et al., 1975; Guadagnoli & Lee, 2004).

In some cases, improved speech intelligibility may not be a realistic goal. Certain neurologic conditions such as Parkinson's disease and multiple sclerosis are progressive and require that the treatment be aimed at slowing down the gradual deterioration of a client's speech. Sometimes, the dysarthria is so severe or the disease process is so rapidly degenerative that speech cannot be the primary mode of communication. Within a social model of disability, clinicians design programming to reduce barriers to successful communication rather than improve speech production skill. In this context, the main goal of therapy is to provide a functional alternative method of conveying messages.

This may include use of gestures, communication boards, or speech synthesizers. Use of augmentative/alternative communication as well as relevant training for others in the client's environment should be considered for individuals with ataxia and dysarthria when reduced speech intelligibility has a substantial impact on functional communication (Alhinti et al., 2020; Bates et al., 2016).

The Dysarthrias

The dysarthrias represent a group of related motor-speech disorders characterized by impaired muscular control over the speech mechanism as a result of central or peripheral nervous system damage. Whereas **apraxia** is a deficit in the planning and sequencing of movement, **dysarthria** represents an impaired ability to execute motor movement. Clients with either of these disorders will demonstrate inaccurate and/or labored performance on tasks that require rapid, repetitive movement of the articulators, such as **diadochokinesis**.

The lack of neurological control with dysarthria can affect the motor-speech subsystems of respiration, phonation, resonance, articulation, and prosody. Unlike apraxia, the dysarthrias involve paralysis, weakness, decreased tone, or incoordination of the speech musculature. Muscles can be impaired with respect to range, direction, strength, endurance, speed, or timing. Dysarthria can be manifested as a paucity or an excess of any of these parameters (e.g., reduced range of motion versus involuntary or uninhibited movement). Dysarthria is a consequence of damage to the cortex, cerebellum, brainstem, or peripheral nervous system. Of particular significance are the cranial nerves, which consist of 12 pairs of neuron bundles emerging from the brainstem. Table 8–1 provides a list of the cranial nerves and their function. The major causes of dysarthrias include stroke, brain tumors, head trauma, toxins, and neuromuscular diseases, many of which are degenerative (e.g., Parkinson's, multiple sclerosis, myasthenia gravis). The degree of impairment secondary to dysarthria can range in severity from quite mild to devastatingly profound.

Impairment of the articulators (lips, tongue, mandible, velum) has a greater negative impact on speech intelligibility than do disruptions of the respiratory or laryngeal systems. In dysarthria, the primary contributors to reduced intelligibility are distorted or omitted consonants and vowels, prolonged phonemes, and erratic articulation performance (McAuliffe et al., 2017; Rosenbek & LaPointe, 1985).

Classification of the Dysarthrias

The most frequently cited classification system for the dysarthrias is based on the Mayo Clinic research studies conducted by Darley et al. (1969a, 1969b, 1975). This work has resulted in the identification of the following seven major types of dysarthria, based on differential patterns of neurological impairment and associated speech characteristics: (a) flaccid, (b) spastic, (c) ataxic, (d) hypokinetic, (e) hyperkinetic, (f) mixed, and (g) unilateral upper motor neuron. Table 8–2 presents a comparative outline of the dysarthrias.

No spontaneous recovery is associated with certain dysarthria etiologies, such as amyotrophic lateral sclerosis (ALS), Parkinson's disease, and Huntington's chorea. However, some neuromuscular diseases, such as multiple sclerosis, do exhibit periods of remission in which symptoms abate. Prognosis for individuals with dysarthria is affected by many of the same variables that are associated with aphasia and apraxia recovery. In addition, there are two dysarthria-specific factors that significantly influence prognosis: (a) if the underlying neuropathology of the dysarthria involves a degenerative disease process, the prognosis for significant improvement is poor; and (b) the existence of a severe co-occurring aphasia will interfere with a client's ability to benefit from dysarthria therapy.

Table 8–1

Cranial Nerves

	Nerve	Function	Type
I	Olfactory	Smell, taste	Sensory
II	Optic	Vision	Sensory
III	Oculomotor	Eye, eyelid, and pupil movement	Motor
IV	Trochlear	Eye movement	Motor
V	Trigeminal	Jaw movement; sensation from jaw, face, and mouth	Mixed
VI	Abducens	Eye movement	Motor
VII	Facial	Facial movement, sensation from anterior tongue	Mixed
VIII	Acoustic (vestibulocochlear)	Balance; hearing	Sensory
IX	Glossopharyngeal	Pharyngeal and palatal movement; sensation from posterior tongue	Mixed
X	Vagus	Movement and sensation from larynx, pharynx, esophagus, and internal organs; branches into inferior and superior laryngeal nerves	Mixed
XI	Spinal accessory	Larynx, chest, shoulder, and neck movement	Motor
XII	Hypoglossal	Tongue movement	Motor

Sources: Adapted from Brookshire, R. H. (2014). *Introduction to neurogenic communication disorders* (8th ed.). Mosby.; Duffy, J. R. (2019). *Motor speech disorders: Substrates, differential diagnosis, and management* (4th ed.). Mosby.

Treatment Efficacy/Evidence-Based Practice

Experimental and clinical evidence indicates that therapeutic intervention is generally effective for individuals with dysarthria (Finch et al., 2018). Yorkston (1996), Kent (2000), Yorkston et al. (2003), and Muñoz-Vigueras et al. (2021) published summaries of group-treatment studies, single-subject studies, and case profiles that offer the following conclusions regarding treatment efficacy with various types of dysarthria:

- Individuals with Parkinson's disease derive greater benefit from treatment that targets both respiratory (breath support for speech) and phonatory function (loudness) than treatment that focuses on respiratory function alone.

- Speech rate control results in improved sentence intelligibility but not phoneme intelligibility.

- Short, intense doses of intervention based on neuroplasticity principles can result in improved speech intelligibility in patients with dysarthria

Table 8-2
Classification of the Dysarthrias

Type	Cause	Site of Lesion	Neuromuscular Status	Speech Characteristics
Flaccid	Bulbar palsy, myasthenia gravis	Lower motor neuron	Weakness, low muscle tone	Indistinct and labored articulation; hypernasality; breathy voice quality
Spastic	Pseudobulbar palsy	Upper motor neuron	Increased muscle tone; reduced range of motion, strength, and speed	Slow, imprecise articulation; hypernasality; strained, strangled, harsh voice quality; monotonous pitch and loudness; short phrasing
Ataxic	Cerebellar disorders	Cerebellum	Inaccurate range, timing, and direction; low muscle tone; reduced speed of movement	Excess and equal stress; irregular articulatory breakdown; slow, inaccurate articulation; rhythm disturbances; phoneme prolongations; some excess loudness
Hypokinetic	Parkinsonism	Extrapyramidal (substantia nigra)	Markedly reduced range and speed of movement; marked muscle rigidity; rest tremors	Monopitch and monoloudness; slow speaking rate with short rushes of speech; long, inappropriate pauses; articulation accuracy fluctuates greatly
Hyperkinetic				
Quick	Chorea, Tourette's syndrome, Huntington's chorea	Extrapyramidal	Rapid, jerky, uncontrolled tic movements	Imprecise articulation; variable rate and loudness; harsh voice; inappropriate pauses; abrupt grunts and barks
Slow	Athetosis, dystonia, dyskinesia	Extrapyramidal	Slow, twisting, writhing movements and postures; variable muscle tone	Irregular articulatory breakdown; monopitch and monoloudness; harsh voice quality
Tremor	Organic voice tremor, myoclonus	Extrapyramidal	Involuntary, rhythmic movements	Voice tremors with rhythmic phonation breaks; choked, strained voice quality

Table 8–2
continued

Type	Cause	Site of Lesion	Neuromuscular Status	Speech Characteristics
Mixed	Amyotrophic lateral sclerosis (ALS), multiple sclerosis (MS), Wilson's disease	Multiple motor systems	Muscular weakness; reduced range and speed of motion; some intention tremors	*ALS*: severely defective articulation; slow rate; noticeable hypernasality; harsh voice quality; marked prosodic disturbances *MS*: harsh voice quality; inconsistent rate; inconsistent articulatory precision *Wilson's disease*: similar to hypokinetic dysarthria without sudden bursts of speech
Unilateral upper motor neuron	Stroke	Posterior frontal lobe	Lower facial weakness; hemiparesis	Imprecise consonants; irregular articulatory breakdown; harsh voice

Sources: Adapted from *Motor Speech Disorders*, by F. L. Darley, A. E. Aronson, & J. R. Brown, 1975, Philadelphia, PA: Saunders; "Treating Apraxia of Speech," by J. C. Rosenbek & L. L. LaPointe, 1985, in *Clinical Management of Neurogenic Communicative Disorders* (pp. 97–152), by D. Johns (Ed.), Boston, MA: Little, Brown; *Motor Speech Disorders: A Treatment Guide*, by J. P. Dworkin, 1991, St. Louis, MO: Mosby Year Book; *Motor Speech Disorders: Diagnosis and Treatment* (2nd ed.), by D. Freed, 2012, Clifton Park, NY: Delmar, Cengage Learning.

- The benefits of therapy for prosody impairment are difficult to determine at this time due to the paucity of information available.

- Various behavioral therapy approaches are effective for individuals with stroke or traumatic brain injury, including feedback of acoustic information, respiratory and speech rate control, and physiological strategies such as biofeedback and reaction times (Bakker et al., 2019).

- Devices such as palatal lifts result in gains in muscle strength and speech intelligibility for individuals with stroke or traumatic brain injury.

- Further research is needed to determine which intervention approaches are best suited for various types of dysarthria. Treatment studies using randomized clinical trials are required to generate reliable and valid efficacy/outcome information.

- Advanced measurement techniques such as neuroimaging should be increasingly utilized in efficacy studies with larger patient populations.

Treatment for the Dysarthrias

The overall goal of dysarthria therapy is to improve intelligibility and, if possible, speech-motor control. Ultimately, goal setting is influenced by the type and degree of dysarthric impairment. For severely impaired individuals, establishing functional communication through the use of augmentative or alternative systems may be the focus of intervention. In contrast, the aim of therapy for clients with mild dysarthrias is to reestablish speech patterns that closely approximate normal production. Spencer et al. (2003) provide a flowchart to guide clinicians through the assessment and treatment of dysarthria, focusing on the impact of respiratory and phonatory impairments on speech production. The flowchart presents different treatment options and strategies for deficits in respiratory control, phonation, and overall coordination for speech. Even if nonspeech tasks or other supports (e.g., postural changes, prosthetic devices) are incorporated into treatment, the authors emphasize the inclusion of speech tasks for relevance and carryover of skills. If intervention results in progress, therapy may be continued in a follow-up nature, especially in cases of progressive disorders; if sufficient progress has not been made with regard to speech intelligibility and/or communicative effectiveness, the clinician may need to consider exploring augmentative and alternative communication (AAC) options.

Types of Treatment

As outlined in Table 8–2, there are several different types of dysarthria with distinctive speech symptoms. However, the basic issues and approaches to treatment are similar across the dysarthria classifications. In general, there are four basic approaches to dysarthria therapy:

- *Behavioral:* This is the traditional approach in which progressively more difficult activities and feedback are used to improve client performance on both nonspeech and speech tasks. This may include use of verbal reinforcement, metronome pacing, biofeedback, delayed auditory feedback, and pacing boards. Biofeedback involves electronic monitoring devices that are used to help a client gain some voluntary control over previously unconscious body functions such as respiration, nasality, and extraneous oral movements. **Delayed auditory feedback (DAF)** is a system in which a client's words are returned to him or her through headphones after an imposed electronic delay of a few milliseconds. A **pacing board** (Helm, 1979) is a series of divided colored squares used to reduce speech rate by requiring a client to touch one square per syllable or word uttered.

- *Prosthetic devices:* The use of an artificial device or appliance to replace the function of a missing or impaired part of the speech mechanism. The most common prosthesis used in the treatment of dysarthria is a palatal lift. This is a mechanical device that elevates the soft palate toward the posterior pharyngeal wall to decrease hypernasal resonance in clients with velopharyngeal incompetence (VPI).

- *Medical and surgical procedures:* The use of drugs and/or surgical procedures to ameliorate deficiencies in the speech production system. A pharyngeal flap and phonosurgery are examples of surgical intervention approaches. **Pharyngeal flap surgery** joins soft tissue from the posterior pharyngeal wall to the soft palate to improve velopharyngeal closure during speech. This procedure is used primarily with hypernasal clients for whom behavioral therapy and prosthetic interventions have been unsuccessful. Three types of **phonosurgery** are associated with treatment for unilateral vocal fold paralysis or paresis: (a) Teflon or Gelfoam injection, in which material is injected into the compromised fold to increase its bulk; the additional mass shortens the distance that the healthy fold must travel across midline to make contact with the paralyzed fold; (b) repositioning of the impaired fold toward midline through surgical insertion of a plastic implant; and (c) reinnervation of the thyroarytenoid muscle through implantation of a nerve-muscle pedicle taken from an intact omohyoid muscle. (See Klein & Johns [2009] for a detailed discussion of phonosurgical procedures.)

Deep brain stimulation (DBS) is a surgical procedure used to treat a variety of disabling neurological symptoms—most commonly Parkinson's disease. DBS uses a surgically implanted, battery-operated device—similar to a heart pacemaker—to electrically stimulate the targeted areas in the brain that control movement (Knowles et al., 2018; Morello et al., 2020). When newer, more promising treatments develop in the future, the DBS procedure can be reversed, allowing individuals to still pursue other treatments as they are developed (National Institute of Neurological Disorders and Stroke, 2010).

- *Augmentative/alternative devices:* Nonvocal modes of communication to supplement or replace speech. These may include communication boards, alphabet boards, gestural systems, computers, and speech synthesizers.

Dysarthria is an impairment that may affect all motor speech subsystems. Treatment of dysarthria is generally based on the hierarchical organization of these subsystems: respiration, phonation, resonance, articulation, and prosody. Following is a brief discussion of basic treatment programming for each of the subsystems.

Respiratory Subsystem

The main respiratory problem of clients with dysarthria is inefficient use of the breath stream for speech, rather than a reduction of vital capacity (total volume of air in the lungs). (*Note:* The normal rate of respiration is 16 breaths per minute.) The goal of intervention for this subsystem is to establish consistent, controlled exhalation of air to support speech production. Following is one basic treatment progression for behavioral training:

1. Establish a stable base for respiratory function through muscle relaxation and adjustments of body posture. For example, (a) progressive relaxation techniques (see Table 9–1 in the next chapter) can be used to decrease muscle stiffness; and (b) a supine (lying face up) position may facilitate loudness. (*Note:* Modifications of posture and seating should always be implemented in consultation with other health care professionals such as physical therapists, occupational therapists, or physicians.)

2. Decrease shallow inhalation and improve control of sustained exhalation by manipulating inspiratory and expiratory cycles in nonspeech breathing. For example, (a) ask the client to take a deep breath and hold it as long as possible while the clinician applies light counterpressure on the abdominal wall; (b) provide visual feedback of the client's expiratory pressure and duration through the use of devices such as manometers or oscilloscopes.

3. Further improve exhalation control by establishing adequate loudness and voice quality while producing speech of increasing length and duration (beginning with isolated phonemes and progressing gradually to longer segments). For example, (a) ask the client to produce and sustain a single phoneme (e.g., /s/) for as long as possible, gradually progress to consonant series (e.g., /s-s-s-s-s-s/), and add vowels and other consonants (e.g., /sa/, /sap/); and (b) practice sound sequences with varying patterns of loudness, stress, and intonation, progressing systematically to the level of conversation.

Phonatory Subsystem

Individuals with dysarthria exhibit a wide range of phonatory abnormalities, which vary according to dysarthria type and underlying neurological damage. These problems can be classified into three main patterns of vocal fold movement: hyperadduction, hypoadduction, and incoordination. **Hyperadduction** refers to excessive laryngeal tension and overly forceful closure of the vocal folds, which produces a harsh or strained-strangled voice quality. **Hypoadduction** involves reduced laryngeal muscle tension and inadequate closure of the vocal folds, resulting in a breathy, hoarse voice quality with decreased loudness and pitch control. **Incoordination** can be defined as inconsistent fluctuations of vocal fold vibration cycles that can result in *aphonia* (no voice), asynchronous onset of exhalation and phonation, and inappropriate pitch and loudness breaks. In general, hyperadduction and incoordination of vocal fold movement have less overall impact on speech intelligibility than hypoadduction and are usually not the primary intervention targets for this subsystem.

The aim of intervention for hypoadduction is to achieve efficient vocal fold closure during speech. This goal may be accomplished through phonosurgical procedures or behavioral training. A behavioral training approach can proceed according to the following sequence:

1. Increase control of glottal closure through sustained breath holding. For example, instruct the client to take a deep breath and hold it for as long as possible with a closed-mouth posture.

2. Improve voluntary control of vocal fold abduction-adduction through physical maneuvers that elicit glottal closure (e.g., lifting, pushing, and pulling). For example, (a) instruct the client to assume a seated position, exhale slowly, and at each clinician signal, pull up as hard as possible on the sides of the seat while deliberately attempting to stop the exhalation; and (b) introduce phonation by asking the client to produce /a/ at a comfortable loudness level on exhalation and employ the glottal closure maneuver described previously on each clinician signal.

3. Refine the client's control of vocal fold valving through the use of a continuum of speech activities. For example, (a) ask the client to use a physical maneuver to induce reflexive glottal closure (e.g., pull up on the seat) and, on clinician instruction, release glottal closure and produce an isolated vowel with a hard phonatory attack; and (b) repeat this procedure with speech stimuli of increasing length and duration (e.g., syllable, word, phrase, sentence, conversation).

One specific technique that addresses both phonatory and respiratory dimensions is the Lee Silverman Voice Technique (LSVT; Finch et al., 2018; Fox et al., 2012; Lowit et al., 2020; Sapir et al., 2013). This intensive approach is designed to improve the perceptual characteristics of voice by targeting loudness. LSVT focuses on increasing phonatory effort, vocal fold adduction, and respiratory support. This 4-week daily program teaches clients to "think loud" in order to produce high-effort, loud phonation. Clients also continuously monitor their vocal loudness and effort. Tasks occur in the context of sustained vowel phonation and progress from reading simple texts to conversation. The overall focus of LSVT is not on the modification of specific speech patterns, but rather on amplifying speech loudness. A similar program called Speak Out also focuses on producing speech that is deliberate with strong intent (Boutsen et al., 2018). Studies have found that increased vocal loudness can alter acoustic aspects of speech (e.g., increasing vowel duration, raising fundamental frequency), and these alterations have a positive impact on speech intelligibility (Mahler & Ramig, 2012; Tjaden & Wilding, 2011).

Resonance Subsystem

The two main symptoms of dysarthric impairment in this subsystem are hypernasality and accompanying nasal air emission due to impairment of the velopharyngeal musculature. The overall goal of intervention for resonance problems is to decrease hypernasality through the use of procedures designed to improve a client's ability to generate intraoral air pressure. Behavioral, prosthetic, and surgical approaches can be used to accomplish this goal. A behavioral regimen is most effective with clients who demonstrate mild resonance problems. Following is a basic behavioral treatment sequence:

- Improve awareness of the degree of nasal resonance through the use of biofeedback devices. For example, instruct the client to produce single sustained vowels alternating between greater and lesser degrees of jaw opening while using an instrument that measures and visually displays the differential amounts of nasal resonance.

- Improve the ability to generate intraoral air pressure during production of consonant-vowel (CV) syllables that contain initial plosives. For example, instruct the client to alternately produce pairs of CV syllables that differ in the nasality of the initial consonant (e.g., *me/be; no/go; my/pie*).

- Further refine control of velopharyngeal function during connected speech using biofeedback information. For example, instruct the client to maintain the target range of resonance while producing speech of increasing length and complexity (i.e., isolated words, short phrases, sentences, conversational speech).

For clients with moderate to severe impairments that significantly impact speech intelligibility, a prosthetic or surgical approach may be recommended. A **palatal lift** is considered a reasonable treatment alternative under the following conditions: relatively isolated paresis or paralysis of the velum, lack of excessive spasticity or increased reflex activity in the velopharyngeal area, and adequate dentition to anchor the appliance. **Pharyngeal flap** surgery is generally instituted when behavioral and/or palatal lift approaches have been unsuccessful and when an adequate degree of lateral pharyngeal wall movement is available (see Dworkin [1991]; Johnston et al., [2021]; and Yorkston et al. [1988] for detailed discussions of these procedures). Prosthetic and surgical interventions usually do not result in the restoration of "normal" function. Improvements gained from a palatal lift or pharyngeal flap must be considered in relation to a client's comorbid impairments in other speech subsystems.

Articulatory Subsystem

The overriding aim of articulation therapy for clients with dysarthria is to achieve improved speech sound production within the constraints of the underlying neuromuscular impairment. Intervention for the dysarthrias is similar to traditional articulation therapy with respect to both programming and procedures. However, the neuromuscular involvement associated with dysarthria necessitates an additional emphasis on oral-motor training (Solomon et al., 2017). The following strategies can be used to facilitate improved function in the articulation subsystem:

- Oral-motor exercises to normalize muscle tone and increase strength and mobility of articulatory musculature (e.g., lip retraction and pursing, tongue elevation and depression, jaw opening and closing)

- Phonetic placement through explanation, modeling, and tactile stimulation of correct positioning of the articulators (see Appendix 3–A on the companion website and Dworkin [1991] for specific training activities)

- Phonetic shaping that entails the use of intact articulatory movements associated with one phoneme (e.g., /t/ to shape a different phoneme, such as /n/)

- Overarticulation of speech sounds through exaggeration of some characteristic feature of a specific phoneme (e.g., aspiration, stridency, voicing) or the exaggerated production of a particular consonant in medial or final word position (e.g., *hotel, happen, sock, mud*)

- Negative practice through the use of minimal pair stimuli (e.g., *mat/pat, mob/mop, cook/took*)

- Accented speech approaches such as the accent-based music speech protocol (AMSP; Kim & Jo, 2013) resulted in changes in all of the speech subsystems, including improvements in articulation. This approach requires clients to produce targeted phonemes in a variety of contrasting manners (e.g., while performing stretches, while hand-drumming and producing accented productions). The accented or exaggerated productions were found to increase voicing skills as well as to result in clearer oral-motor movements and thus more defined speech productions.

The pattern of articulatory errors and, therefore, the specific targets selected for treatment will vary according to the type of dysarthria. One basic sequence that can be considered in the selection of articulation targets mirrors the order of phoneme acquisition with regard to place of articulation. Therapy may begin with vowels and progress in the following sequence: bilabials → labiodentals → linguadentals → lingua-alveolars → culminating with linguapalatals.

The following task hierarchy can be used to train identified phoneme targets (e.g., /b/; LaPointe & Katz, 2002):

Final position of VC syllables:	/ab/
Final position of CVC syllables:	/tab/
Medial position of VCV syllables:	/aba/
Initial position of CV syllables:	/ba/
Initial position of CVC syllables:	/bag/

Varying positions in multisyllabic words and short phrases

Varying positions in sentences and conversational speech

Some clients with dysarthria may experience extreme difficulty producing particular phonemes (e.g., those that require tongue tip elevation). In such cases, it may be necessary to begin articulation therapy at the isolated phoneme level and/or develop compensatory movements to produce adequate approximations of these speech sounds.

Prosody Subsystem

The speech of clients with dysarthria is often characterized by prosodic and suprasegmental (e.g., stress, pitch) disturbances. Common manifestations include monopitch, monoloudness, excessive and equal stress on each word, inappropriate phrasing and intonation contour patterns, and a tendency to attempt maintenance of premorbid speech rate even when no longer appropriate. (*Note:* The normal speaking rate for adults is 150 to 250 words per minute or 4.4 to 5.9 syllables per second [Goldman-Eisler, 1968]. Table 8–3 presents comparative data regarding normal speech rate.) The ultimate aim of intervention with any symptom in this subsystem is to increase a client's overall speech intelligibility. Following are basic intervention strategies for prosody problems:

- Improve stress and intonation patterns through contrastive drills. This technique employs identical pairs of stimuli that change in emphasis or meaning as a result of differences solely in stress or intonation. Compound words, sentences, or longer units of connected language can be used. For example, "sun shine" versus "sunshine"; "Bill likes *baseball*" versus "*Bill* likes baseball"; or "Bill likes baseball" versus "Bill likes baseball?"

- Reduce monopitch and monoloudness through the use of negative practice drills. In this procedure, a client is required to intentionally produce a target behavior using a habitual error pattern, thus highlighting the contrast between the habitual error and the desired response. For example, instruct the client to alternate between habitual and target productions of word pairs with respect to pitch or loudness (e.g., movie versus MOVIE). Stimuli can be systematically programmed to include more complex units of language. Negative practice drills can be used to highlight any aspect of prosody.

Table 8–3
Normal Speaking Rates for Adults and Children

Task	Average Speaking Rate	Study
Adults		
Uninterrupted discourse	220–240 words per min (wpm)	Weiner (1984)
Conversational speech	270 wpm	Calvert & Silverman (1983)
	4.4–5.9 syllables per sec (sps)	Goldman-Eisler (1961)
Oral reading	160–180 wpm	Calvert & Silverman (1983)
	150–190 wpm	Darley & Spriestersbach (1978)
Responses to questions	115–165 wpm	Andrews & Ingham (1971)
	150–250 wpm	Goldman-Eisler (1968)
Children		
Responses to questions	Age 3 years: 116–163 syllables per min (spm)	Pindzola, Jenkins, & Lokken (1989)
	4 years: 117–183 spm	
	5 years: 109–1823 spm	
Conversational speech	First grade: 125 wpm	Purcell & Runyan (1980)
	Fifth grade: 142 wpm	

Note. Discrepancies in speaking rates are due to variations in calculation methods (e.g., wpm versus spm) and task differences.

- Modify speaking rate through manipulation of the number and duration of pauses rather than attempting to alter the articulatory movements required for speech sound production. This can be accomplished through the use of metronomes, pacing boards, DAF, or tapping. In each of these strategies, the client modifies his or her habitual speech rate by producing each syllable or word in unison with the imposed beat or tempo. Speech rate also can be modified by requiring the client to write the initial letter of each word uttered. In theory, modifications to speech rate, such as a reduction in rate, can promote greater speech intelligibility by providing the speaker with more time to focus on articulatory precision and by providing the listener with more time to process the utterance (Lansford et al., 2011). However, reductions in speech rate can alter the acoustic signal of the utterance in a manner that negatively affects the intelligibility of the message (Tjaden & Wilding, 2011).

Example Profiles

Following are three profiles that characterize the speech disturbances exhibited by individuals with different types of dysarthria (flaccid, hypokinetic, and ataxic). These examples have been designed to illustrate the selection of intervention targets as well as specific therapy activities and materials. Most of the chosen activities can be implemented in either individual or group therapy settings.

PROFILE 1: FLACCID—75-YEAR-OLD

Mr. Patel, a 75-year-old male, suffered a brainstem stroke 2 weeks ago. He presents with mild paresis of all limbs, intact receptive and expressive language skills, and a moderate flaccid dysarthria. Assessment of the speech musculature indicates reduced strength and range of motion of the velum, tongue, and lips. Laryngeal movement is judged to be less affected. Respiratory support for speech appears to be within normal limits as measured by his ability to adequately sustain the vowel /a/. Mr. Patel's speech output is characterized by marked hypernasality; breathy voice quality; and slowed, labored articulation. The prosodic features of Mr. Patel's speech are unremarkable. Overall speech intelligibility is rated as 50% to 65% when the context is unknown to the listener.

Selection of Therapy Targets. The subsystems to be targeted for therapy are resonance and articulation. The first two areas were selected because the degree of Mr. Patel's hypernasality and his slow, imprecise articulation contribute most significantly to a reduction in perceived speech intelligibility.

Sample Activities

Resonance

1. Employ a Nasometer, which is a computerized instrument that calculates and visually displays the ratio of nasal acoustic energy versus oral acoustic energy. (Consult the *Nasometer Instruction Manual*, Kay Elemetrics Corporation, Pine Brook, New Jersey.) Develop a list of 80 stimuli that include 20 CV, VC, CVC, and VCV syllables containing low or mid vowels and liquid consonants (e.g., CV: *yo* and *ro*; VC: *all* and *air*; CVC: *war* and *roll*; VCV: *olo* and *airo*). Set the threshold line on the Nasometer to indicate an acceptable percentage of nasal resonance. Instruct the client to produce each syllable three times while closely watching

the computer screen. Explain that the visual display of the client's valving behavior should consistently fall within the targeted range of resonance. The threshold line can be reduced in 5% steps as the client demonstrates increased mastery of velopharyngeal valving. If the client has difficulty achieving success at a particular percentage level, the threshold line can be raised 10%.

Articulatory

2. Instruct the client to elevate the tongue tip to the alveolar ridge and then raise the tongue tip outside the mouth beyond the upper lip. Provide a mirror for visual feedback. Repeat this elevation movement pattern three times and then pause. Continue the activity by gradually increasing the number of repetitions between each pause. To strengthen this lingual movement, use a tongue depressor to push against the tongue tip to provide resistance that the client must overcome during tongue elevation.

Prosody

3. Make a list of 25 sentences, 7 to 10 words in length, and type them on a sheet of paper. Double-space the sentences and leave large spaces between the words in each sentence. Sample sentences include the following:

> I really enjoyed my vacation last month.
> I don't know what you mean by that.
> The people are walking in the park.
> Sometimes I watch TV in the evening.
> Do you want spaghetti for dinner tonight?
> My family visited the museum in London last year.
> I saw your wife at the store yesterday.
> What time do you usually get home from work?
> I am sad to hear that you are not coming.
> I heard there is a big sale at the mall.

Take a piece of paper with the approximate dimensions of a 12-in. ruler and cut a slit in it that is the length and height of the longest word in the sentence set (e.g., *spaghetti* or *yesterday*). The clinician places the slit card over the first sentence and moves it slowly across the paper. Instruct the client to read each word aloud as it is revealed by the slit in the card. After each sentence is completed, remove the card and instruct the client to read the sentence again, maintaining the slowed speech rate of the first production.

PROFILE 2: HYPOKINETIC—58-YEAR-OLD

Mrs. Fields, a 58-year-old female, presents with a moderate hypokinetic dysarthria that is secondary to Parkinson's disease. Her overall status (including speech musculature) is characterized by muscle rigidity, limited range of movement, and rest tremors (involuntary, rhythmic movements exhibited when muscles are at rest). Voice quality is breathy with monopitch and decreased loudness due to limited capacity and control of the respiratory musculature. Resonance is judged to be unaffected. Mrs. Fields's articulatory precision is mildly to moderately affected and is marked by short bursts of hurried speech separated by grammatically inappropriate and abrupt pauses. She demonstrates reduced prosody of speech. Her speech intelligibility is rated as moderately unintelligible, primarily as a result of vocal abnormalities with a more modest contribution from her articulation errors. Language abilities appear to be within normal limits.

Selection of Therapy Targets. The areas to be targeted are the respiratory, phonatory, and articulatory subsystems. These were selected according to the subsystem hierarchy. The first two were chosen based on Mrs. Fields's vocal symptoms of breathiness and reduced pitch and loudness. The third was targeted in an effort to increase her intelligibility to its maximum level. Respiration was selected as the initial focus of therapy, because it serves as the foundation for all other speech subsystems.

Sample Activities

Respiratory

1. Instruct the client to inhale deeply and hold the breath as the clinician slowly counts to three. Tell the client to exhale slowly while producing rhythmic patterns of a voiceless fricative (e.g., /s/). Sound productions of long and short duration comprise the rhythmic patterns. Following are sample series:

   (_____ = long sound: ____ = short sound):

   ____ _____ ____ _____ ____ _____

   _____ ____ ____ _____ ____ _____

   _____ _____ ____ ____ _____ _____ ____

   ____ ____ ____ _____ ____ ____ ____ _____

   _____ ____ _____ ____ _____

   Remind the client that each series must be produced on a single exhalation. This activity can be implemented with any rhythmic pattern and can be extended to gradually introduce additional voiceless fricatives, such as /f/, /θ/, and /ʃ/.

Phonatory

2. Write the numbers 1 to 10 on 20 index cards. Highlight various combinations of numbers on each card by using bold print or type. Instruct the client to read the digit series on each card with increased loudness on the boldface numbers. Sit within 5 ft of the client and encourage her to project her voice without excessive muscular tension. Use the following series:

1	**2**	3	**4**	5	**6**	7	**8**	9	**10**
1	2	**3**	4	5	**6**	7	8	**9**	10
1	2	3	4	5	6	**7**	**8**	9	10
1	2	3	**4**	5	**6**	7	8	**9**	**10**
1	**2**	**3**	4	**5**	6	**7**	**8**	9	**10**

Increase the level of difficulty of this activity by gradually expanding the distance between the client and clinician.

Articulatory

3. Identify the client's articulation errors that result from limited range and strength of the oral musculature. Develop compensatory phonetic placements that affect acceptable approximations of the target sounds. Examples include the following:

Error Sound	Compensatory Placement
/p, b/	Place upper teeth on lower lip and abruptly drop the lower jaw to produce the desired plosive air burst.
/m/	Touch upper teeth to lower lip and produce sound with nasal resonance.
/t, d, l, s, z, n/	Elevate tongue blade to touch alveolar ridge while maintaining tongue tip in lower position.

PROFILE 3: ATAXIC—45-YEAR-OLD

Mr. Seymour, a 45-year-old male, presents with a mild to moderate ataxic dysarthria as a result of a tumor that caused localized damage to the cerebellum. His current condition is marked by hypotonia, slow and jerky voluntary movements, and inaccurate direction of movement. Mr. Seymour's breath support for speech appears to be adequate. His voice quality, although slightly harsh and monotone, is judged to be within normal limits. Resonance is unremarkable. In spontaneous speech, Mr. Seymour exhibits transient articulatory breakdowns characterized by imprecise consonants and distorted vowels, prolongations of phonemes, and dysprosody of speech due to excessive and equal stress of syllables and words. Overall speech intelligibility is rated at approximately 65% to 75% when the context is unknown to the listener.

Selection of Therapy Targets. The areas to be targeted are articulation and prosody. These were selected because Mr. Seymour's reduced speech intelligibility is caused primarily by deficits in these two subsystems.

Sample Activities

Articulation

1. Develop three word lists for an intelligibility drill, each of which contains 10 CVC words that are similar except for a single phoneme. Sample word lists follow:

Paul	beer	ban
ball	dear	pan
call	fear	can
mall	near	man

wall	cheer	ran
gall	tear	Dan
fall	gear	tan
tall	we're	wan
hall	hear	fan
doll	mere	van

Print each word on an index card and shuffle the cards so that the words are in random order. Instruct the client to select a card from the deck, keeping it out of the clinician's visual field, and read it aloud. The clinician is unaware of the specific word being produced and must guess the identity of the utterance based solely on the client's intelligibility. The client indicates the accuracy of the clinician's guess. If the clinician's first guess is incorrect, the client repeats the target word once. If the clinician's second guess is erroneous, the clinician reads the index card and models the correct production of the word. The client imitates this model five times, returns the index card to the pile, and draws another card.

Prosody

2. Develop a set of 25 identical sentence pairs that contain at least a subject, verb, and object. Write each pair on a separate index card and underline or boldface a different word in each sentence. Explain that this activity focuses on the ways in which changes in prosody affect sentence meaning. Further explain that the clinician will ask a stimulus question that the client must answer by reading aloud the prosodically appropriate sentence from a corresponding index card. Instruct the client to choose one index card, listen to the stimulus question, and read aloud the correct version, using exaggerated intonation to highlight the boldface word. Examples of pairs of stimulus questions and response sentences include the following:

Question	*Response*
What did you open?	I opened the **door**.
What did you do?	I **opened** the door.
Did she read the email?	She **wrote** the email.
Who wrote the email?	**She** wrote the email.
Whose car is John driving tomorrow?	John is driving **my** car tomorrow.
Is Phil driving your car tomorrow?	**John** is driving my car tomorrow.
What dance is Sadie doing?	Sadie is dancing the **tango** with Mel.
Who is she dancing with?	Sadie is dancing the tango with **Mel**.
Does Tom call Judy often?	Tom **always** calls Judy on her birthday.
When does Tom call Judy?	Tom always calls Judy on her **birthday**.

Prosody

3. Gather several reading passages and highlight the syllables and words that receive primary stress. (*Note:* Stress patterns may vary according to regional dialect.) Instruct the client to read each passage aloud while concentrating on stress, rhythm, and intonation. Explain that

this can be achieved by *strongly* emphasizing the boldface portions. Examples of reading materials include the following:

The Little Girl and the Wolf
(From *The Thurber Carnival* by James Thurber, 1945)

One after**noon** a big **wolf wait**ed in **a dark for**est for a **little girl** to come a**long carry**ing a **bas**ket of **food** to her **grand**mother. **Fin**ally a **little girl did** come a**long** and **she** was **carrying a bas**ket of **food.** "**Arc** you **carry**ing that **bas**ket to your **grand**mother?" **asked** the **wolf.** The **little girl** said **yes**, she **was.** So the **wolf asked** her **where** her **grand**mother **lived** and the **little girl told** him and he **dis**appeared into the **woods.**

When the **little girl o**pened the **door** of her **grand**mother's **house,** she **saw** that there was **some**body in **bed** with a **night**cap and **night**gown on. She had **approached** no **near**er than **twen**ty-five **feet** from the **bed** when she **saw** that it was **not** her **grand**mother but the **wolf,** for even in a **night**cap a **wolf** does **not** look any **more** like your **grand**mother than the **M-G-M li**on looks like **Calvin Coo**lidge. So the **little girl** took an auto**matic** out of her **bas**ket and **shot** the **wolf dead.**

Moral: It is **not** as easy to **fool little girls now**adays as it **used** to be.

Oh When I Was ...
(From *A Shropshire Lad* by A. E. Housman, 1896)

Oh when **I** was in **love** with **you,**

Then I was **clean** and **brave,**

And **miles around** the **won**der **grew,**

How **well** did I be**have.**

And **now** the **fancy passes by,**

And **noth**ing will re**main,**

And **miles around** they'll **say** that **I**

Am **quite** my**self** again.

Helpful Hints

1. It is important to avoid the tendency to simply instruct a client to slow down, speak up, or try harder. Explicit and intensive drills are required to successfully modify the prosodic features of a client's speech.

2. Verbal instructions for therapy activities may have to be simplified for clients who present with language deficits due to a concomitant aphasia.

3. Mirrors, audio recordings, and video recordings are useful adjuncts for developing a client's self-monitoring skills for speech production.

4. When working with adults, it is extremely important to explain why a given task is being implemented rather than merely describing how the task should be performed.

5. Clinicians should be aware that a client's reluctance to perform speech tasks may be related to fears about cosmetic changes (e.g., facial asymmetry, drooling) resulting from oral-facial sensory deficits.

6. Family education is an integral part of therapy programming for clients with dysarthria. For useful handouts about the nature of dysarthria and tips for effective communication strategies, see Yorkston et al. (2004) and Tanner (2008).

7. Given the recent advances in technologically based therapy, clinicians are encouraged to stay abreast of these new approaches.

Apraxia of Speech

Apraxia is an inability to plan and execute volitional motor movements due to central nervous system damage despite intact muscle strength and coordination. This deficit can affect any system that requires purposeful sequences of muscle movement. In a **limb apraxia**, voluntary movements of the extremities are affected in gestures such as waving good-bye or making a fist on command. An **oral apraxia** involves difficulty with nonspeech movements of the oral mechanism such as tongue protrusion and lip pursing on command.

Apraxia of speech (AOS; or verbal apraxia) is a neurologically based articulation disorder characterized by difficulty in positioning speech muscles and sequencing muscle movements for the voluntary production of speech. This disorder is not associated with weakness, slowness, or incoordination of these muscles during automatic and reflexive acts (McNeil et al., 1997). Verbal apraxia is a motor speech disorder; therefore, language comprehension and the grammatical system are not affected. However, it should be noted that apraxia frequently co-occurs with aphasia. It is also important to note that the term apraxia of speech is distinct from the motor speech disorder childhood apraxia of speech (CAS). (For information on CAS, see Chapter 3 and Allison et al., 2020.) Apraxia results from a lesion in the left frontal lobe near Broca's area. The main causes of apraxia are quite similar to those associated with aphasia and include cerebrovascular accident (CVA), trauma, tumors, and disease processes such as Alzheimer's.

Severity of apraxia ranges along a continuum from very subtle articulatory errors to completely unintelligible speech. At the most extreme level of impairment, an individual may be unable to initiate phonation volitionally. Following are the most significant characteristics of verbal apraxia (Croot, 2002; Duffy, 2020; Wertz et al., 1991):

- Highly unpredictable and inconsistent errors are made, even on repeated attempts at the same word. For example, an individual with apraxia may produce the following sequence in an attempt to produce the word *escalator:* elescat, lator, scalator, lescatator, lescator, elescator.

- Substitutions and transpositions are the most frequent type of speech production errors, but omissions and distortions are also common.

- Complex consonant blends are often substituted for simpler phonemes (e.g., "strondo" for *tornado*).

- There is difficulty initiating speech as evidenced by frequent stops, restarts, long pauses and hesitations, and repetition of initial sounds and syllables.

- Articulatory accuracy deteriorates as word length increases.

- There are visible and audible groping behaviors in which the speaker struggles to achieve appropriate placement of the articulators through trial and error.

- Automatic speech generally contains fewer articulatory errors than purposeful productions. For example, rote recitation of the months of the year may be relatively error free (i.e., January, February, March . . .), whereas meaningful production of any of these words is likely to include numerous articulation errors (e.g., In response to the clinician's question, "When are you going to visit your daughter?" the client says, "Ferry . . . ferrary . . . fruary . . . befuary").

- Client may be aware of the articulation errors but is unable to correct them on subsequent attempts.

- Prosody of speech is atypical with respect to rhythm, word stress, and intonational contour.

- Speech rate is slowed.

As discussed in the previous chapter, a period of spontaneous recovery follows the initial neurological insult. This period may continue for up to 6 months, with the most significant improvement occurring during the first 8 weeks. The prognosis is determined by many of the same factors that affect recovery from aphasia, including size, location, and etiology of lesion, age at onset, and overall health of the client. However, there are certain apraxia-specific indicators that are associated with a less favorable prognosis. These include (a) presence of an accompanying oral apraxia, particularly lasting more than 2 months; and (b) the severity and duration of an accompanying aphasia.

Although apraxia and dysarthria are both motor-speech disorders, their symptomologies are considerably different. Table 8–4 presents the differentiating characteristics of these disorders.

Table 8–4
Differential Characteristics of Apraxia and Dysarthria

Apraxia	Dysarthria
Articulation is better in involuntary/automatic speech; periods of error-free speech may exist.	Automatic and voluntary speech are similarly impaired; there are no periods of error-free speech.
Errors are unpredictable and highly inconsistent.	Errors are predictable and highly consistent.
Substitution and transposition errors predominate.	Distortion and omission errors predominate.
There is significant difficulty with the initiation of speech, evidenced by hesitations, pauses, restarts, and repetitions.	Initiation of speech is usually not affected.
Visible and audible groping postures of the articulators are evident.	There are no visible or audible groping postures of the articulators.
Deficits occur primarily in articulation and prosody.	All speech processes are involved, including respiration, phonation, articulation, prosody, and resonance.

Sources: Adapted from Wertz, R. T., LaPointe, L. L., & Rosenbek, J. C. (1991). *Apraxia of speech in adults: The disorder and its management.* Singular.; LaPointe, L. L., & Katz, R. C. (2002). Neurogenic disorders of speech. In G. H. Shames & N. B. Anderson (Eds.), *Human communication disorders* (6th ed., pp. 472–509). Allyn & Bacon.; Duffy, J. R. (2019). *Motor speech disorders: Substrates, differential diagnosis, and management* (4th ed.). Mosby.

Treatment Efficacy/Evidence-Based Practice

Few studies have been conducted that directly address either efficacy or outcome issues in apraxia of speech. Van Heugten et al. (2000) investigated the effect of a functional treatment program with 33 stroke patients with apraxia and 36 stroke patients without apraxia. Their results suggest that traditional prognostic variables such as cognitive impairment, motor impairment, and advanced age were not related to treatment outcome. McNeil et al. (2010) conducted a study with two individuals with acquired apraxia of speech to determine the effect of augmented feedback on treatment outcomes. Feedback from clinicians as well as visual, biofeedback sources were both found to improve performance on speech tasks. Ballard's (2001) critical review of the existing literature suggests that response generalization effects are slight, especially in the application of trained behaviors to novel situations. Wambaugh et al. (2006) conducted a treatment literature review, with the overall conclusion that individuals with apraxia of speech may show improvement in speech production even when the impairment is chronic. The strongest evidence was found for treatments that focus on the articulatory aspects of speech production. An updated systematic review was conducted by Mauszycki and Wambaugh (2011), citing studies that found evidence for using articulatory-kinematic and rate/rhythm control treatment approaches with AOS.

Treatment for Apraxia of Speech

The ultimate aim of intervention for apraxia of speech (heretofore referred to simply as apraxia) is to increase a client's voluntary control over the articulatory movements necessary for accurate speech production to the limits imposed by the neurological impairment (Wambaugh, 2021). For clients with severe to profound apraxia, intelligible speech may not be a realistic goal. Within a social model of disability, intervention in this context may focus on reducing barriers to successful communication along with training for others in the client's environment rather than targeting speech production skills. This may incorporate use of augmentative or alternative means of communication (AAC). The Modified Diadochokinesis Test (MDT) is a psychometrically sound assessment tool for measuring treatment gains, although clinicians are advised to implement informal measures (e.g., conversational level speech) for a more holistic view of patient improvement (Hurkmans et al., 2012). Many traditional approaches to intervention for apraxia can be discussed from two basic perspectives: structure (how to teach) and function (what to teach). Information can be found in the following sections.

Structure

Intervention programs for apraxia can be structured in several different ways. The central feature of nearly all approaches is the use of drill; motor learning is dependent on repeated opportunities to practice desired movement patterns.

One well-known paradigm for structuring apraxia therapy is the eight-step task continuum developed by Wertz et al. (1991). This continuum incorporates Milisen's (1954a) concept of "integral stimulation," which emphasizes simultaneous input in multiple modalities, especially auditory and visual. This paradigm utilizes imitation as the primary teaching strategy and attempts to facilitate increased voluntary articulatory control through systematic, gradual fading of clinician cues. Following are the eight steps:

| Step 1 | Clinician presents integral stimulation (i.e., "Watch me"; "Listen to me"); clinician and client then produce target utterance in unison. |

Step 2	Clinician presents integral stimulation; and then clinician offers visual cue only (i.e., mouths each utterance without sound) while client simultaneously produces the target utterance aloud.
Step 3	Clinician presents integral stimulation; and then client imitates target utterance independently.
Step 4	Repeat Step 3, but require the client to produce target utterance several times in a row without any intervening clinician model.
Step 5	Clinician presents written stimuli, which client reads aloud.
Step 6	Clinician presents and then removes written stimuli; client attempts target utterance.
Step 7	Clinician presents a question designed to elicit target utterance and client responds.
Step 8	Clinician engages client in role-play situations to elicit target utterance. (This step is most appropriate for target behaviors at the word level and beyond.)

Content

The preceding section on structure presents guidelines for "how to teach" or structure a therapy program. This section focuses on "what to teach," or the content of an intervention program for apraxia. In 1975, Darley et al. recommended a basic treatment progression. This protocol was adapted for discussion in this chapter because of its simplicity and its suitability for almost any degree of apraxic impairment. The point in the progression at which therapy is initiated depends on an individual client's capabilities.

Phase I: Initiate Phonation. Instruct the client to do the following:

- Produce a cough or sigh.

- Prolong exhalation and shift from a cough or sigh to phonation.

- Induce phonation through humming (or singing) in unison with clinician.

- Overlay a variety of mouth opening and tongue configurations to produce vowels and diphthongs.

Phase II: Increase Smoothness and Length of Speech

- Use automatic speech such as TV jingles, the Pledge of Allegiance, rotely memorized poems and songs, and everyday expressions—such as, "How are you?" or "I feel fine"—to experience the feel of easily produced speech.

- Use highly familiar or automatic speech patterns to provide a base for establishing propositional vocabulary; for example, "salt and _____" or "roses are _____."

Phase III: Phonemic Drill. Individuals with apraxia exhibit the least amount of difficulty with vowels, glides, and nasal sounds; more difficulty with plosives; increased difficulty with fricatives and affricates; and the most difficulty with consonant clusters. This hierarchy of difficulty with respect to manner of production can guide the selection of therapy targets for drill work. Once a target phoneme has been identified, voluntary motor control can be increased using Darley et al.'s (1975) suggested 10-step therapy sequence.

Step 1	Hum the phoneme in isolation: /nnnnn/.
Step 2	Add a vowel to the consonant target and produce the syllable 20 times (e.g., /na/). Repeat this drill with other vowels.
Step 3	Produce a series of five or six different CV syllable combinations: nu, na, ny, now, naw.
Step 4	Produce reduplicative syllables first in isolation (nana, nana, nana; nini, nini, nini) and then in succession (nana, nini, nunu).
Step 5	Add the target phoneme as the final consonant to form a CVC syllable: nan, nin, nown. As in Step 4, first practice in isolation and then in succession.
Step 6	Produce the target phoneme in short words with simple phonetic environments: *new, nine, nap, nag, nod, nail, bin, bone, run, loan, dune.*
Step 7	Produce two-word phrases with the target phoneme in the initial position of both monosyllabic words: *not now, no news, near noon, nice night, north nook.*
Step 8	Repeat Step 7 with target phoneme in the final position of words: *down town, dine in, main man, one gown, lean on.*
Step 9	Produce two-word utterances in which the target phoneme is in the initial position of the first word and the final position of the second word: *knee pain, need ten, new phone, need loan.*
Step 10	Produce multiword utterances with some polysyllabic words, gradually expanding them into sentences: *Natalie won the honor; Nan lives near Ned; Napoleon Bonaparte; nutmeg and cinnamon; north of Jefferson County.*

Once a client has mastered the production of several different target phonemes, introduce them in minimal word pairs to facilitate accurate articulatory transition from one target phoneme to another across word boundaries. Examples include *name-game, run-rut, banner-backer.*

Throughout phonemic drill training, encourage the client to anticipate upcoming phonemes in an utterance and plan or mentally rehearse appropriate articulatory postures. As the client's voluntary control over articulatory movements improves, foster more natural sounding speech by increasing speech rate and highlighting other prosodic features.

Wambaugh et al. (2006) and Van Sickle (2016) present perspectives on categorization of treatment approaches for apraxia of speech: articulatory/kinematic, rate and/or rhythm, intersystemic/reorganization, and alternative/augmentative.

Articulatory/Kinematic

- Emphasizes regaining adequate points of articulation and sequencing of articulatory gestures
- Often focuses on improving spatial and temporal aspects of speech production
- Includes teaching strategies, such as modeling and placement cues

Rate and/or Rhythm

- Focuses on modifying the temporal patterning of speech

- Emphasizes reduced rate of speech to provide additional time for motor planning

- May utilize metronomes, pacing boards, computers, and other devices

Intersystemic/Reorganization

- Utilizes intact modality (e.g., gestures, signing) to facilitate speech production

Alternative/Augmentative

- Utilizes nonspeech communication strategies (e.g., spelling, drawing, gestures, symbols, pictures, writing) to substitute for speech production on a temporary or permanent basis

Two additional AOS treatment approaches that focus on content at the speech sound and/or phrase level are described next.

Sound Production Treatment (Bislick, 2020; Kallhoff & Wambaugh, 2021; Mauszycki & Wambaugh, 2020; Mozeiko et al., 2020; Wambaugh et al., 2021; Wambaugh et al., 2020)

- Studies have evaluated sound production treatment (SPT) with a range of AOS severities. Treatment targets are individualized based on a client's error patterns; minimal pairs are selected based on the speech sounds produced incorrectly during baseline measures.

- Speech sound errors are addressed according to a hierarchy of support provision.

- Feedback is given after every client production, with further supports provided only if errors persist.

- The frequent co-occurrence of AOS and aphasia warrants a treatment that addresses both motor planning and linguistic deficits.

- The SPT hierarchy progresses from minimal prompting to maximal prompting as follows:
  - Verbal modeling of targets (say ball . . . tall); client imitation of targets
  - Verbal modeling while pointing to letters corresponding to targets; client imitation
  - Integral stimulation with error sound or target word (watch me, listen to me, and say it with me; say ball); client imitation
  - Verbal modeling of the incorrect word in segments (say b . . . all); client imitation
  - Verbal cues as to articulatory placement (start with your lips closed for the /b/), followed by verbal model; client imitation

- If the individual still has difficulty at the highest level of prompting, the next minimal pair is targeted and the cycle is repeated. This approach stresses the motor principles of blocked and random practice of targets through the use of repetitive articulation drills with varying speech targets.

Script Training (Youmans et al., 2011)

- Although developed for people with aphasia, script training has been used with individuals with concomitant apraxia of speech to facilitate greater ease in producing phrase-level speech.

- Training principles remain the same when using script training with AOS.

- Strong emphasis is placed on providing feedback so that the individual does not learn incorrect speech patterns.

- Due to the nature of apraxia, the client's speech will continue to contain errors when using scripted phrases, although the frequency of error productions may be reduced.

- However, gains are expected in speaking confidence, ease, and fluidity.

Example Profiles

Following are two profiles that are representative of the speech characteristics of individuals with apraxia. These examples have been designed to illustrate the selection of intervention targets as well as specific therapy activities and materials. Most of the chosen activities can be implemented in either individual or group therapy settings.

PROFILE 4: SEVERE APRAXIA—65-YEAR-OLD

Mrs. Elizondo, a 65-year-old female, exhibits a severe apraxia after surgery to remove a tumor localized in the left frontal lobe. She demonstrates no volitional speech but occasionally produces undifferentiated CV or VC syllables and some automatic utterances (e.g., "Oh my goodness"; "I don't know"). Mild to moderate oral and limb apraxia is present, with no evidence of an accompanying aphasia or hemiparesis. Currently, her sole means of communication is through writing.

Selection of Therapy Targets. Therapy will focus on ensuring the availability of an alternative mode of communication, the initiation of voluntary phonation, and the facilitation of propositional speech. An alternative system will be implemented to provide Mrs. Elizondo with an immediate means of communicating with others. The severity of her verbal apraxia dictates that treatment begin at the most basic level, which involves elicitation of volitional phonation. Because the only intelligible speech in her repertoire consists of sporadic automatic phrases, this type of utterance will be used to stimulate the production of propositional speech at the single-word level.

Sample Activities

Alternative Means of Communication

1. The prognosis for significant improvement in speech production is difficult to determine so early in the recovery process. Therefore, the clinician should provide Mrs. Elizondo with a functional and reliable way of communicating. Many forms of alternative communication systems are available, including picture boards, alphabet boards, electronic devices, and digitized speech. It is the clinician's responsibility to review the available options and select the method within the client's linguistic and motoric capabilities that is (a) most flexible, allowing for the expression of the broadest possible range of messages; and (b) generates messages that are most easily understood by listeners.

Given Mrs. Elizondo's current status, writing is judged to be the optimal choice for a nonvocal communication system. This selection was based on the fact that her language skills are essentially unimpaired and that the limb apraxia does not significantly impede her ability to write. At this stage in Mrs. Elizondo's recovery, it is not known whether writing will serve as an interim method of communication or eventually become a true alternative to speech as her permanent, primary mode of communication.

Volitional Phonation

2. (Step 1 of Rosenbek and LaPointe's [1985] structural hierarchy and Phase I of the Darley et al. [1975] content hierarchy.) Explain that the clinician will model a vocal behavior (i.e., a cough or sigh) two times. For the first trial, instruct the client to watch and listen carefully. On the second trial, instruct the client to attempt the cough or sigh in unison with the clinician's production. Repeat this sequence until the client can produce a cough on volition. Progress through the next three tasks in Phase I, using the same "integral stimulation-unison production" training paradigm. These tasks consist of (a) prolonging exhalation to transition from the cough or sigh to phonation, (b) extending phonation through humming, and (c) superimposing mouth opening and different tongue positions over the humming to produce vowels.

Propositional Speech

3. (Adaptation of Step 7 of Rosenbek and LaPointe's [1985] structural hierarchy and Phase II of the Darley et al. [1975] content hierarchy.) Develop a set of 25 familiar or high-probability phrases. Examples include the following:

   Salt and _____ (pepper)

   Cup of _____ (coffee)

   Knife and _____ (fork)

   Look before you _____ (leap)

   Birds of a _____ (feather)

   Shoes and _____ (socks)

   Turn over a new _____ (leaf)

   Paper and _____ (pencil)

   Peaches and _____ (cream)

   Bacon and _____ (eggs)

   Bread and _____ (butter)

   The early bird catches the _____ (worm)

   Gather pictures that represent the missing word in each fill-in-the-blank phrase. Explain that the clinician will say a phrase aloud while presenting the corresponding picture. Instruct the client to listen carefully, look at the picture, and produce the target word as quickly as possible. If the client is unsuccessful in the first attempt, the clinician can provide additional cues by demonstrating the appropriate placement of the first phoneme or by modeling the first phoneme aloud.

PROFILE 5: MODERATE APRAXIA—58-YEAR-OLD

Mr. Collins, a 58-year-old male, sustained a left frontal lobe CVA 1 year ago, which resulted in a moderate apraxia with an accompanying mild to moderate nonfluent (Broca's) aphasia. He presents with a mild right-sided weakness with no significant oral or limb apraxia. Mr. Collins demonstrates good language comprehension for relatively simple oral and written material. With respect to expression, his utterances are pragmatically appropriate and consist of short, effortful phrases marked by morphological and syntactic errors. Mr. Collins exhibits the ability to imitate verbal utterances; however, his performance deteriorates as utterance length and complexity increase. His speech is characterized by unpredictable articulation errors consisting mainly of sound substitutions and transpositions of plosives, fricatives, and affricates. These errors occur more frequently in multisyllabic utterances. Errors on nasal consonants are noted in connected speech. Speech melody is atypical with respect to stress and intonation; struggle behaviors to achieve accurate articulation placement were clearly visible. Overall, speech is rated as moderately unintelligible, particularly in unknown contexts. Mr. Collins recognizes the inadequacy of his communication skills and is frustrated by them.

Selection of Therapy Targets. The areas to be targeted are the /m/, /p/, and /s/ phonemes as well as the prosodic feature of stress. These sounds were selected according to the hierarchy of difficulty identified by Darley et al. (1975) based on their experience with apraxic individuals. Stress, particularly at the phrase level, was chosen as a means of increasing Mr. Collins's speech intelligibility.

Sample Activities

1. (Adapted from Steps 5 and 6 of Rosenbek and LaPointe's [1985] structural hierarchy and Step 9 of the Darley et al. [1975] phonemic drill sequence.) Develop a list of 25 two-word phrases in which /m/ is in the initial position of the first word and the final position of the second word. Select short words with simple phonetic environments. Write each phrase on an index card, and place the pile face down on the table. Examples include the following:

make time	meet him
my room	miss Tom
mail them	more gum
made ham	meal time
men came	moon beam

   Instruct the client to select the top card and read the phrase aloud. Remove the card and tell the client to repeat the same phrase three times. Following the last production, provide feedback—such as, "You did a nice job saying /m/ in 'make time'"—to expose the client to a clearly articulated indirect model of the target sound. The difficulty of this activity can be increased by gradually incorporating polysyllabic words that contain the target sound into longer phrases and sentences.

2. (Step 4 of Rosenbek and LaPointe's [1985] structural hierarchy and Step 3 of the Darley et al. [1975] phonemic drill sequence.) Write the target phoneme in the center of a large

index card or sheet of paper and surround it with four vowels or diphthongs (e.g., ɑ, o, ɔ, ə). Arrange the vowels as follows, using traditional spelling rather than phonetic symbols.

$$
\begin{array}{ccc}
 & \text{ah} & \\
 & \uparrow & \\
\text{aw} \leftarrow & \text{p} & \rightarrow \text{o} \\
 & \downarrow & \\
 & \text{uh} &
\end{array}
$$

Explain to the client that this activity is designed to improve his or her ability to transition quickly from one syllable to another. Instruct the client to watch and listen (integral stimulation) as the clinician models CV syllables at a relatively rapid rate. This is accomplished by pairing the target consonant with each of the four vowels in a clockwise progression from ah to aw. Client imitates the clinician's model of the syllable series 10 times. This activity also can be used to provide intense drill work on all other target phonemes.

3. Create a set of 20 pairs of phrases or short sentences in which manipulations of stress and pause time alter meaning. Examples include the following:

The sky is falling.	This guy is falling.
An ice man.	A nice man.
A man eating shark.	A man-eating shark.
Oranges have a peel.	Oranges have appeal.
He's a gentle man.	He's a gentleman.
What a dark room!	What a darkroom!
I don't like cross words.	I don't like crosswords.

Each phrase/sentence is written on separate index cards, which are then shuffled and placed in a pile face down on the table. Instruct the client to select one card, keeping it out of the clinician's view, and read it aloud using the appropriate stress pattern. The clinician guesses the utterance based on the client's prosody and coarticulation cues and writes it down on a blank index card. The two cards are then compared to determine whether the client successfully communicated the intended message. If the cards do not match, the clinician models both stress patterns. The client is asked to identify the target pattern and imitate it.

Helpful Hints

1. To avoid or minimize client confusion during the initial stages of phonemic drill training, the clinician should select successive sound targets that are maximally different from one another.

2. A client's success on imitation tasks is sometimes facilitated by the clinician's use of an exaggerated stress or intonation when modeling stimuli.

3. To facilitate the concept of errorless learning, clinicians can provide cueing and/or feedback as promptly as possible in order to promote relearning of correct speech patterns and to prevent acquiring error patterns. See Mauszycki et al. (2017) for more information on the relationship between error awareness and word production.

4. A metronome is a particularly effective temporal cue for regulating the pace of a client's speech.

5. For some clients, a productive strategy for promoting speech initiation or output is to encourage them to pair a gesture with a word.

6. Melodic intonation therapy (MIT; Helm-Estabrooks & Albert, 2004) can be used successfully to promote speech output; the rhythmic nature of intoning a melody facilitates production for some clients with apraxia.

7. Counseling must frequently address the fact that other individuals may negatively judge a client's intellectual/language comprehension skills based on poor speech intelligibility.

8. Families may require considerable education regarding the nature of apraxia to ensure that the client's inconsistent speech errors are not misperceived as signs of laziness or lack of motivation.

Conclusion

This section has presented basic information, protocols, and procedures for dysarthria and AOS intervention at an *introductory* level. This material is intended only as a starting point in the reader's clinical education and training. For more in-depth coverage of these areas, the following readings are recommended.

Brookshire, R. H. (Ed.). (2014). *Introduction to neurogenic communication disorders* (8th ed.). Elsevier Mosby.

Duffy, J. R. (2020). *Motor speech disorders: Substrates, differential diagnosis, and management* (4th ed.). Elsevier Mosby.

Freed, D. (2018). *Motor speech disorders: Diagnosis and treatment* (3rd ed.). Plural Publishing.

Webb, W. G., & Adler, R. K. (2016). *Neurology for the speech-language pathologist* (6th ed.). Elsevier Mosby.

Yorkston, K. M., Miller, R. M., Strand, E. A., & Britton, D. (2013). *Management of speech and swallowing in degenerative diseases* (3rd ed.). Pro-Ed.

Additional Resources

Dysarthria and Apraxia of Speech

The Source for Dysarthria, Second Edition
A comprehensive manual that includes information about dysarthria such as the different types; etiologies; evaluation and treatment planning options; and treatment objectives for respiration, phonation, resonance, articulation, and prosody. Also includes examples of documentation and sample reports.

The Source for Apraxia Therapy

A resource that combines a visual-auditory-kinesthetic approach to improve intelligibility in clients with mild, moderate, or severe apraxia. It is divided into three sections, which focus on production of words and simple sentences, articulation, fluency, phrasing, and paralinguistic drills.

Just for Adults Apraxia Cards

A set of 300, 7 × 5 in. cards with photos and illustrations pertaining to 12 themes (e.g., kitchen, clothing, holidays). The cards are organized by phonetic complexity, from CV and VC through multisyllable words. Each card has prompts, such as responding to questions and completing sentences, to help increase client's speech intelligibility.

The Apraxia of Speech Stimulus Library

Includes a research-based manual, four boxed sets of stimulus cards, and reproducible data collection sheets. Uses high-interest words (depicted graphically or by pictures) and practical phrases to improve production of phonemes and phoneme sequences.

Dysarthria Treatment Manual

Imaginative treatment approach emphasizing self-monitoring and self-reliance. Its practical exercises target oral-motor skills, resonance, relaxation, respiration, prosody, and intelligibility. It offers client and family handouts, a simple communication board, and home practice activities.

Lingraphica Apps

Lingraphica offers several video apps within its SmallTalk app series that provide visual supports of oral-motor movements needed to produce speech, from the phoneme level up to words. The Phonemes app and Consonant Blends app focus on individual speech sounds, whereas the Days, Months, Dates app and Letter, Colors, Numbers app provide visuals of the oral-motor movements needed to produce words in those categories. There is also a Common Phrases app of functional phrases for individuals to practice connected speech.

Tactus Therapy Solutions

Speech FlipBook

This app enables you to create monosyllabic target words by selecting the speech sounds you want to target in each syllable position. Therapy can be programmed to increase the complexity of syllables from CV or VC up to consonant clusters. It has a recording feature that enables users to practice the targets and then view their performance.

Dysphagia

Dysphagia is a swallowing disorder characterized by difficulty moving food from mouth to stomach, including all the behavioral and physiological aspects of the process (Clark et al., 2009; Groher & Crary, 2020; Panebianco et al., 2020; Thiyagalingam et al., 2021). Dysphagia occurs in all age groups and may result from a variety of structural or physiological abnormalities. The onset of dysphagia can be acute (e.g., resulting from a stroke) or characterized by gradual deterioration (e.g., resulting from a progressive disease process such as amyotrophic lateral sclerosis). Difficulties can occur in any of the four stages of the normal swallow, which correspond to the approximate location of the food bolus as it moves through the system: (a) preparatory (chewing), (b) oral (back of mouth), (c) pharyngeal (throat), and (d) esophageal (toward stomach). See Edgar (2003) for an extensive review of research on swallowing in normal adults. Intervention designed for preparatory and/or oral stage problems is generally referred to as "feeding" techniques, whereas pharyngeal stage intervention is described as "swallowing" therapy. The role of a speech-language pathologist (SLP) in treatment is generally limited to difficulties in the first three stages of swallowing; problems in the esophageal stage are usually managed medically or surgically.

SLPs have an important role to play in the treatment of swallowing and feeding disorders. Their education and clinical background in the anatomy and physiology of respiration, swallowing, and speech prepare them to perform a variety of functions, including the following:

- Developing and implementing treatment plans for individuals with dysphagia

- Providing education and counseling to patients and their families

- Serving as members of a multidisciplinary/interdisciplinary management team

- Advocating for services for individuals with dysphagia

- Advancing the knowledge base on swallowing and feeding disorders through research activities

Treatment for Dysphagia

The two paramount goals of dysphagia management are: (a) prevention of aspiration, malnutrition, and dehydration; and (b) reestablishment of oral intake of food and liquid. Traditionally, these aims are targeted using approaches such as retraining muscle function, teaching new sequences of muscle activity, or stimulating increased sensory input (Logemann, 1998). A more recent approach, the application of neuromuscular electrical stimulation (NMES) to head and neck muscles, is being currently explored, typically as an adjunct to traditional treatment approaches (Langdon & Blacker, 2010). Clinical decision-making is often carried out through a multidisciplinary team, which may include a physician, dietitian, radiologist, or occupational therapist (Krekeler et al., 2020).

Intervention for feeding and swallowing disorders can be categorized into two main approaches: *compensatory strategies* or *rehabilitative strategies*. The goal for compensatory strategies is to eliminate or reduce abnormal symptoms without changing the underlying physiology of the client's swallow. This approach requires minimal cognitive or physical effort from the client and largely involves manipulation of variables such as head postures and bolus presentations.

The goal of rehabilitative strategies is to effect change in the client's swallow pattern. This approach generally focuses on range of motion and coordination/timing of movement. In addition to targeting the mechanical aspects of the swallow, clinicians also consider neurologic principles to determine ways to improve swallowing (e.g., techniques to stimulate nerves or the provision of sensory stimulants; Miller, 2008). Clients must be able to follow instructions and have the capacity to practice exercises independently. Intervention may be implemented indirectly with just saliva or directly with food/ liquid. This decision should be made solely on the basis of aspiration findings from radiographic studies (Logemann, 1998).

A discussion of strategies for dysphagia intervention follows. For additional information, refer to the systematic reviews conducted by Bahia and Lowell (2020), Cheng et al. (2022), and Teasell and Foley (2016). Please see Appendix D on the companion website for a schematic of the vocal tract structures discussed in this section. Additional helpful schematics can be found in Murray et al. (2020).

Postural Techniques

- *Chin down:* The downward placement of the chin decreases both the distance between the tongue base and the pharyngeal wall and the airway opening. This postural technique is used with patients who have dysphagia due to a tongue base disorder, a pharyngeal phase delay, or compromised airway protection (Park & Hwang, 2021).

- *Chin elevated:* This posture uses gravity to move the bolus from an elevated position downward through the oral cavity when sufficient lingual pressure is not present. This posture poses an aspiration risk if the patient has concomitant pharyngeal phase delays. It is typically used with patients whose dysphagia is due to oral tongue factors, such as surgical removal of the tongue or amyotrophic lateral sclerosis (ALS).

- *Head turn:* In cases of unilateral damage to the pharyngeal wall and/or larynx, turning the head to the weaker side enables the patient to isolate and utilize the stronger side for a safer transportation of the bolus.

- *Head tilt:* This posture also is used in cases of unilateral damage to the oral cavity or pharyngeal wall. In contrast to the head turn technique, this posture requires tilting the patient's head to the undamaged side to direct the bolus toward the stronger side.

- *Lying down:* If damage is bilateral or if laryngeal elevation is reduced, the combination of lying down to swallow with a follow-up swallow will move the bolus and any accompanying residue into the esophagus. The horizontal position of the larynx is intended to reduce the risk of aspiration because gravity will work to accumulate residue that can be controlled and then cleared into the esophagus with the follow-up swallow.

Maneuvers

- *Supraglottic swallow:* The patient is instructed to hold his or her breath throughout the entire swallow (before, during, after); holding one's breath causes the vocal folds to close, sealing off the opening of the trachea. Once the swallow is completed, the patient voluntarily coughs and swallows a second time to clear any residue. This maneuver is used with reduced airway protection and/or with patients who have demonstrated aspiration.

- *Super-supraglottic swallow:* The "super" part of the maneuver denotes the use of extra effort during the supraglottic swallow approach, typically by pushing down on a hard surface with one's hands. The extra effort may facilitate the use of the false vocal folds via arytenoid movement as additional airway protection.

- *Effortful swallow:* Extra effort is applied as patients are instructed to squeeze the muscles involved in swallowing hard while completing a swallow. The resulting increase in movement of the tongue base should assist patients with tongue retraction or with clearing residue from the valleculae (two spaces or pockets located in the throat just below the root of the tongue).

- *Mendelsohn maneuver:* This maneuver requires self-awareness and the ability to voluntarily segment a swallow into stages. The patient places a hand on his or her throat to feel the laryngeal elevation that occurs in swallowing while taking practice swallows. Once familiar with the concept of laryngeal elevation, the patient is instructed to hold the position of laryngeal elevation for several seconds before completing the swallow and allowing the larynx to drop back to the starting position. The rationale for this maneuver is the increased laryngeal movement and coordination in patients where these abilities are diminished, such as after a brainstem stroke. The Mendelsohn maneuver also may increase duration of upper esophageal sphincter opening, thus facilitating movement of the bolus into the final swallowing phase.

- *Masako maneuver:* After firmly holding the tongue tip in place between teeth, the patient then completes a swallow, making sure not to let the tongue release from between the teeth. This maneuver forces the glossopharyngeal muscle to contract with greater effort and is helpful for patients who have reduced pharyngeal contraction.

Exercises *(Balou et al., 2019; Krekeler et al., 2021)*

- *Shaker exercises:* This series of movements is meant to target both hyolaryngeal movement and upper esophageal opening. While lying down, instruct the patient to raise his or her head while keeping the shoulders on the ground and the mouth closed. The patient holds this position for approximately 1 min, relaxes the head back down for approximately 1 min, and then repeats this cycle three more times. This same cycle of holding and relaxing is then repeated 30 times at a faster pace of lift-lower-lift-lower. These exercises can be repeated several times during the day.

- *Tongue exercises* (McKenna et al., 2017): In cases of oral phase dysphagia, tongue exercises may be used to target swallow efficiency and strength. Exercises include holding the tongue in a retracted position (horizontal) for several seconds, gargling, and moving the tongue in a horizontal manner anteriorly and posteriorly.

- *Transference of treatment effects:* Russell et al. (2010) conducted a systematic review of the literature to see if exercises targeting one function of the cranial sensorimotor system (e.g., swallowing, voice, speech) would result in gains to other functions, since there is an overlap of anatomical structures. Several studies indicated positive findings for transference, including one study that found that an LSVT approach resulted in improvements in both voice and swallowing abilities in patients with Parkinson's disease.

Sensory Stimuli

With patients who have dysphagia due to decreased sensation in the oral and/or pharyngeal regions (e.g., delayed oral onset of swallow), there are sensory stimuli that can be applied to heighten sensation to these regions. Foods and liquids can be altered for taste (e.g., made more sour), volume (e.g., larger bolus), temperature, or carbonation to increase the sensation of their presentation. In a similar manner, thermal tactile stimulation involves the application of a cold stimulus to increase sensation and to promote a swallow response; thermal tactile stimulation may be more beneficial as a short-term compensatory strategy (Schwarz et al., 2018). Another commonly used sensory technique is the application of increased pressure (e.g., spoon placed on tongue surface) to heighten sensation and facilitate preparation for the presentation of a bolus (Rizzo et al., 2016).

Dietary Changes

Various food textures and consistencies can be implemented on a trial basis to determine which diet reduces aspiration risk and helps with swallow efficiency (Nagshabandi et al., 2023). Options for altering food textures include pureeing solid foods and adding thickeners to liquids (Beck et al., 2018). Publications such as the national dysphagia diet (American Dietetic Association) can be consulted for planning therapeutically appropriate dietary choices.

Medical

Three main types of surgical procedures are associated with medical treatment for dysphagia. The first type aims to protect the airway by improving vocal fold function (i.e., injecting the vocal folds with biomaterials to improve their ability to close adequately during a swallow). The second type also targets airway protection but involves making the tracheal and esophageal segments more distinct (e.g., laryngectomy, stent placement). The third type targets the functioning of the **pharyngoesophageal segment (pes)**. The pes can be dilated to make it larger or can be injected with botulinum toxin to decrease tension. An additional medical treatment for dysphagia is **neuromuscular electrical stimulation (NMES)**. Designed for pharyngeal phase dysphagia, NMES involves electrode placement on the surface of the throat to elicit the muscle contractions needed to swallow (Bulow et al., 2008; Carnaby et al., 2020). Furthermore, the purported goal of NMES is to rewire the swallow pattern at the level of the cortex by retraining the muscles at the level of the pharynx (Bulow et al., 2008). One study investigating NMES and neurologic changes found that even though swallow function increased, no changes were noted cortically over a 5-day treatment period (Gallas et al., 2010). A systematic review of literature on NMES found some positive findings. However, the research design of these studies was not robust. One tentative finding from NMES efficacy studies is that patients with mild to moderate dysphagia seem to benefit the most from NMES because there is still some remaining volitional muscle movement (Langdon & Blacker, 2010). However, this treatment approach continues to generate much debate and more information is needed to determine the actual efficacy of this treatment approach (Alamer et al., 2020).

Pediatric Dysphagia

It is important to acknowledge that dysphagia with pediatric populations is not the same as adult dysphagia. It includes additional factors such as latching, sucking, feeding, and breathing. Five phases of swallowing in young patients are described as follows:

- Preoral: important considerations include alertness, food selection, and manner of food introduction

- Oral: suckling, sucking or chewing, and transfer of the bolus to posterior of the oral cavity

- Pharyngeal: swallowing reflex is triggered by contact with tonsillar pillars

- Esophageal: muscular relaxation of patient's esophagus

- Gastro-esophageal: lower portion of the esophagus relaxes to allow bolus to move to the stomach

For more comprehensive discussion of anatomy/physiology and dysphagia in this population, see Murray et al. (2020).

Ethical Considerations

Intervention for feeding and swallowing disorders can have life-and-death consequences. Ethical issues in this area are complex and extremely serious (Sharp & Bryant, 2003). At this point, no universal guidelines exist for acceptable amounts of aspiration (i.e., entry of food/liquid into airway below level of the vocal folds). Radiographic evaluation is *absolutely* required to identify the existence, severity, and cause of aspiration. Logemann (1998) suggests oral intake of a given food consistency be prohibited if a client aspirates more than 10% of each bolus despite the use of optimal intervention techniques. However, clinicians should be aware that the wishes of clients and/or their families may run contrary to therapeutic recommendations. An instructive example involves a terminally ill client for whom the clinician has determined that oral intake be prohibited due to excessive aspiration under all conditions. Yet the client and family insist on continuing to eat by mouth. The clinician's ethical dilemma is whether to provide information/training on the least harmful way to swallow within a range of life-threatening alternatives. Speech-language pathologists can refer to their professional organization (e.g., ASHA's Code of Ethics; see Appendix A on the companion website) for guidance in dealing with ethical dilemmas. In addition, a survey of speech-language pathologists revealed five elements commonly considered when addressing ethical problems: (a) client well-being and quality of life, (b) professional scope of practice (e.g., roles and responsibilities), (c) establishment of professional relationships with other team members as well as the client and family, (d) economic need to balance resources to provide appropriate services, and (e) acknowledgment that personal and professional value systems may differ (Kenny et al., 2010).

Helpful Hints

1. If the client's progress plateaus for at least 4 weeks, active therapy can be terminated until/unless status changes.

2. Clinicians must carefully consider the eligibility question: "Will this client benefit from intervention?" Individuals with severe cognitive limitations or advanced motor neuron disease may not be considered good candidates for swallowing treatment.

3. Several factors may complicate the treatment of patients with dysphagia. For example, reduced hearing ability or cognitive decline may make it more difficult for patients to follow directions during treatment, and, thus, additional supports (e.g., text, diagrams) may be beneficial.

4. Patient education through the use of visual supports of the swallowing anatomy and/or biofeedback measures (e.g., ultrasound) may help patients to understand their disorder as well as help them to perform certain treatment exercises.

5. Oral care is extremely important for individuals with dysphagia because there is a risk of aspirating bacteria from the oral cavity. Frequent teeth brushing, gargling, and adequate hydration can help to maintain oral care.

6. The patient's family can learn the various safe swallowing strategies available to help promote independence. These strategies include an upright posture, taking small bites, and alternating bites and sips.

7. Molds are available to make pureed foods more closely resemble the intended food item, which may increase the patient's motivation to eat.

8. Some individuals with dysphagia (e.g., a patient with head/neck cancer who has undergone radiation treatment) have a condition known as xerostomia (excessive dry mouth). Products are available to help patients to replace the saliva and moisture in their mouth.

9. Keep in mind that sharing food is a highly valued social construct in many cultures. Effective clinicians use their awareness of the patient's cultural background to bring positivity into the context of swallowing therapy.

Conclusion

This section presented basic information, protocols, and procedures for intervention with dysphagia at an *introductory* level. This information is intended only as a starting point in the reader's clinical education and training. For more in-depth coverage of this area, the following readings are recommended:

Daniels, S. K., Huckabee, M.-L., & Gozdzikowska, K. (2019). *Dysphagia following stroke* (3rd ed.). Plural Publishing.

Groher, M., & Crary, M. (2020). *Dysphagia: Clinical management in adults and children* (3rd ed.). Mosby.

Leonard, R., & Kendall, K. (2018). *Dysphagia assessment and treatment planning: A team approach* (4th ed.). Plural Publishing.

Logemann, J. A. (1998). *Evaluation and treatment of swallowing disorders* (2nd ed.). Pro-Ed.

Murry, T., Carrau, R. L., & Chan, K. (2020). *Clinical management of swallowing disorders* (5th ed.). Plural Publishing.

Additional Resources

Dysphagia

The Source for Dysphagia, Fourth Edition
This 305-page workbook includes Medicare changes related to swallowing treatment; detailed educational handouts for physicians, patients, and staff; information on fiberoptic endoscopic evaluation of swallowing (FEES); new information on how to perform and interpret a modified barium swallow; and descriptions of new therapy techniques and references to document their efficacy.

The Source for Pediatric Dysphagia, Second Edition
This resource provides information on feeding, swallowing, and treatment goals for young patients. The techniques also can be applied to older children with cerebral palsy, neurological disorders, or any swallowing disorder. From diagnosis through treatment, chapters cover anatomy and physiology,

diagnostic procedures, infant feeding techniques, behavioral feeding disorders, goals and treatment objectives, and tools for feeding.

Pre-Feeding Skills: A Comprehensive Resource for Mealtime Development, Second Edition

This program for infants to adolescents discusses normal development, limitations, and management of tube feeding, cleft palate, drooling, prematurity, and feeding in autism. It covers evaluation, treatment, oral stimulation, positioning, oral-motor limitations, and nutritional factors. It features reproducibles, mealtime exercises, and Spanish translations of parent questionnaires.

Swallow Right: An Exercise Program to Correct Resting Posture and Swallowing Patterns, Second Edition

Comprehensive exercise manual for evaluation and treatment of oral myofunctional disorders. Suitable for individual, group, or carryover programming. Program covers theory, treatment, and tracking charts for the three main stages of swallowing.

Speechmark Working With Dysphagia

This workbook is designed to provide information on a variety of disorders associated with dysphagia as well as a variety of settings in which an SLP would work with clients with dysphagia. In addition to assessment and treatment, the text also provides information on related topics such as tracheostomies, ethical issues, and nutritional needs.

Swallow Safely: A Caregiver's Guide to Dysphagia

Provides information in a manner that is beneficial in counseling both the client and the family about dysphagia. It includes information on signs to look for that indicate swallowing difficulties, related problems that may occur, and the treatment options that are available. It also discusses swallowing and how the process can become disordered.

Lingraphica: SmallTalk Dysphagia App

The SmallTalk Dysphagia App was designed to enable individuals with swallowing disorders to explain their disorder to others, primarily those responsible for their care and/or medical treatment. It utilizes icons as well as spoken phrases so that individuals can communicate the safe swallowing strategies they need implemented while eating and drinking.

Northern Speech Services: Dysphagia App

This app is meant for educational purposes. It provides videos of normal swallowing as well as disordered swallowing, with a variety of disorders and swallowing complications to choose from. Videos include "Impairment of Bolus Transport," "Impairment of Pharyngeal Contraction," and "Example of Penetration with Aspiration."

Chapter 9

Intervention for Stuttering

NOTE: *Use of person-first language ("person who stutters") or identity-first language ("stutterer") is an individual choice expressed by many in the disability community (Dunn & Andrews, 2015). Both are used in this chapter.*

The focus of this chapter is on **stuttering**, the major type of disfluency exhibited by children and adults. Cluttering, an associated fluency disorder, is beyond the scope of this chapter. Readers who are interested in this topic are referred to Myers et al. (2012), Scaler Scott et al., (2022), and Ward and Scott (2011).

Stuttering is characterized by an abnormally high frequency and/or duration of stoppages in the forward flow of speech (Andrews & Harris, 1964; Bloodstein et al., 2021; Manning, 2010; Tetnowski et al., 2021; Wingate, 1964; Yaruss, 1998). Studies indicate that prevalence under age 6 years is considerably higher than in later periods in life and that stuttering occurs in approximately 0.72% to 1% of the population; however, Yairi and Ambrose (2013) suggest that this percentage is substantially higher in subgroups of the population, particularly males. Many theories have been proposed regarding the cause of stuttering, ranging from genetic and other organic explanations to learned, environmental, or linguistic accounts. Certain theories emphasize differences in cerebral dominance (Travis, 1931), disruptions of speech motor timing (Kent, 1984; Van Riper, 1982), or anticipatory struggle to avoid communicative failure (Bloodstein, 1987; Sheehan, 1958). The covert repair hypothesis proposed by Kolk and colleagues (Howell, 2007; Kolk, 1991; Kolk & Postma, 1997; Postma, 2000; Vasic & Wijnen, 2005) suggests that stutterers may be prone to errors in phonological planning; their attempts to edit these errors prior to producing the utterance are manifested as disfluencies.

In addition, several multifactorial theories have emphasized the interaction between stuttering and a variety of intrinsic/extrinsic factors. One account is the capacities and demands model, which posits that stuttering results from demands for performance that exceed the speaker's capacities in one or more domains (i.e., linguistic, motor, cognitive, or emotional; Starkweather & Gottwald, 2000). The three-factor hypothesis (Wall & Myers, 1995) claims that a combination of psycholinguistic, psychosocial, and physiological factors is involved in the phenomenon of stuttering. The Packman model (2012) is multifactorial and includes the following components: (a) underlying deficit in neural processing for spoken language; (b) triggers inherent in spoken language, such as variable syllable stress and linguistic complexity; and (c) modulation factors unique to each individual, such as emotional reactivity and environmental stressors. In their multifactorial-dynamic model, Smith and colleagues (Smith, 1999; Smith & Kelly, 1997) argue that interaction among these factors occurs on multiple nonlinear levels and that stuttered moments should be viewed as dynamic rather than static events. Similarly, Chang et al. (2011), De Nil and Kroll (2001), Giraud et al. (2008), and Watkins et al. (2008) interpret the interactionist approach to stuttering by emphasizing that all environmental and intrinsic factors are ultimately filtered through the stutterer's neurophysiological system.

Recently, Kang (2021) identified specific gene mutations correlated with stuttering. These mutations involve metabolic deficiencies in the body's ability to process certain enzymes. Epidemiologic studies are being developed to determine the proportion of the world's population that carries these mutations and how many of them are identified as stutterers.

Jackson et al. (2012) discussed the prevailing view of stuttering as a disorder defined by listener-based perceptions of acoustic interruptions. They argued that the disorder is actually more complex than these surface features (e.g., repetitions, prolongations, blocks) and encompasses crucial speaker-based perceptions of "loss of control" along with powerful cognitive and affective variables. Their proposed definition for stuttering includes consideration of a neurobiological lack of integration of the processes of planning and producing language and speech that, upon verbal execution, can lead to interruptions in the acoustic speech signal and physical struggle (e.g., tension). The underlying features may lead to surface behaviors as well as emotional and cognitive reactions. Individuals may experience severe difficulties in communication, with a highly adverse impact on their quality of life (Tichenor et al., 2022; Usler, 2022). Healey et al. (2004) proposed the CALMS model of stuttering, which includes cognitive, affective, linguistic, motor, and social components. This model accounts for individual differences across the five components and how an individual's overall communication ability is influenced by changing demands (Westby, 2019).

The specific interactions among linguistic, motor, cognitive, genetic, emotional, and social factors are yet to be determined as is their influence on the variable nature and complexity of stuttering. (See Bloodstein & Ratner [2008] and Bloodstein et al., [2021] for a review of different theoretical positions.)

The onset of stuttering usually occurs between 2 and 5 years of age and may emerge in a sudden or severe manner (Yairi & Ambrose, 1999). Some researchers report that approximately 80% of children who stutter will spontaneously recover before the age of puberty (Andrews & Harris, 1964; Yairi & Ambrose, 1999). Some evidence suggests that spontaneous recovery is a gradual process that may begin within the first year of stuttering and not reach completion until 3 or 4 years postonset (Yairi & Ambrose, 1999). Differences in terminology, methodology, and interpretation of data make it difficult to compare results (Bothe et al., 2006; Ingham & Bothe, 2001; Onslow & Packman, 1999a, 199b; Prins & Ingham, 2009; Yairi & Ambrose, 1999, 2001, 2013). Many clinicians use a rule of thumb that 50% to 80% of children who stutter will recover with or without treatment (Guitar, 2019). For individuals who continue to stutter, the characteristics of the disorder may gradually change over time. Several viewpoints regarding the development of stuttering have been proposed. Bloodstein (1960) describes a four-phase model that progresses from mild episodic disfluencies to severe, chronic stuttering accompanied by fear and avoidance reactions. Van Riper (1982) suggests a three-stage progression that includes primary, transitional, and secondary phases. A third hypothesis put forth by Starkweather (1987) indicates that the development of stuttering fluctuates as a result of an individual's changing capacity to accommodate environmental demands for communicative performance. Finally, longitudinal data on preschool stutterers suggest that severity of stuttering at onset may remain unchanged up to 3 years postonset (Sawyer & Yairi, 2010; Throneburg & Yairi, 2001).

Categories of Stuttering Behaviors

Two main categories of characteristics are associated with stuttering: core behaviors and secondary behaviors.

Core Behaviors

Core behaviors are the basic manifestations that seem beyond the voluntary control of the stutterer and include the following:

- Repetitions of sounds, syllables, or whole words (e.g., c-c-cat; ba-ba-balloon; we-we-we are going)

- Prolongations of single sounds (e.g., sssssoap; fffffishing)

- Blocks of airflow/voicing during speech (inappropriate stoppage of air or voice at any level of the vocal tract)

Secondary Behaviors

Secondary behaviors develop over time as learned reactions to the core behaviors and are categorized as **escape** or **avoidance** behaviors. Escape behaviors occur during a stuttering moment and are attempts to break out of the stutter. Common examples of escape behaviors include head nods, eye blinks, foot taps, and jaw tremors. In the more advanced stages of stuttering, these behaviors may be accompanied by visible struggle and muscular tension. Avoidance behaviors occur in anticipation of a stuttering moment and are attempts to refrain from stuttering. Typical avoidance behaviors are circumlocutions (substitutions of less feared vocabulary words), unfilled pauses without accompanying tension and struggle within or between words, and use of "um" or other interjections to postpone speaking.

Developmental Disfluencies Versus Stuttering

Most typically developing children between 2 and 4 years of age display some of the following relatively effortless disfluencies during the normal course of language acquisition (Coleman, 2013; Pellowski & Conture, 2002; Zebrowski, 1994):

- Hesitations (silent pauses)

- Interjections of sounds, syllables, or words (e.g., "Um, I went to school"; "Did you, *you know*, find her?")

- Revisions/repetitions of words, phrases, or sentences (e.g., "You have to touch, *no, turn* it"; "I have some . . . *I want you to look at* these baseball cards")

- Normal rhythm and stress patterns

- No tension or tremors noted

It is important to differentiate between these normal disfluencies and the atypical disfluencies in the following list, which are often the early signs of stuttering:

- Three or more *within-word* disfluencies per 100 words (especially fragmentation of syllables)

- Disfluencies on more than 10% of syllables spoken

- Predominant use of prolongations, blocks, and part-word repetitions (as opposed to interjections and whole-word or phrase repetitions)

- Presence of secondary behaviors/increased tension

- Vowel neutralization (schwa) during repetitions (e.g., buh-buh-beat)

- Duration of single instance of disfluency that exceeds 2 s

- Uncontrolled or abrupt changes in pitch or loudness

Ambrose and Yairi's (1999) large-scale study of preschool children provides strong evidence that stuttering can be differentiated from normal disfluency on the basis of three main characteristics: (a) part-word repetition, (b) single-syllable word repetition, and (c) disrhythmic phonation (i.e., prolongations, blocks, and broken words). This differential pattern of disfluency types was significant even at the early stages of stuttering. Pellowski and Conture (2002) also found that the speech of children who stutter (CWS) could be differentiated from the speech of children who do not stutter (CWNS). Specifically, CWS produced approximately 2.5 to 4 times as many total disfluencies as the CWNS. Also, CWS produce an average of 2.0 extra repetition units (per instance of part- or whole-word repetition) than their typically developing counterparts. Zebrowski (1997) suggests that clinical decision-making regarding intervention should be influenced by whether the child demonstrates five important characteristics that are associated with a high probability of recovery:

- 18 months to 3 years of age at onset

- no family history of stuttering or a small number of affected relatives who recovered in childhood

- female

- few to no associated behaviors

- no coexisting phonological or cognitive problems

In addition, Walsh et al. (2018) suggest that performance on a nonword repetition task may predict persistence in childhood stuttering. Howell and Davis (2011) conducted a longitudinal study that indicated that severity of stuttering at 8 years was the single-most predictive factor for the persistence or recovery of stuttering in adolescence.

Treatment for Fluency Disorders

Regardless of theoretical orientation, the ultimate aim of most stuttering therapy programs is spontaneous fluency. Fluency can be described as consisting of four primary components: rate, continuity, rhythm, and effort (Andrews et al., 2012; Starkweather, 1985, 1987). Accordingly, spontaneous fluent speech is smooth, relatively rapid, and melodic (as opposed to monotonous) and appears free of conscious physical or mental effort. For people who demonstrate severe stuttering behavior, spontaneous fluency may not be considered a realistic goal. Controlled fluency or acceptable levels of stuttering may be identified as the ultimate goal of treatment for these individuals, depending on the clinician's philosophy of the general nature of stuttering. The stutterer's cultural and linguistic background, as well as preferences and priorities, also may influence the choice of general approach to intervention. In addition, it is important to recognize that, unlike most other speech and language disorders, relapse is a common phenomenon in stuttering. Stutterers frequently experience periods of increased disfluency after treatment has been terminated. For this reason, periodic follow-up sessions should be an integral part of an effective fluency treatment program. For example, Blood (1995) advocates a cognitive-behavioral relapse management program for adolescents that is instituted following the completion of a traditional course of fluency therapy. This program provides training in five basic areas: problem-solving, general communication skills, assertiveness, coping strategies, and establishment of realistic expectations. More recently, Druker et al. (2019) and Druker et al. (2020) found that combining parent-administered resilience/self-regulation training with standard stuttering treatment resulted in positive treatment outcomes that were sustained at follow-up.

Individuals who stutter have been shown to demonstrate performance differences in some language and phonological skills when compared with typical speakers (Anderson & Conture, 2004; Anderson et al., 2006; Cuadrado & Weber-Fox, 2003; Melnick et al., 2003). Recently, Brundage and Bernstein-Ratner (2022) summarized the existing literature on the linguistic aspects of stuttering such as features associated with increased stuttering frequency, whether stutterers exhibit language differences/deficits, and language factors that may influence recovery from early stuttering. Stuttering also can occur concomitantly with other communication problems such as language or phonology disorders, particularly in preschool and school-age children (Gregory, 2003). Multiple authors (Brent & Yairi, 2012; Smith et al., 2010) have investigated the association of stuttering with phonology disorders and have come to the conclusion that children with persistent stuttering are at increased risk for phonological and articulation disorders. There are at least four programming alternatives for treating coexisting impairments (Ratner, 1995):

Discrete: A certain amount of therapy time is allotted to treat each disorder in isolation. For example, in a 1-hr therapy session, a clinician may devote 20 min to fluency goals and the remaining 40 min to articulation goals. Alternatively, a twice-weekly therapy schedule can be divided to spend one session on each disorder area.

Modified cycles: Treatment for one disorder is implemented for a specified block of time (e.g., 6 weeks) and then discontinued. An equivalent time period is then devoted to treatment of the other communicative impairment. This cycle is alternated until long-term goals are achieved for each disorder.

Blended: Therapy goals for one disorder are incorporated into the therapy activities for a second disorder. For example, during articulation activities, the clinician can encourage fluency-enhancing behaviors such as slower speaking rate and increased pause time between conversational turns.

Lagged: This is a modified form of the blended approach that incorporates an initial time delay. Specifically, a period of initial therapy focuses on attaining a predetermined level of mastery in the concomitant disorder area (e.g., phonological or linguistic). Once the child has reached this level of mastery, fluency therapy can begin using the recently mastered phonological/linguistic forms as the basis for practice. Fluency therapy continues to be programmed at comfortable levels of phonological/linguistic demand as the child progressively masters new objectives in the concomitant disorder area.

Treatment Efficacy/Evidence-Based Practice

Efficacy in the area of stuttering therapy is particularly difficult to measure because its definition must incorporate three interrelated factors: (a) objective measures of frequency and duration of stuttered moments, (b) client emotions and attitudes, and (c) the client's amenability to participate in communicative interactions with a variety of partners. The importance of treatment outcomes has been increasingly addressed in the stuttering literature. Prins and Ingham (2009) developed definitional and operational guidelines that facilitate the clinician's ability to critically evaluate different approaches to stuttering treatment for young children and adults (Blood & Conture, 1998; Finn, 2003; Ingham, 2003). In 2001, the World Health Organization (WHO) presented a multidimensional classification scheme for describing health status and the experience of disability. This paradigm—the International Classification of Functioning, Disability, and Health (ICF; WHO, 2001)—has been adapted by Yaruss (2010) and Coleman and Yaruss (2014) to describe the speaker's experience of the disorder of stuttering and its implications for assessment and treatment. Specifically, this can involve negative affective, behavioral, and cognitive reactions (both from the speaker and the listener) as well as significant limitations in the speaker's ability to participate in daily activities and a negative impact on the speaker's overall quality of life. They advocate for the use of the ICF as a framework for measuring treatment outcomes for persons who stutter. Brignell et al. (2021) conducted a recent systematic review of treatment efficacy studies in stuttering in children and adolescents. Results indicate that direct (e.g., Lidcombe) and indirect (Demands-Capacity Model) are effective for preschool age stutterers. In addition, service delivery in a teletherapy format was non-inferior to traditional in-person treatment. No high-level evidence of treatment effectiveness was noted for school-age and adolescent stutterers. Several authors have conducted systematic reviews of the treatment literature for both children and adults (Baxter et al., 2016; Bothe et al., 2006; Conture, 1996; Herder et al., 2006; Prins & Ingham, 2009). The overall conclusion is that treatment for fluency disorders is generally effective across age ranges. The findings from these reports, presented in the following points, are organized according to four age groups: preschoolers, school-age children, adolescents, and adults. (For a comprehensive summary of the treatment literature in stuttering, see Bloodstein & Ratner [2008] and Bloodstein et al. [2021].)

- Preschool children benefit from initiation of therapy in the early stages of stuttering.

- Response-contingent intervention is the most well-documented approach for preschoolers who stutter.

- Efficacy information for school-age children and adolescents is scant, although preliminary data are emerging regarding predicting and/or minimizing relapse after treatment.

- Studies of adults indicate that prolonged speech, gentle onsets, monitoring, and modeling are among the most effective treatment strategies for remediating stuttering.

- For both children and adults, an increased amount of intervention contact time does not appear to be directly correlated with better treatment outcomes (i.e., dose-response relationship).

- Future efficacy research is needed to address several critical issues, including the relationship between reduced stuttering and naturalness of speech, attitudinal changes, and long-term outcomes (e.g., more than 5 years) of intervention.

An interesting development in the field of treatment efficacy includes the notion of "common factors." First proposed in the field of psychology (Ahn & Wampold, 2001; Wampold, 2015), this model suggests that efficacy data often show little difference across treatment regimens but that variance related to other factors does exist. The alliance between the therapist and the client as well as the quality of clinician expertise seem to have significant influence on treatment effect sizes. This finding was corroborated by a meta-analysis of stuttering treatment conducted by Herder et al.

(2006). They came to the conclusion that what is critical for successful treatment outcomes may not be the intervention itself but rather the knowledge and skill of the clinician. Johnson et al.'s (2016) systematic review offers a welcome focus on qualitative outcomes associated with therapeutic interventions for stuttering. Evidence suggests that attention to emotional, situational, and practical needs facilitates successful intervention outcomes in stuttering therapy.

Intervention Techniques

Various techniques are used in the treatment of stuttering as comprehensively discussed in Bloodstein et al. (2021). Some classic examples of therapy approaches include Shames and Florance's (1980) stutter-free speech program, Ryan's (1974) graduated increase in length and complexity model, computer-aided fluency establishment training (Goebel, 1986), Bloodstein's (1975) anticipatory struggle program, and Shine's (1980) systematic fluency training—to name just a few. Frequently, the client's age is a critical factor in determining how intervention will be implemented.

Onslow and colleagues (Arnott et al., 2014; Onslow & Andrews, 1994; Packman et al., 2014) developed the Lidcombe program: a response-contingent approach to stuttering intervention for young children. The central component of this fluency-shaping program is the presentation of verbal contingencies for stuttered versus stutter-free speech (i.e., praise versus corrective feedback). It incorporates a strong focus on parental participation as well as a structured maintenance phase.

Philosophically, all of the different approaches can be divided into two primary schools of thought: fluency shaping and stuttering modification/management.

Fluency Shaping

Fluency shaping is based on the assumption that stuttering is a learned behavior. The primary goal of fluency shaping is to eliminate disfluencies and gradually change the speaker's habitual speaking pattern to one of fluent speech. This is accomplished through the use of several fluency-enhancing techniques:

- **Easy onset/prevoice exhalation:** The speaker is taught to exhale slightly before beginning phonation and reach conversational loudness gradually.

- **Decreased speaking rate (prolonged speech):** The speaker is trained to stretch out the sounds (primarily vowels) in his speech and produce words at a slower-than-normal speaking rate while maintaining normal stress and intonation.

- **Light articulatory contacts:** The speaker is taught to move the articulators in a loose and relaxed manner.

- **Continuous phonation:** The speaker is trained to reduce all breaks between words by maintaining voicing continuously until he naturally needs to take a breath.

The ultimate aim of programs based on a fluency-shaping philosophy is to completely change speech behavior by teaching clients to use these techniques at all times, not just during disfluent moments. These techniques are designed to interfere with the stuttering behaviors, thus reducing them. Overall, most fluency-shaping programs can be categorized according to which parameter of communicative interaction is the focus of change: phonation, speech rate, length of utterance, or provision of contingent feedback. Therapy sessions focus solely on acquisition of fluency-enhancing behaviors and generally do not address a client's secondary behaviors or the negative feelings and attitudes that may be associated with the stuttering.

Delayed Auditory Feedback (DAF)

This fluency-shaping technique has been widely used in the treatment of stuttering. A speaker's own words are returned through headphones after an imposed electronic delay of a few milliseconds. For normal speakers, the discrepancy between expected and received auditory feedback disrupts the smooth flow of speech and results in a significant breakdown in fluency. DAF has the opposite effect on the speech of many individuals who stutter; it decreases their speech rate and reduces the number of notable disfluencies. As a general rule, therapy is initiated at a delay time of approximately 250 ms. The time delay is then reduced in 50-ms intervals (i.e., 200 ms, 150 ms, 100 ms, and so on) as the client stabilizes fluency skills at each level. (See Ham [1999]; Hudock & Kalinowski [2014]; and Saltuklaroglu [2012] for detailed information on the implementation of DAF as a clinical procedure.) In a 2008 study, Daliri et al. found that adults and children who stutter responded differentially to DAF. According to the authors, these data indicate that stuttering in adults is associated with managing the discrepancies between predicted and received auditory feedback, but not in children. Use of DAF in stuttering therapy has been recommended by many authors, including Webster et al. (1970), Van Riper (1973), and Shames and Florance (1980). Proponents of this technique suggest that it tends to generate increased fluency in the early stages of therapy. DAF also is believed to enhance the speaker's ability to monitor oral-sensory feedback cues from his own speech mechanism. Finally, it facilitates a slower speaking rate by increasing a client's syllable duration and phonation time. However, other writers have cautioned about the possible drawbacks of DAF (Sheehan, 1968; Wingate, 1976). Among the most commonly cited disadvantages are difficulty in weaning clients from the DAF equipment and the development of a "DAF voice" (slow, labored, lacking in inflection and stress variation). For a detailed review of the literature on the effects of DAF, see Bloodstein and Ratner (2008) and Bloodstein et al (2021).

Numerous **assistive devices** have been developed to treat stuttering from a fluency-shaping perspective. Some devices, such as SpeechEasy, use **frequency-altered feedback** (FAF) as well as DAF to promote fluent speech (Foundas et al., 2013; Stuart et al., 2004). In FAF, digital technology allows speech signal frequencies to be adjusted without changing a client's speech rate. Other portable devices, such as the Edinborough Masker, permit clients to turn on masking noise in anticipation of a disfluency (Block et al., 1996). With the rapid advances in digital technology, other portable devices are likely to become available. The way in which these devices are incorporated into intervention should be determined by the clinician on a case-by-case basis.

Stuttering Modification/Management

Stuttering modification is based on the premise that stuttering may involve a physiological predisposition. The primary goals of stuttering management are to modify each disfluent moment by stuttering more easily and to eliminate struggle and avoidance behaviors (Van Riper, 1973). Gregory (1979) called this the "stutter more fluently" approach. In essence, the strategy is to minimize a client's reaction to loss of speech control rather than to eliminate the disfluencies themselves. These goals are accomplished through the use of a combination of the following techniques:

- **Self-analysis:** Increase the client's awareness of the type, severity, and loci of disfluencies as well as any accompanying secondary behaviors. Attention also may be given to increasing the client's self-awareness of the characteristics of his nonstuttered speech and monitoring his proprioceptive awareness of the oral musculature.

- **Relaxation:** Reduce the client's anxiety and muscle tension through relaxation training (Table 9–1 lists specific steps).

- **Desensitization:** Reduce negative emotions associated with stuttering (e.g., fear, frustration, embarrassment) by decreasing sensitivity to core behaviors and listener reactions through activities such as voluntary stuttering or voluntary exaggeration of a stuttered moment.

In this philosophy, therapy outcomes are not defined strictly by decreases in stuttering frequency counts. Rather, progress is measured along a qualitative continuum as the nature of stuttering shifts from high-struggle speech with syllable fragmentations to less effortful, forward-moving speech. A notable example of this is avoidance reduction therapy, which was originally developed by Sheehan (1958, 1970). In this model, secondary behaviors that listeners perceive as stuttering (e.g., eye blinks, facial grimacing, pitch breaks) are the result of the conflict between the individual's desire to speak and the simultaneous urge to hide the stuttering. Avoidance reduction therapy focuses on achieving a more comfortable forward-moving form of stuttering (see Sisskin [2018] for a comprehensive discussion of this treatment approach to fluency). Clinicians who employ a stuttering modification/management approach work with clients to identify hierarchies of feared speaking situations.

Table 9–1
Progressive Relaxation Training

Step 1	Ensure that the client is seated comfortably.
Step 2	Explain that this procedure involves the deliberate contracting and relaxing of various muscles to help the client recognize and discriminate between muscular tension and relaxation.
Step 3	Starting at the level of the abdomen, instruct the client to tightly contract his stomach muscles for at least 5 sec and then relax them. Encourage the client to concentrate on how his muscles feel when they are in a tensed versus relaxed state. Require the client to perform this activity three to five times.
Step 4	Repeat the contraction–relaxation sequence with other muscle groups moving progressively toward the head (i.e., arms, shoulders, neck, face). The clinician should periodically check the client's level of relaxation during the release phase by placing one hand on the target muscle group and pushing slightly to determine the degree of muscle resistance. Noticeable resistance indicates an insufficient degree of relaxation.
Step 5	At the level of the face, instruct the client to perform each of the following movement sequences three to five times: clench the mandible against the upper molars and release; pucker and release the lips; push the blade of the tongue strongly against the hard palate and release; tightly close both eyes and then open; frown in an exaggerated manner and relax.

Note. The aim of teaching progressive relaxation is to enable the person who stutters to consistently identify instances of excessive muscular tension during speech and to immediately transition into a relaxed state without having to work through the entire stepwise progression. Adapted from *The Modification of Stuttering,* by E. Brutten and D. Shoemaker, 1967, Englewood Cliffs, NJ: Prentice Hall; *Progressive Relaxation,* by E. Jacobson, 1938, Chicago, IL: University of Chicago Press; *Techniques of Stuttering Therapy,* R. Ham, 1986, Englewood Cliffs, NJ: Prentice Hall.

These hierarchies are valuable tools for a variety of therapeutic purposes: (a) developing clients' self-awareness and ability to analyze their behavior, (b) recognizing variations in clients' stuttering patterns across different settings, and (c) facilitating development of sequential behavioral objectives and collection of data. (Figure 9–1 presents sample hierarchies.)

The following stuttering modification/management techniques are generally intended to be used as a three-part sequence in the following order (Van Riper, 1973):

- **Cancellations:** When experiencing a disfluency, the speaker is encouraged to *complete* the intended word without attempting to break out of the disfluency. After the disfluency has been produced, the speaker is instructed to pause and mentally rehearse a technique for producing the word more fluently (or with an easier stutter) and then repeat the word.

- **Pull-outs:** When experiencing a disfluency, the speaker is taught to stop in the *middle* of the stuttering moment, mentally rehearse the intended word using a fluency-enhancing technique (or easier stuttering pattern), and then reproduce it.

- **Preparatory sets:** The speaker is encouraged to anticipate an imminent disfluency and pause briefly to mentally rehearse fluent (or gentle stuttering) production *before* the word is attempted.

The ultimate aim of programs based on a stuttering modification/management philosophy is to modify stuttering behaviors to an acceptable level rather than eliminate them entirely. The client's negative attitudes and feelings toward his or her stuttering are typically identified and monitored

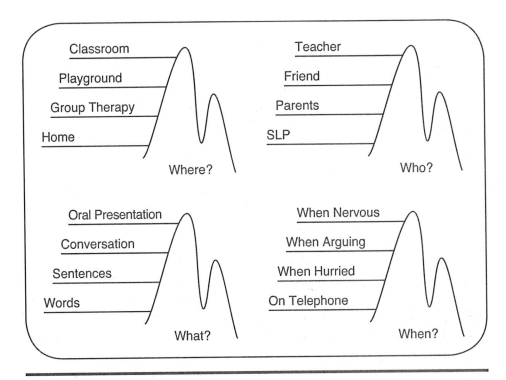

Figure 9–1
Climbing the fear hierarchy. Used with permission of V. Sisskin, University of Maryland.

over time through the administration of attitudinal scales. Therapy sessions also give considerable attention to the reduction of speech fears and secondary behaviors as a means of minimizing the impact of stuttering. Elementary school-age children and adolescents are particularly vulnerable to teasing and negative self-image. Effective therapy programs incorporate activities such as role-playing and brainstorming to proactively address these issues. Detailed information on related counseling techniques can be found in Chapter 11.

Guitar (2019) suggests that long-term fluency goals and clinical methods are two important treatment issues that differentiate fluency shaping and stuttering modification/management approaches. With regard to fluency goals, the three possible outcomes of therapy are spontaneous fluency, controlled fluency, and acceptable stuttering. The outcome of choice for both therapy approaches is spontaneous fluency, with a secondary goal of controlled fluency.

Yairi and Seery (2021) suggest that therapists consider three major alternatives when designing long-term treatment for people who stutter: increased fluency, reduced stuttering, and improved cognitive-emotional adjustment. Guitar (2019) and others advocate the integration of fluency shaping and stuttering modification/management techniques in the treatment of stuttering. They believe that stuttering results from an interaction of physiologic factors and learned behaviors. Therefore, facets of each approach are viewed as essential components of an effective treatment paradigm. Likewise, the CALMS model (Healey et al., 2004) can serve as an effective framework for integrating fluency shaping and stuttering modification techniques as needed on an individualized basis.

Example Profiles

Four profiles representative of fluency problems exhibited by clients of different age ranges (i.e., preschool, school age, and adult) are presented in this section. These examples are designed to illustrate the selection of intervention targets, specific therapy activities, and materials. Implementation of both fluency shaping and stuttering modification/management approaches is demonstrated for each profile.

PROFILE 1: PRESCHOOL—3-YEAR-OLD

Eli is 3 years old, and his speech is characterized by hesitations, whole-word or whole-phrase repetitions, and interjections of syllables/words (e.g., "um," "well") with no accompanying struggle behaviors. Analysis of a 200-syllable spontaneous speech sample indicated that 20% of the syllables uttered were disfluent. By parental report, Eli appears to exhibit no awareness of his communication difficulties. Receptive and expressive language abilities as well as other developmental skills appear age appropriate.

Selection of Therapy Targets. The overall communicative profile demonstrated by Eli is consistent with that of a child experiencing normal disfluencies, except for the relatively high frequency of the disfluencies. Based on Eli's disfluency rate and his young chronological age, an indirect approach to treatment is selected. An indirect approach focuses on the modification of the communicative environment rather than on treating the disfluencies themselves. The child's family is taught strategies for adapting their communicative behaviors in ways that create an environment conducive to the production of fluent speech. This is particularly important because survey evidence indicates that parents may unknowingly exacerbate children's disfluencies by correcting and/or finishing their utterances. Families are encouraged to do the following:

- Listen attentively to the child's message rather than to his speech pattern.

- Avoid speaking for the child; do not fill in or complete the child's message.

- Avoid communicative stresses such as time pressures.

- Decrease demands for verbal performance (e.g., "Tell Aunt Suzie what you did in school today.").

- Avoid interrupting the child or allowing siblings or friends to interrupt (emphasize the rules for turn taking in conversation).

- Avoid the predominant use of questions that demand lengthy or complex responses in favor of those that require simple one- or two-word answers.

- Avoid using an excessively rapid speech pattern; be sure to model smooth, relaxed speech when talking with the child (Guitar & Marchinkoski, 2001).

- Avoid labeling disfluencies as stuttering.

- Maintain natural eye contact while the child speaks, even during disfluencies.

- Avoid correcting the child's mispronunciations of speech sounds.

An important aspect of the indirect approach is to facilitate parental awareness of the child's fluency status in the home environment. This can be accomplished through use of a fluency observation chart (Form 9–1) in which parents keep a record of each disfluency exhibited by the child at home and the factors that surround it.

It is essential to maintain regular contact with the family to monitor the effectiveness of these strategies in ameliorating the child's disfluencies. A more direct treatment approach should be considered when no significant improvement is reported after a predetermined time period (e.g., 3 to 4 months), or more immediately if the child's communication performance deteriorates (i.e., demonstrates a higher frequency or longer duration of disfluencies, emergence of struggle behaviors).

Helpful Hints

1. Video recordings of natural family interactions (e.g., birthday party, family vacation, family reunion) can be helpful in identifying the communication patterns used by different family members with the child.

2. The effectiveness of an indirect treatment approach can be enhanced by preparing simple, clear materials that outline the desired communication strategies listed previously. These materials can be given to individuals with whom the child has regular contact (i.e., day care providers, preschool teachers, babysitters, grandparents, and so on).

3. For families that seem overly sensitive to their child's disfluencies, it may be helpful to have them chart the type and number of disfluencies that occur naturally in everyday conversations among normally fluent speakers.

4. Parents often express feelings of guilt regarding a child's disfluencies. It is important to assure parents that they did not cause the fluency problem and that their consistent use of the recommended communication strategies can be the most powerful, positive facilitator of fluent speech for their child. (Refer to Chapter 11 for additional information on counseling strategies.)

5. Clinicians may need to make parents aware that the severity of their child's stuttering can vary considerably from one day to the next. This inconsistent behavior is typical of stuttering and should not be interpreted as voluntary in nature or indicative of permanent change in fluency status.

6. In their attempts to minimize disfluent moments, families may inadvertently reduce or alter the amount/variety of verbal exchanges with their children. Clinicians should encourage family members to maintain natural levels of communicative interactions that typically occur in the home environment.

7. For older children, a hybrid format of individual plus group sessions may be useful. Individual sessions can target specific skills and feelings, while group sessions help students realize that "you are not alone . . . other people struggle with this too."

Form 9-1. HOME FLUENCY OBSERVATION CHART

Child's Name: _____ Informant: _____

INSTRUCTIONS: Over the next week, write down at least five situations in which your child experiences disfluency. Please indicate the circumstances in which the disfluency occurs by recording the following information. It is recommended that a separate recording chart be maintained by each observer.

Date/ Time	Situation/ Topic	Type of Disfluency	Child's Reaction to Disfluency	Listener Name/ Reaction to Disfluency	What Triggered the Disfluency

For each of the remaining profiles, two sets of therapy targets will be presented: one based on a fluency-shaping approach and the other on stuttering modification/management. The sample activities that are included were designed to illustrate how each of these treatment paradigms can be implemented.

PROFILE 2: PRESCHOOL—3 YEAR-OLD

Kate is 3 years old and her speech is characterized by hesitations, whole-word/phrase repetitions, and interjections of syllables/words. Unlike Eli in Profile 1, Kate also demonstrates occasional word-initial syllable repetitions, accompanied by the incipient secondary behaviors of eye blinks and head nods. Analysis of a 200-syllable spontaneous speech sample indicated that 23% of the syllables uttered were disfluent. According to her parents, Kate is extremely frustrated by her disfluencies and often states, "I can't say that word." Her receptive and expressive language abilities as well as other developmental milestones appear age appropriate.

Selection of Therapy Targets Using a Fluency-Shaping Approach. The behaviors to be targeted are decreased speech rate and easy onset of phonation. These techniques were chosen because they are relatively easy for a young child to conceptualize and generally yield a marked decrease in disfluencies. In addition, the use of easy onset is particularly appropriate because it tends to inhibit the production of word-initial disfluencies.

Sample Activities

Easy Onset of Phonation and Decreased Speaking Rate

1. Fill a large bag or pillowcase with 25 to 30 small toys and objects. Collect pictures of one slow-moving and one fast-moving animal (e.g., whale and rabbit). Point to each picture while modeling the animals' special voices. Demonstrate the whale's voice by producing simple sentences using an exaggerated slow speech rate (approximately three to four syllables per second) and easy onset of phonation. Repeat the same sentences to demonstrate the rabbit's voice with an extremely rapid speech rate and abrupt onset of phonation.

   Select a carrier phrase that begins with a vowel, such as "I have a _____." Tell the child that she should close her eyes and pick one object from the bag. Have the child say the carrier phrase five times, including the name of the chosen object, using the preferred "whale voice" (e.g., "I have a *ball*"). As each utterance is produced, the clinician identifies the child's speech pattern by pointing to one of the animal pictures. Whenever the child's utterance is more like the rabbit's voice, the clinician provides another model of the whale's smooth, easy speaking voice and asks the child to imitate it. The child is then given a brief opportunity to play with the selected toy before repeating the sequence with another toy.

Decreased Speaking Rate and Light Articulatory Contact

2. Obtain an empty coffee can and punch 20 holes (approximately the diameter of a pencil) in the plastic lid. Place a small toy or other prize inside the can. Gather 20 lengths of colored yarn (each approximately 12 in. long) and tie a large knot at one end of each piece. Put the knotted ends of the strings at the bottom of the can and replace the lid on the can with unknotted ends of each piece protruding slightly through a hole in the lid. Select a book

that contains pictures of common objects and activities with which the child is familiar. The clinician shows the child the first picture in the book and models simple three- to five-word sentences (e.g., There's a doggie; I see a baby; The man is running; The house is red) using a very slow, easy speaking voice. The child is required to imitate the sentence using the same speech pattern while pulling one string of yarn through the coffee can lid in a correspondingly slow and gentle manner (until the yarn is stopped by the knot). Model a different sentence for each successive picture until all of the yarn pieces are "sprouting" from the can. After the last string has been pulled, the child may remove the lid to find the prize hidden inside.

Selection of Therapy Targets Using a Stuttering Modification/Management Approach. Stuttering modification may be of limited usefulness with a child of this age because many of the techniques employed in this approach require relatively advanced cognitive skills beyond the grasp of a 3-year-old child (e.g., self-analysis, cancellations, pull-outs). However, parents can be encouraged to minimize their child's anxiety by using appropriate vocabulary for casual reference to disfluencies (e.g., bumpy speech) and modeling expressions that mirror their child's feelings (e.g., "That one was really tough to say"). One aspect of this approach that can be extremely effective with very young disfluent children is desensitization. Therefore, the goal is to lessen the child's sensitivity to her own disfluencies.

Sample Activities

Desensitization

1. Obtain two simple puzzles and a deck of 25 cards depicting different agent + action relationships. Give one puzzle to each player and place the card deck face down on the table. Introduce a "Catch Me if You Can" game by explaining that each person will take a turn picking a card from the deck, placing it face up on the table, and describing it. The clinician should be prepared to pseudo-stutter (pretend to be disfluent) using the child's habitual pattern on about half of her turns. The child is instructed to listen carefully for any instances of "bumpy" (disfluent) speech during the clinician's or her own turn and to immediately slap the picture as soon as she hears it. The clinician provides feedback regarding the smoothness or bumpiness of every production. The player who correctly slaps the picture first earns a chance to put a piece in the puzzle. Repeat this sequence until the card deck is depleted.

2. Gather three puppets with movable mouths. One is for the clinician; the others are given to the child. Select a storybook that has a repetitive refrain or story line (e.g., *Green Eggs and Ham*, *The Little Red Hen*, and so on). Explain to the child that her puppets both have "bumpy" voices but that "Snappy" has more trouble with his words and gets stuck more often than "Max." The clinician uses her puppet to model both voices. The bumpier voice should reflect the child's habitual disfluency pattern in a slightly exaggerated manner and be accompanied by the child's secondary behaviors. The other voice is produced with just a few easy whole-word repetitions. Tell the child that the clinician's puppet is going to read a story out loud alternately using one or the other of her puppets' voices. The child's puppets will supply the refrain or repetitive line. The child must identify which voice the clinician's puppet is producing by making either Snappy or Max say the refrain in the same voice as the clinician's model. The clinician should gradually increase the frequency with which Max's less bumpy voice is presented as a model for imitation.

PROFILE 3: SCHOOL AGE—9-YEAR-OLD

Susan is 9 years old and her speech is characterized by part-word repetitions, whole-word repetitions, prolongations of initial sounds (approximately 2 to 3 s), and phrase revisions. She was noted to demonstrate several secondary behaviors, of which she did not seem consistently aware. These included excessive leg movements, lip tremors, and eye gaze aversion. Analysis of a 200-syllable spontaneous speech sample indicated that 29% of the syllables uttered were disfluent. According to parental report, Susan is extremely anxious about her speech difficulties. Developmental history is unremarkable, and her academic performance is appropriate for her grade level.

Selection of Therapy Targets Using a Fluency-Shaping Approach. The behaviors to be targeted are easy onset of phonation, light articulatory contacts, and decreased speaking rate. An analysis of Susan's disfluency profile indicates that her most severe stuttering characteristics are initial sound prolongations and part-word repetitions. Easy onset and light articulatory contacts were chosen because they are effective in addressing these types of disfluencies, especially when they occur in the word-initial position. Decreased speaking rate is considered a basic intervention technique that generally results in an immediate observable decrease in frequency of stuttering and thus provides the child with success in the very early stages of therapy.

Sample Activities

Easy Onset of Phonation and Light Articulatory Contacts

1. Play a modified version of an "I Spy" game in which the clinician is "it." Before beginning the game, teach the fluency-enhancing techniques of easy onset of phonation and light articulatory contacts. Instruct the child to release a little bit of air before starting her voice and to move her tongue and lips gently during speech. The clinician models each of the target techniques in single words. As soon as the child demonstrates some mastery of these behaviors (e.g., five consecutive correct responses), the I Spy game can be initiated. The clinician thinks of an object in the room and gives the child clues to its identity by describing its attributes one at a time (e.g., "I spy something black," "I spy something heavy," and so on), employing a slightly exaggerated rendition of both techniques. After each clue, the child takes one guess at identifying the object (at the single-word level) using both fluency techniques. Continue to present clues until the object is named. In the early phases of therapy, a slight modification of the game is recommended when the child takes his turn to be "it." Following the child's selection of an object, the clinician supplies the carrier phrase, "I spy something . . . ," for the child to complete with a single-word clue using the target fluency techniques.

Decreased Speaking Rate

2. Obtain a book/digital list of Mad Libs. Mad Libs are stories or vignettes in which specific parts of speech (e.g., noun, proper noun, adverb, adjective, and so on) have been omitted. When the missing parts are filled in, the result is a semantically absurd and funny text. The clinician selects one of the stories and says, "Give me an example of a _____" for each of the omitted parts of speech. These utterances should be produced with a slightly decreased speaking rate to highlight the target behavior. The child provides a word or phrase, which the clinician inserts into the written story. When all of the blanks have been

filled in, the child is instructed to read the whole story aloud using a predetermined slow rate of speech. The child then takes a turn choosing a Mad Lib and asks the clinician to supply the missing parts, remembering to use her slow speech rate. Instruct the child to read the completed story aloud to give her maximal opportunities to practice the target behavior. (This task is best used with children who have already demonstrated initial mastery of decreased speaking rate at the level of imitation.)

Selection of Therapy Targets Using a Stuttering Modification/Management Approach. Based on Susan's fluency profile, the therapy targets are her secondary behaviors, prolongation of initial sounds, and part-word repetitions. The secondary behaviors were selected because Susan shows little awareness of them and because these behaviors are highly distracting to conversational partners. The prolongations and part-word repetitions were identified as therapy targets because they represent Susan's most severe disfluency types.

Sample Activities

Self-Analysis

1. Obtain a 20- to 30-min video sample of the child's connected speech that represents her typical pattern and level of disfluencies. Explain to the child that when she stutters, she often exhibits some extra body movements and tends to look away from the listener. Tell her that she and the clinician will review the video to increase her awareness of the occurrence of these accompanying behaviors (i.e., leg movements, lip tremors, and eye gaze aversion). Select one of the secondary characteristics and tell the child that she and the clinician will watch the tape carefully for instances of that behavior. The first person to notice an occurrence of the target should signal by raising her hand. The person who signals correct identifications most frequently is declared the winner. Particularly clear examples of the behaviors may be played again to reinforce the child's understanding of the nature of the secondary characteristic. The initial stages of this activity should entail the use of brief segments of video (about 1 min), which can be gradually increased as the child demonstrates greater facility with the task.

Cancellations

2. Compile a list of 25 animal riddles (e.g., Q: Why do chimpanzees like bananas? A: Because they have a-peel). Underline one word in the question part of each riddle, being sure to vary the location of the underlined word in the sentence. Tell the child that she is going to read the riddles to the clinician using cancellations.

   Before beginning this activity, review this stuttering modification/management technique with the child. Remind the child that whenever she gets stuck on a word, she should complete the stutter without trying to start the word or sentence again. Once the word is finished, the child should pause to think about what went wrong, using the self-analysis skills learned in previous stages of therapy. The child should plan how to correct it by silently rehearsing how it would feel to say the word fluently. Then, have the child repeat the word in a smooth, prolonged manner. Provide the child with several opportunities to practice the technique by modeling some disfluencies and cancellations for her to imitate.

   Instruct the child to read the first part of each riddle and to deliberately stutter on the underlined word in the question. Each disfluency should be modified using cancellation.

Once the cancellation has been successfully completed, the child can finish reading the whole riddle. Any spontaneous disfluencies that occur on words other than the underlined target should also be canceled.

 PROFILE 4: ADULT—29-YEAR-OLD

Patrick is 29 years old, and his speech is characterized by laryngeal blocks and prolongations of initial sounds. Duration of blocks ranges between 2 and 20 s, whereas prolongations tend to last 3 to 5 s. Patrick was observed to demonstrate numerous secondary behaviors, including head jerks, jaw tremors, eye blinks, and audible inhalation. Analysis of a 200-syllable spontaneous speech sample indicated that 35% of syllables uttered were disfluent. During the case history interview, Patrick stated that stuttering has been a problem since childhood and that he is currently seeking treatment because his disfluencies are interfering with career advancement as well as interpersonal relationships.

Selection of Therapy Targets Using a Fluency-Shaping Approach. The behaviors to be targeted are easy onset of phonation and continuous phonation. These techniques were chosen because they require an open vocal fold posture and therefore inhibit the production of laryngeal blocks, Patrick's most severe type of disfluency.

Sample Activities

Easy Onset of Phonation

1. Draw a graphic representation of two breath curves, like the ones shown in Figure 9–2. Explain that the first drawing represents the usual pattern of speaking, in which voicing (the dotted line) is initiated at the same time as the onset of exhalation (the solid line). Explain to the client that his attempts to use this pattern often result in complete involuntary closure of the vocal folds (i.e., laryngeal blocks). Introduce the second drawing and tell him that it illustrates an alternative phonation pattern that will help prevent these blocks. Explain that the solid line again represents the point at which inhalation ends and exhalation begins and

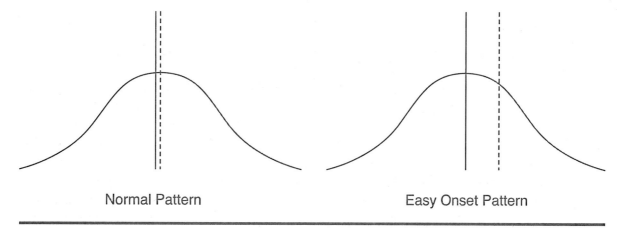

Normal Pattern   Easy Onset Pattern

Figure 9–2
Breath curves.

that the dotted line has been moved to indicate that his voice should start *after* exhalation has begun. Using the easy onset graph, instruct the client to place his finger at the beginning of the breath curve. Tell him to move his finger slowly along the curve as he inhales. When his finger reaches the solid line, he should begin to exhale slowly and continuously. As his finger reaches the dotted line, the client should *maintain* his open vocal fold posture and smoothly produce an isolated vowel, such as /o, a, uh/. Once the client can easily initiate phonation without blocking, the task can progress hierarchically from isolated vowels to h-initial words and then to more complex units of speech. (See Appendix 9–A companion website for sample phrases, questions, and monologue topics.)

Continuous Phonation

2. Prepare a list of 50 simple three-word phrases (see Appendix 9–A on the companion website). Introduce the technique of continuous phonation by explaining to the client that he should keep his voice turned on even between words, but without increasing his habitual speech rate. Model use of the technique by first producing an audible yawn, which is characterized by continuous voicing. Produce the yawn a second time, and overlay a four-word utterance that lasts throughout its duration. Stress the idea that speaking over the yawn results in a smooth, unbroken utterance stream. Instruct the client to produce several audible yawns to heighten his awareness of how it feels to produce smooth, flowing streams of phonation. Read phrases from the prepared list, and have the client imitate each stimulus phrase using the yawn technique to emphasize the production of continuous phonation.

Selection of Therapy Targets Using a Stuttering Modification/Management Approach. Based on Patrick's fluency profile, the therapy targets are his secondary behaviors, laryngeal blocks, and prolongations of initial sounds. The secondary behaviors were chosen because their bizarre nature tends to invoke severe listener penalty. Patrick's two main disfluency types were selected because both blocks and prolongations interfere significantly with his ability to communicate.

Sample Activities

Desensitization

1. Help the client to generate a list of anxiety-producing speaking situations and arrange them hierarchically from least to most feared. Teach the client a tension reduction procedure such as progressive relaxation (Jacobson, 1938). This technique can be modified specifically for stutterers by using the steps outlined in Table 9–1. Once the client demonstrates the ability to consciously achieve a relaxed state, explain that relaxation will be used to desensitize him to the previously identified feared speaking situations. Beginning with the least feared situation in the hierarchy, instruct the client to use visual imagery to imagine himself in that situation. Tell him to monitor his overall level of muscle tone for any significant increase in tension. Whenever the client identifies an occurrence of excessive tension, he is instructed to employ the relaxation skills learned in progressive relaxation training. Continue to have the client focus on the same speaking situation until he demonstrates the ability to remain relaxed throughout the entire visualization. Once the client can maintain a relaxed state at

this level with minimal discernible effort, move to the next situation in the hierarchy. Repeat the visualization–relaxation sequence for each successive entry until the client is effectively desensitized to the thought of all the feared speaking situations in the hierarchy. Once the client can consciously induce a relaxed state, progress to more difficult environments such as including strangers in the therapy session and going outside the clinic setting (e.g., a store or library).

Voluntary Stuttering

2. Introduce the technique of **voluntary stuttering** and the rationale for its use in the treatment process. Explain that this technique requires clients to stutter on purpose and then analyze their own feelings as well as listener reactions. The goal of voluntary stuttering is to reduce/minimize the stutterer's feelings of fear or embarrassment associated with disfluent moments. Model easy repetitions and prolongations for the client during a short conversational interaction. Then instruct the client to produce at least five of these voluntary stutters on nonfeared words during another 3-min conversation. Provide visual cues (e.g., hand gestures), as necessary, to prompt the client's use of easy repetitions and prolongations. Following the conversation, the client should rank feelings of anxiety on a 5-point scale. Once the client is comfortable with this technique in the clinical setting, the task can be implemented gradually in real-world situations with other conversational partners. In addition, the rating scale can be expanded to rank degrees of negative listener reactions.

Freezing

3. Introduce the concept of **freezing**, which involves purposefully extending the moment of stuttering to increase the client's tolerance for and control over core stuttering behaviors. Instruct the client to read aloud lists of short phrases (e.g., those in Appendix 9–A on the companion website). Explain that when a disfluency occurs, the clinician will signal the client to continue the stutter. The client should maintain the same disfluency pattern (prolongation, repetition, or block) until the clinician signals to release it.

Pull-Outs

4. Obtain a board game suitable for adults that generally requires the production of multi-word responses, such as Jeopardy. Explain the rules of the game and inform the client that he will assume the role of contestant. Tell him that each of his responses must contain at least one pseudo or real disfluency that he will modify using pull-outs. Review this stuttering modification/management technique by reminding the client that whenever he gets stuck on a word, he should (a) stop in the middle of the disfluency; (b) pause to mentally rehearse how it would feel to produce that word fluently; (c) say the word a second time in a smooth, prolonged manner; and (d) complete the rest of the intended utterance without going back to the beginning of the sentence. Provide several opportunities to practice this technique by modeling some disfluencies and pull-outs for him to imitate. Begin the game by instructing the client to choose a topic category and a difficulty level. Read the designated "answer" to which the client must respond in the form of a question that contains a pull-out. Provide the opportunity for the client to produce at least 50 "questions" during the game.

Helpful Hints

1. For each of the activities listed, the difficulty of the task can be manipulated systematically with regard to utterance length using the traditional hierarchy of single words, carrier phrase, sentence, two- to four-word sentences, and conversation. Provision of consistent clinician models should be faded gradually until all client responses are spontaneously generated without any model.

2. As therapy progresses, introduce activities that simulate natural speaking situations. For young children, these might include asking for a turn to play with a toy, asking for assistance in completing a puzzle, describing pictures in a book, playing house or tea party, telling stories, and negotiating the rules of a game. For older children and adults, activities may involve talking on the telephone, ordering food at a restaurant, asking for directions, interviewing for a job, and giving presentations in class or at work.

3. Fluency shaping and stuttering modification/management techniques can be combined within the same therapy session. It is best to begin the session with stuttering modification techniques and then move on to fluency shaping. If implemented in the reverse order, carryover from fluency-shaping practice may significantly decrease the number of disfluencies the client produces during the treatment visit. The reduced frequency of stuttering may not provide the client with adequate opportunities to learn and practice stuttering modification/management techniques later in the session.

4. Once the target concepts and techniques have been established in individual sessions, group therapy can be particularly effective for strengthening and refining clients' fluency skills.

5. It is essential for the clinician to monitor her or his reactions to client disfluencies. Even subtle indications of discomfort (e.g., averted eye gaze) may adversely affect the therapeutic relationship between client and clinician.

6. A client's feelings about his stuttering can be monitored over the course of therapy by periodic readministration of a stuttering attitude checklist (see Form 9–2). Such scales are not intended to be scored quantitatively along a continuum of severity but rather to provide descriptive information about changes in the client's emotions and attitudes.

7. Families should be encouraged to avoid a conspiracy of silence regarding stuttering. Open acknowledgment and discussion can minimize the feelings of isolation and shame often experienced by individuals who stutter. (Refer to Chapter 11 for additional information on counseling strategies.)

8. Avoidance reduction therapy frequently results in a noticeable increase in observable disfluencies as the client begins to relinquish habitual avoidance strategies. The focus of counseling at this point is twofold: (a) to help the client understand that this stage of therapy is temporary and (b) to provide consistent and direct support as the client confronts feared speaking situations during this phase.

9. Clinicians should be aware that older students and adolescents (i.e., between approximately 10 and 17 years of age) frequently demonstrate extreme resistance to any type of fluency therapy. Parents may require considerable counseling support to accept the fact that their child may not be emotionally ready to benefit from direct intervention during this period. Clinicians should also reassure parents that willingness to participate in therapy reemerges with increased maturity.

10. Individuals with a long-standing history of severe stuttering often limit their participation in social interactions, resulting in a relative lack of practice with conversational skills in both speaker and listener roles. Clinicians can incorporate pragmatic language goals into the fluency treatment plan in order to facilitate maximal communicative effectiveness.

11. Even if a person who stutters makes no change in the frequency of disfluencies, a significant reduction in the use of postponements and starters (e.g., "uhm," "you know," "well, let me see") can improve the listener's perception of speech.

12. Clinicians should monitor client progress over time and be aware of the difference between a "lapse" (a small slip or mistake) and "relapse" (cessation of newly learned behaviors with a return to previous performance levels).

Form 9–2. STUTTERING ATTITUDE CHECKLIST

INSTRUCTIONS: Respond to the following by circling "Y" to indicate that "Yes, I agree" or "N" to indicate "No, I do not agree" with each statement. Record your initial reaction rather than analyzing or deliberating over each statement.

1.	Y	N	I often feel that stuttering is my own fault.
2.	Y	N	I find it easy to talk to people in authority such as my teacher or my employer.
3.	Y	N	Sometimes I wonder if I stutter on purpose to get attention.
4.	Y	N	I have more trouble saying some words/sounds than others.
5.	Y	N	Most people think that stutterers are not quite as smart as people who do not stutter.
6.	Y	N	People always seem comfortable when I am talking to them.
7.	Y	N	I think that stuttering is caused by some kind of mental or emotional problem.
8.	Y	N	My stuttering keeps me from doing the kind of work that I would really like to do.
9.	Y	N	I sometimes think that other people are responsible for having caused my stuttering.
10.	Y	N	The way I talk does not embarrass me.
11.	Y	N	Stuttering is my biggest problem.
12.	Y	N	Even when I know the right answer to a question, I often keep silent because of my stuttering.
13.	Y	N	I think speech therapy can help me a great deal.
14.	Y	N	My stuttering would go away if I stopped worrying about it all the time.
15.	Y	N	I feel that I should be able to stop my stuttering without help from anyone else.

Sources: Adapted from "Stuttering Therapy: The Relation Between Changes in Symptom Level and Attitudes," by G. Andrews & J. Cutler, 1974, *Journal of Speech and Hearing Disorders, 39*(3), 312; *Cooper Personalized Fluency Control Therapy for Adolescents and Adults: Clinician's Manual,* by E. Cooper & C. Cooper, 2003, Austin, TX: Pro-Ed.; "Overall Assessment of the Speaker's Experience of Stuttering (OASES): Documenting Multiple Outcomes in Stuttering Treatment," by J. S. Yaruss & R. W. Quesal, 2006, *Journal of Fluency Disorders, 31*(2), 90–115.

Conclusion

This chapter presented basic information, protocols, and procedures for intervention with fluency disorders at an *introductory* level. This information is intended only as a starting point in the reader's clinical education and training. For more in-depth coverage of this area, the following readings are recommended:

Amster, B. J., & Klein, E. R. (2018). *More than fluency: The social, emotional, and cognitive dimensions of stuttering.* Plural Publishing.

Bloodstein, O., Ratner, N., & Brundage, S. (2021). *A handbook on stuttering* (7th ed.). Plural Publishing.

Guitar, B. (2019). *Stuttering: An integrated approach to its nature and treatment* (5th ed.). Wolters Kluwer.

Manning, W. H. (2017). *Clinical decision making in fluency disorders* (4th ed.). Plural Publishing.

Yairi, E., & Seery, C. (2021). *Stuttering: Foundations and clinical applications* (3rd ed.). Plural Publishing.

Additional Resources

50 Great Activities for Children Who Stutter: Lessons, Insights, and Ideas for Therapy Success (E-Book Option)

This practice manual contains 50 activities, most including several possible adaptations. The activities are divided into five categories and include reproducible homework and handouts: identifying and exploring stuttering, practicing speech tools, learning the facts, uncovering feelings, and targeting language and stuttering goals.

The Lidcombe Program Treatment Guide

This concise pdf is written for clinicians to provide detailed information on the method and implementation of the Lidcombe Program: a parent-conducted, behavioral treatment for stuttering that is designed for children younger than age 6 years. The guide is available to access online for free.

Easy Does It for Fluency: Preschool/Primary and Intermediate Sets

This series provides a manual and a workbook for therapists and students to use during therapy. It provides a direct approach to intervention and addresses the motor, linguistic, and psychosocial aspects of stuttering. The workbook is divided into six levels: getting ready, analyzing, modifying speech production, desensitizing, transferring, and maintaining. The series includes a CD for access to forms, such as parent and teacher letters and home assignments.

The Source for Stuttering and Cluttering

This comprehensive resource for ages 7 to 18 years includes all phases of the therapeutic process, from assessment through diagnosis and treatment. Tools, tips, activities, and strategies to help develop skills including planning and implementing therapy, providing "real-world" practice, working effectively with parents and teachers, and much more is provided.

The Child and Adolescent Stuttering Treatment and Activity Resource Guide, Second Edition

This guide provides specific, hands-on activities that can be used in the evaluation of fluency disorders in children. It offers specific decision-making information to help clinicians choose goals to address and gives ideas on activities and strategies that can be used to meet these goals.

Stuttering and Your Child: Help for Parents

Appropriate for viewing in any home, day care, clinical, or educational setting, this 30-min video provides parents with up-to-date information about what stuttering is, what is thought to cause and worsen childhood stuttering, and what parents can do to help their child. Visit the Stuttering Foundation of America's website to view the video online.

Effective Counseling in Stuttering Therapy

This book helps the clinician have a better understanding of the counseling aspect of therapy and suggests ways to use it effectively.

The School-Age Child Who Stutters: Working Effectively With Attitudes and Emotions

This resource focuses on assessing and treating feelings/beliefs in school-age children who stutter. It contains practical, concrete ideas for documentation and strategies to achieve change.

The Power R Game!

This resource uses a game board format to change attitudes and feelings about stuttering. It contains 94 game cards with 564 statements for directing discussions about stuttering and an additional 50 cards containing diversion scenarios. The second edition provides an updated manual with additional resources and references.

Miscellaneous

Stuttering Home Page (web.mnsu.edu/comdis/kuster/stutter.html)

This is a comprehensive site for individuals who stutter and the professionals who work with them. The site includes information about research and treatment as well as support organizations and conferences.

Chapter 10

Intervention for Voice and Alaryngeal Speech

This chapter addresses impairments in phonation (traditionally referred to as voice disorders) as well as alaryngeal speech resulting from surgical removal of the larynx. To competently diagnose and treat phonatory disorders, clinicians must be well acquainted with the mechanisms involved in normal voice production. The reader is referred to Aronson and Bless (2009), Boone et al. (2019), Seikel et al. (2015), and Zemlin (1998) for detailed discussions of laryngeal anatomy and physiology.

Voice Disorders

A voice disorder is a disturbance of pitch, loudness, or quality in relation to an individual's age, gender, and cultural background. Voice disorders are identified on the basis of a listener's judgment rather than by any absolute or standardized criteria for normal voice production. The term **dysphonia** refers to any deviation in phonation, whereas **aphonia** is a term used to indicate the absence of audible phonation. Payten et al. (2022) present a scoping review of the research on terminology and definitions for voice disorders.

Appendix D on the companion website provides a schematic of the vocal tract structures relevant to phonation. In the normal production of voice, the airstream is generated by the lungs. As the air passes through the larynx, the vocal folds are set into vibratory motion, which results in the production of sound (i.e., phonation). The sound continues to travel through the upper vocal tract and is modified by the resonating characteristics of the pharynx and oral and nasal cavities. Loudness and pitch are controlled by different physiologic mechanisms. Loudness is the perceptual counterpart to amplitude (the height of a sound wave). It is determined primarily by the amount and speed of subglottal air pressure. A voice becomes louder when there is an increase in the volume and velocity of the airstream as it passes through the glottis. Pitch is the perceptual correlate of frequency (number of vibratory closing and opening cycles per second). The relative length and thickness of the vocal folds determine voice pitch. The voice becomes higher in pitch when the vocal folds are elongated with a concurrent decrease in mass and an increase in elasticity of the vocal folds. The pitch most frequently used by an individual speaker during spontaneous speech production is known as **fundamental frequency** or **habitual pitch**. The fundamental frequencies used by normal speakers of different ages and genders are shown in Table 10–1.

Normal voices function in at least three pitch ranges or **voice registers**. These are the **pulse** (the lower range of fundamental frequencies), **modal** (the range of fundamental frequencies used in normal speech), and **loft** (the highest range of fundamental frequencies) registers. Each register is characterized by a distinct pattern of vocal fold approximation. The vocal folds vibrate in the same manner throughout a given pitch range; the pattern of vibration changes as the maximum limit for the range is exceeded and a new voice register is entered.

Table 10–1
Normal Fundamental Frequencies for Males and Females

Age in Years	Fundamental Frequency (Hz)	
	Male	Female
1–2	400	400
3	300	300
4	285	285
5–7	265	265
8	250	255
9–13	235	240
14	175	225
15	165	220
16	150	215
17	135	210
18–19	125	205
20–29	120	227
30–39	112	214
40–49	107	214
50–59	118	214
60–69	112	209
70–79	132	206
80–89	146	197

Sources: Adapted from "Normative Voice Data for Younger and Older Adults," by H. Goy, D. N. Fernandes, M. K. Pichora-Fuller, and P. van Lieshout, 2013, *Journal of Voice,* 27(5), 545–555; *Clinical Voice Disorders* (4th ed.), by A. E. Aronson and D. Bless, 2009, New York, NY: Thieme Medical Publishers.

Voice quality is difficult to define but can be described as the aspects of a voice that differentiate it from another voice at identical pitch and loudness levels. It is regulated, at least in part, by the manner and force with which the vocal folds approximate one another. For example, if the folds are loosely approximated during phonation, the resulting voice quality is generally labeled as breathy, whereas overly tense vocal fold approximation is generally associated with a harsh, strained voice quality.

Resonance is another factor that affects voice production. The sound generated at the laryngeal level is amplified or filtered as it passes through the resonating cavities of the upper vocal tract (i.e., pharynx, oral and nasal cavities). Vocal resonance can be affected by a variety of neurological and structural factors. Information regarding voice symptoms and resonance problems associated with various kinds of dysarthrias was discussed in Chapter 8; resonance problems that accompany cleft palate were described in Chapter 3.

The incidence of voice disorders is estimated to occur in approximately 3% to 9% of the general population including children and adults (Ramig & Verdolini, 1998; Roy et al., 2005). An epidemiologic study investigating voice disorders in adults estimated the prevalence of voice disorders at approximately 7% of this population (Roy et al., 2005). The percentage of adults reporting a past history of voice disorders is higher, around approximately 30%, reflecting the typically transient nature of voice disorders (Roy et al., 2005).

Prevalence data for voice disorders are influenced by factors such as gender, age, and occupation (Martins et al., 2016). With regard to gender, voice disorders are more commonly reported in boys than girls. This gender distribution flips in adult populations with a ratio of 1.5 females to every 1.0 male. With regard to age, higher prevalence rates are reported for elderly adults, with estimates ranging from 5% to 30% (de Araújo Pernambuco et al., 2015). In the pediatric population, voice disorder prevalence data ranges from 1.4% to 6% (Black et al., 2015). Populations most at risk for developing voice disorders include teachers, factory workers, salespersons, and singers (Cohen et al., 2012).

Classification of Voice Disorders

Traditionally, voice disorders have been classified as either organic or functional (Aronson & Bless, 2009; Boone et al., 2019). **Organic** voice disorders result from pathology or disease that affects the anatomy or physiology of the larynx and other regions of the vocal tract. **Functional** voice disorders are dysphonias related to vocal abuse/misuse or psychogenic factors in the absence of an identifiable physical etiology. The distinction between these two diagnostic categories is not always clear. For example, a pattern of long-term vocal abuse may eventually lead to organic pathology of the vocal folds. The most common voice disorders are functional in nature and involve faulty habits of vocal usage (Boone et al., 2019). However, several organic etiologies have a significant impact on voice production.

The speech-language pathologist (SLP) should be familiar with the range of possible organic and functional etiologies and their implications for treatment planning. Table 10–2 lists the most common organic and functional voice problems.

Organic

Many organic factors alter the mass of vocal folds and result in lowered pitch, decreased loudness, and a breathy, hoarse voice quality. These alterations affect the shape, the mobility, and/or the muscular tension of the vocal folds. Lower pitch is a result of the inability of the vocal folds to be lengthened and thinned. Reduced loudness and a breathy, hoarse voice quality will occur if the folds cannot achieve adequate closure (adduction). Examples of these organic factors include the following:

- **Edema** (swelling) related to **laryngitis** (inflammation of the folds and other regions of the larynx, usually caused by bacterial infection)

Table 10–2
Organic and Functional Voice Problems

Organic	Functional
Vocal fold paralysis	Abuse/misuse
Laryngeal webs	Vocal nodules
Papilloma	Contact ulcers
Edema	Ventricular dysphonia
Tumor	Psychogenic
Granuloma	Conversion dysphonia
Neurologic/endocrine disease	Mutational falsetto
Spasmodic dysphonia[a]	

[a]Several varieties have been described; etiology is not known.

- Mass lesions, such as **tumors**, large **granulomas**, and **papillomas**

- **Neurologic** or **endocrine disorders** (e.g., degenerative diseases such as parkinsonism and hypothyroidism)

- **Laryngeal webs** (membranes that extend from one vocal fold to the other and partially occlude the airway)

- **Vocal fold paralysis** due to impairment in the recurrent or superior laryngeal nerves that innervate the larynx

Functional

Functional voice disorders arise from faulty voice usage or psychogenic factors. Symptoms range from a breathy, whispered voice to a strained, tight voice with inappropriate loudness and pitch.

Vocal abuse/misuse is directly related to excessive muscle tension (i.e., laryngeal hyperfunction). In laryngeal hyperfunction, the pattern of vocal fold closure is abrupt and forceful. The most common types of abuse/misuse include shouting, screaming, and excessive talking as well as excessive coughing or throat clearing. Initiation of phonation is accomplished by **hard glottal attack**, which is characterized by tight glottal closure, increased subglottal air pressure, and explosive abduction (opening) of the folds. Consistent use of faulty patterns can result in pathology (e.g., chronic laryngitis, vocal nodules, or contact ulcers). **Vocal nodules** are benign, whitish protuberances that occur at the junction of the anterior and middle thirds of the vocal folds, the area of maximum impact during vocal fold closure. These calluslike formations prevent complete adduction of the folds and result in a lower pitch and breathy, hoarse voice quality. **Contact ulcers** are benign, bilateral, sorelike lesions on the posterior third of the vocal folds caused by habitual use of hard glottal attacks and excessively low pitch. Symptoms include hoarseness and laryngeal pain. Another example of vocal misuse is **ventricular**

dysphonia. This disorder involves the use of the ventricular folds (false vocal folds) as the primary source of phonation while the true folds are held in an abducted position.

Psychogenic voice disorders arise from emotional or mental factors such as anxiety, depression, or personality disturbance that interfere with voluntary control over voice production (Aronson & Bless, 2009; Tezcaner et al., 2019). These disorders may develop subsequent to an occurrence of physiologic changes in the larynx, such as laryngitis, and persist long after the physical symptoms have disappeared. Two primary examples of psychogenic voice disorders are conversion dysphonias and mutational falsetto. **Conversion dysphonias** are the physical manifestations of psychological conflict and range in severity from mild hoarseness to whispering to complete absence of voice (i.e., dysphonia → aphonia → mutism). A **mutational falsetto** is characterized by the continued use of a higher pitched childhood voice into adolescence and adulthood in the presence of a normal laryngeal system. This condition is seen mainly in males and results in a voice that is high pitched, breathy, hoarse, and gives the overall impression of immaturity.

Spasmodic dysphonia (SD) is a voice disorder that resists easy classification. Several different types of these dysphonias have been described, some of which are considered organic and others functional in origin (Aronson & Bless, 2009; Sanuki, 2022; Stemple et al., 2000). However, there is mounting evidence of an underlying neurologic etiology for all types. This growing consensus suggests that SD is a focal dystonia, a condition characterized by involuntary movement in an isolated body part. These abnormal movement patterns occur predominantly during purposeful tasks, such as speech, and may not affect reflexive functions such as coughing, laughing, or sneezing. This disorder involves severe spasmodic movements of the vocal folds that interrupt the normal adduction–abduction cycle of phonation. Hintze et al. (2017) identify a list of factors that may contribute to a differential SD diagnosis, including family history of neurologic impairment, recent viral illness, and heavy voice use. The disorder is traditionally divided into two main categories: **adductor spasmodic dysphonia** and **abductor spasmodic dysphonia**, depending on when the vocal fold spasms occur. In the more common adductor type, glottal closure is so tight that the vocal folds cannot vibrate in the usual sustained fashion. This overadduction results in a voice that can be described as hoarse, strained, and staccato. It is accompanied by periodic cessation in phonation (phonation breaks) and sudden, unpredictable changes in pitch (pitch breaks). Abductor spasmodic dysphonia is less common than the adductor type and is characterized by excessive and spasmodic opening of the vocal folds during phonation. This uncontrolled abduction allows a great deal of unphonated air to pass through the larynx, causing a breathy voice quality.

There is a distinct lack of research data regarding prognostic indicators related to voice disorders. The same factors generally associated with improvement of any communication disorder can also be applied to individuals with vocal abnormalities. A favorable outcome is generally associated with structural adequacy of the speech production mechanism with little or no organic impairment, a high degree of client motivation and cooperation, and a client's ability to discriminate and self-monitor target behavior. A recent systematic review by Rumbach et al. (2022) found that treatment outcomes in spasmodic dysphonia are variable due to the lack of a unified measurement approach. Advances in voice assessment technology such as laryngeal imaging and ambulatory voice monitoring (i.e., wearable data collection devices) have the potential to significantly influence clinical decision-making for the treatment of voice disorders in the next 5 to 10 years (Van Stan et al., 2017).

Treatment Efficacy/Evidence-Based Practice

Desjardins et al.'s (2017) systematic review of the literature indicated that behavioral voice treatment results in positive voice production changes compared to other/no treatment. More recently, Mahoney et al. (2022) reported emergent support for respiratory muscle training, botulinum toxin, and low dose amitriptyline for reducing vocal cord dysfunction symptoms. These authors emphasized the need for a more robust set of randomly controlled trials addressing treatment efficacy. In a much earlier study, Ramig and Verdolini (1998) provided a comprehensive summary of available data on treatment efficacy for voice disorders. They reviewed group and single-subject experimental designs, retrospective analyses, case studies, and program evaluation data. Their overall conclusion was that voice treatment is effective for both functional and organic voice disorders. Their analysis also resulted in several additional conclusions:

- Disorders of vocal misuse and hyperfunction can be effectively treated with a variety of intervention techniques, including biofeedback of laryngeal muscle activity, progressive relaxation, yawn-sigh procedure, and vocal intensity reduction.

- Voice therapy significantly reduces the recurrence of vocal nodules after surgical removal. (See Pedersen & McGlashan [2012] for a discussion of surgery versus behavioral intervention as an initial approach to the management of vocal fold nodules.)

- Voice therapy is effective in reducing or eliminating contact ulcers for most individuals.

- Lee Silverman Voice Treatment (LSVT) successfully increases vocal loudness and functional communication in individuals with Parkinson's disease (Pu et al., 2021).

- A combination of voice therapy and botulinum toxin (Botox) injection significantly improves laryngeal function for clients with spasmodic dysphonia. (See Guglielmino et al. [2018] for a comparative study on the use of botulinum toxin versus propranolol for dystonic vocal tremors.)

Additional studies have been conducted to investigate evidence-based practice (EBP) for specific voice disorders and conditions:

- In a comprehensive review of treatment approaches for vocal fold paralysis, Walton et al. (2017) identified 12 studies that reported positive outcomes for voice therapy. However, the low level of evidence across these studies prevented a recommendation for any particular intervention technique.

- This equivocal finding is echoed in the 2018 clinical practice guidelines published by the American Academy of Otolaryngology–Head and Neck Surgery (Stachler et al., 2018) for treating the vocal symptom of hoarseness.

- Yiu et al. (2017) found a similar lack of persuasive data regarding the relative effectiveness of resonant voice therapy techniques.

- For transgender voice therapy, Davies (2017) identified studies that support the benefit of targeting multiple voice parameters in treatment rather than focusing solely on pitch/ fundamental frequency.

Treatment for Voice Disorders

The goal of treatment for voice disorders is to help a client produce a voice of the best possible pitch, loudness, and quality in relation to the individual's age and gender within the context of his or her cultural and linguistic background. There are three main approaches to voice treatment: (a) medical, (b) indirect/environmental, and (c) direct/behavioral. Medical interventions include surgery, medication, and radiation (e.g., removal of vocal fold polyps). Indirect strategies involve modifying a client's daily surroundings or helping a client adjust to the vocal demands of his or her environment. Three common modifications include (a) education about anatomy/physiology of voice production (Gartner-Schmidt et al., 2013); (b) suggestions for voice amplification (Teixeira & Behlau, 2015); and (c) monitoring of vocally stressful situations (Verdolini Abbott, 2008). Direct strategies target the client's respiration, phonation, resonance, or articulation (Van Stan et al., 2015). Ohlsson et al. (2020) concluded that behavioral voice therapy strategies are most efficacious when delivered via group therapy settings.

The approach to intervention for some organic voice disorders is strictly medical. For example, papillomas (wartlike growths on the inner margin of the vocal folds) are effectively treated only through surgical removal. Other organic disorders are best treated through a combination of medical and behavioral therapies. For instance, treatment for a neurological disorder such as Parkinson's disease generally consists of medications as well as symptomatic voice therapy. Functional voice disorders are usually treated effectively with voice therapy alone.

Numerous intervention techniques for voice disorders have been described in the literature. Certain approaches are applicable to any voice disorder regardless of symptomatology or etiology. These include the following:

- *Listening skills:* These techniques are used to increase the client's awareness of his or her vocal behaviors. The clinician demonstrates and contrasts appropriate and inappropriate vocal behaviors. The client is asked to identify and discriminate between the two in live and recorded samples.

- *Respiratory control:* These strategies are used to optimize respiratory support for voice production. Attention is given to posture, breathing patterns, and expiratory control for phonation. The client may be asked to prolong phonation for as long as possible at a variety of different pitch and intensity levels.

- *Vocal rest:* Reduction or elimination of phonation is sometimes recommended to limit laryngeal irritation and to permit the vocal folds to recover from surgery or misuse. A client may be asked to modify or totally refrain from talking for a specified amount of time (usually 4 days to 2 weeks). Individuals most likely to be placed on vocal rest have (a) fluid-filled lesions that may rupture (e.g., cysts), (b) vascular conditions such as hematoma, or (c) just undergone laryngeal surgery. The strategy of complete voice rest is highly controversial with regard to its value and practicality.

Intervention Techniques

This section is devoted to a discussion of therapy techniques associated with specific voice abnormalities. Although the organic versus functional paradigm was appropriate for a description of voice disorder classification, we find it clinically more useful to organize treatment information according to the following four categories: vocal hyperfunction, vocal hypofunction, psychogenic disorders, and spastic dysphonias.

Vocal Hyperfunction

This category includes any voice disorder characterized by excessive laryngeal tension or overly forceful closure of the vocal folds. It consists primarily of dysphonias related to vocal abuse or misuse. The majority of voice problems encountered by SLPs are related to vocal hyperfunction caused by vocal abuse or misuse. The following techniques are useful in treating symptoms associated with laryngeal hyperfunction (Boone et al., 2019; Prater et al., 1999). The overall aims of these techniques are (a) to reduce muscular tension and (b) to eliminate abusive vocal behaviors.

Relaxing Muscles. Techniques can be directed specifically to the vocal tract musculature or toward relaxation of the whole body. One method of tension reduction for the muscles of the larynx is the adoption of an open-mouth posture during speech, because muscular tension in the jaw area is usually related to tension in the laryngeal musculature. The client visualizes the contrasting mouth postures of a ventriloquist and an opera singer. The client then practices speaking alternately with a closed-mouth and open-mouth posture in front of a mirror. Other vocal relaxation techniques include laryngeal massage and head and neck rolls. (For step-by-step instructions, see Prater et al. [1999].) One of the most common approaches to tension reduction for the whole body is progressive relaxation, which was described in detail in Chapter 9. Muscle relaxation typically is used in conjunction with one or more of the other therapy techniques in this category.

Reducing Loudness. The client reads short phrases or sentences aloud, using a different intensity level for each one. A lower intensity level that is optimal for the client is identified (described by Boone et al. [2019] as the voice to use when not wanting to wake up a sleeping person). This quieter voice is practiced in drills that require reading utterances of increasing length (i.e., single sentences → multiple sentences → short paragraphs).

Softening Glottal Attacks. Several techniques can be used to soften hard glottal attacks:

- *Yawn-sigh:* The client yawns in a natural manner and phonates a gentle sigh on exhalation. Once relaxed phonation is mastered, the client produces words on the exhalation. Begin with single words that begin with /h/ or a vowel and progress to four to five words per exhalation. The eventual goal is for the client to induce easy phonation by imagining the relaxed oral feeling associated with the yawn-sigh approach.

- *Chewing:* The client chews in a natural but exaggerated manner while simultaneously producing phonation (Froeschels, 1952). Start with vowels and gradually increase the length of the utterance on successive exhalations. The client practices variations in pitch and loudness levels while chewing/phonating. Relaxation of laryngeal musculature should be maintained.

- *Easy onset:* The client produces syllable combinations of /h/ + vowel to practice relaxed initiation of phonation. This phoneme sequence establishes airflow through the glottis prior to phonation. Gradually lengthen utterances to polysyllabic words and short sentences. Expand the drills to include other voiceless fricatives and other sound classes.

- *Chant talk:* The client listens to and imitates a recording of chanting—a speaking pattern characterized by the production of words in a continuous unbroken monotone, prolongation of vowels, and lack of syllable stress (e.g., Gregorian chant). Once this speaking style can be reliably produced, the client reads aloud for 20-s periods, alternating between habitual voice and chant talk.

Adjusting Pitch. A habitual pitch that requires the least amount of physical effort and tension results in the most pleasant-sounding voice. The client produces "um-hum" with a closed-mouth posture using a rising inflection. This vocalization should simulate the conversational device that is commonly used to signal agreement with a partner's statement. Once identified, a pitch pipe can be used to provide a model for the client to imitate. Begin with isolated vowels and progress to single words, sentences, and paragraphs. Instrumentation (e.g., Visi-Pitch IV from PENTAX Medical Corporation) can be used to provide visual feedback, which helps the client maintain appropriate pitch use for longer periods of time.

Phonating on Inhalation. The client inhales slowly while attempting to phonate a hum as modeled by the clinician. Once this behavior is reliably established, the client attempts to phonate on exhalation and match the pitch produced during the previous inhalation. Gradually, phonation is produced only on exhalation and at a wide variety of pitch levels. This technique is often used with cases of ventricular phonation, because phonating on inhalation requires the use of the true vocal folds rather than the false folds.

Lessac-Madsen Resonant Voice Therapy (LMRVT). This treatment approach can be used to address both vocal hyperfunction and hypofunction (see the following section on hypofunction). Treatment protocols begin with stretching exercises to position the vocal folds slightly ajar. Clients then perform syllable- and sentence-level tasks while maintaining this vocal fold position. The aim of LMRVT is to produce a strong voice with the minimal amount of intraoral pressure needed. LMRVT is also preventative in nature by tailoring vocal protocols to each client in order to promote the use of treatment exercises and target behaviors in the client's habitual speech pattern. See Yiu et al. (2017), Desjardins et al. (2017), and Verdolini Abbott (2008) for more information on this technique.

Flow Phonation. This treatment method focuses on airflow management as a means of retraining a natural airflow for speech. Clients who have developed maladaptive breathing and/or muscle contraction patterns during speech benefit from flow phonation techniques. Vocal stretching is one of the main components used to retrain natural phonation. The client works from controlled exhalations to adding in voicing to his or her phonation until airflow for speech sounds can be sustained and produced in a balanced manner. See Gartner-Schmidt (2006) for more information on this technique.

Manual Circumlaryngeal Techniques. In this approach, the SLP uses his or her hand to massage and/or to reposture the larynx. Several maneuvers can be used to return the larynx to a more neutral position. The client is directed to phonate when the larynx is in a more neutral position to promote developing awareness of correct vocal positioning and target vocal production behaviors. This approach is used primarily with clients who have muscular tension or organic lesions that have resulted in maladaptive vocal habits. See Gartner-Schmidt (2006) for more information on this technique.

Confidential Voice. This technique focuses on laryngeal muscle relaxation in an effort to reduce vocal fold tension. The client begins by producing a breathy voice quality and builds to normal phonation without decreasing airflow. See Casper (2000) for more information on this technique.

Cough Suppression. In cases of refractory chronic cough, an SLP can provide education as well as treatment to patients to reduce cough frequency. Treatment typically focuses on vocal hygiene and techniques to minimize the cough reflux (e.g., cough suppression swallow and breathing patterns). This approach is nonpharmacological and typically requires only a few sessions of treatment to educate the patient for home practice and implementation of methods. See Ryan et al. (2010) for more information on this technique.

Vocal Hypofunction

This category refers to voice disorders characterized by incomplete closure of the vocal folds. It involves dysphonias resulting from neurologic disorders such as unilateral vocal fold paralysis, myasthenia gravis, and muscular dystrophy. The techniques described next are useful in treating symptoms associated with laryngeal hypofunction (Boone et al., 2019; Schneider, 2019). The main purposes of these techniques are to achieve firmer closure of the vocal folds and/or compensatory movements (e.g., one fold moves across the midline to compensate for the other in unilateral paralysis).

Pushing/Pulling. The client engages in forceful muscular activity that elicits reflexive glottal closure (Froeschels et al., 1955). These activities should be used for short periods of time and discontinued as soon as the client demonstrates an awareness of the "feel" of tighter vocal fold closure. Care must be taken to ensure that an overly hyperfunctional behavior does not occur. In one method, the client sits in in a chair, firmly grasps each side of the seat, and pushes downward with both arms while producing a vowel such as /a/. A variation of this activity requires the client to raise both fists to the level of the chest with the elbows extended outward. The client then pushes both fists downward forcefully while producing a vowel sound as loudly as possible. A third method requires the client to link the fingers of both hands together at the level of the chest and to pull in opposite directions while producing a vowel such as /a/. Length of phonation should be gradually increased while maintaining the improved loudness and voice quality.

Vocal Function Exercises (VFEs). VFEs address the interplay between the four subsystems involved in voice production. This approach utilizes a variety of exercises (i.e., warm-up, stretching, contracting, and power). Phonation time goals are set on an individual basis. See Angadi et al. (2019) and Bane et al. (2019) for more information on this approach.

Increasing Loudness. In some cases, loudness can be improved by establishing a more efficient respiratory pattern (i.e., abdominal-diaphragmatic breathing). The client lies supine and places one hand on the chest and the other on the abdomen. The client inhales through the nose and closely monitors movement of the abdomen (not the chest) while exhaling through the mouth. During subsequent respiratory cycles, the client deliberately relaxes the abdominal muscles during inhalation and tenses the same muscles during exhalation. Once this respiratory pattern has been established, the client begins to produce prolonged vowels on exhalation at an increased level of loudness. Progress occurs from vowels to syllables to words to phrases to sentences. Vocal loudness also can be addressed through the use of the pushing/pulling techniques described in the previous section. In 2017, Darling-White and Huber reported on the impact of expiratory muscle strength training (EMST) in patients with Parkinson's disease. This technique directly targets the respiratory subsystem rather than voice production. Results showed improved airflow measurements of speech breathing patterns, although improvements in utterance length and vocal loudness were not observed.

A programmed approach to remediating reduced vocal loudness in clients with Parkinson's disease is the **Lee Silverman Voice Treatment** (Bryans et al., 2021; Ramig, 1998; Ramig et al., 1995). This approach utilizes high-phonatory-effort tasks to increase vocal fold adduction and respiratory support. The goal of this program is to improve functional speech intelligibility to a realistic level. A minimum of 16 intensive individual sessions within a 4-week period is required regardless of a client's severity of impairment. The program also provides specific guidelines for posttreatment maintenance and reevaluation.

Paradoxical Vocal Fold Dysfunction

There are several theories as to the etiology of paradoxical vocal fold dysfunction—a disorder characterized by aberrant adducting movements of the vocal folds during inhalation and/or exhalation. Possible etiologies include psychological disorders, neurologic factors, possible laryngeal dystonia, and irritation of the laryngeal tract (Mathers-Schmidt, 2001). Patients with paradoxical vocal fold dysfunction often present with asthmalike symptoms such as stridor, dyspnea, and feelings of tightness in the chest or larynx. The SLP serves as part of a team along with other domains, such as psychologists and otolaryngologists, in order to differentially diagnosis this disorder and to determine contributing factors in order to inform the rehabilitation process.

Respiratory Retraining. These techniques are used with clients with paradoxical vocal fold movement disorders. In 2020, van de Wetering-van Dongen et al. reported positive effects for several strategies including inspiratory/expiratory muscle training and "air-stacking" (breathing in slowly, stacking one breath on top of others as tolerance allows, holding breath briefly, then slowly exhaling). In an earlier article, Gartner-Schmidt (2006) recommended making respiration the main focus of therapy, with breathing rhythm used to help retrain clients with a natural breathing pattern to support phonation and speech. Clients perform breathing exercises that require inhalation of air through the nose, passage through a relaxed oral cavity, and then exhalation through a slightly tense labial posture (e.g., the articulatory placement for /s/).

Psychogenic

This category involves voice disorders that arise from psychological or emotional factors. Symptoms associated with psychogenic voice disorders range from mild dysphonia to complete loss of voice and can involve pitch, loudness, or voice quality (Tezcaner et al., 2019). The overall purpose of treatment is to reestablish a client's access to his or her own normal voice. This purpose is generally achieved through three sequential stages of intervention (Aronson & Bless, 2009), as discussed in the following sections.

1. Client Education. The clinician discusses available medical reports with the client and emphasizes that the client's laryngeal anatomy and physiology are intact and, more important, that the client is capable of producing a normal voice.

2. Symptomatic Therapy. The clinician attempts to elicit normal phonation through vegetative vocal functions. The client produces a variety of these sounds (i.e., coughing, throat clearing, laughing, gargling, humming). When normal phonation occurs during one of the vegetative behaviors, it should be brought to the client's attention immediately. The client then extends this normal voice into vowels, single words, and sentences. For clients with mutational falsetto, inhalation phonation (as described in the section on vocal hyperfunction) also may be an effective technique for eliciting normal phonation.

3. Referral. The clinician considers the possibility that voice intervention alone is insufficient to resolve a client's underlying emotional problems and may counsel the client to seek psychological or psychiatric services as needed.

Spasmodic Dysphonia

Sanuki (2022) and Rumbach et al. (2022) provide overviews of treatment options for spasmodic dysphonia. This category encompasses two distinct types of voice disorders characterized by spasms that result in abnormalities of vocal fold approximation. Adductor spasmodic dysphonia has been treated with a variety of surgical and medical interventions. In general, the surgical approach focuses on removal of a small segment (resection) of the recurrent laryngeal nerve to improve vocal fold function (Ryan et al., 2022). More recently, injection of **botulinum toxin (Botox)** into the vocal folds has become the treatment of choice for this type of dysphonia (Faham et al., 2021; Hyodo et al., 2021; Meyer et al., 2021). Botox injections are also used to treat the abductor type of SD, although with somewhat less effectiveness. Spasmodic dysphonias are also treated with symptomatic voice techniques, although voice therapy alone usually does not result in significantly improved voice production. These techniques are similar to those employed for treating laryngeal hyperfunction/hypofunction and are generally used on a trial basis before and after medical intervention. The overall goal of symptomatic voice therapy is to help the client achieve the best possible voice, with the recognition that normal voice quality may never be regained.

Premedical Therapy Techniques. Techniques aimed at reducing laryngeal muscle tension are employed, including chewing, chant talk, yawn-sigh, and easy onset. (See the section on vocal hyperfunction for a description of these techniques.)

Postmedical Therapy Techniques. Techniques aimed at decreasing breathiness, increasing loudness, and establishing a new pitch are employed, including pushing/pulling and abdominal-diaphragmatic breathing. (See the section on vocal hypofunction for a description of these techniques.)

Transgender Voice

Transgender is a broad term that describes individuals whose gender, gender identity, or gender expression is different from that assigned at birth. This difference may lead to marked and lasting incongruence between their sense of self and other people's perceptions of them. Transmasculine is a term that refers to a person who was assigned female at birth but has a male gender identity (Myers & Bell, 2020), while transfeminine refers to a person who identifies more closely with characteristics typically identified as female (Houle et al., 2022). Intervention with transgender clients is a complex and continually evolving topic. Often, SLP training programs do not provide future clinicians with adequate preparation for clinical work in this area. Therefore, it is the SLPs' responsibility to educate themselves regarding the philosophical, technical, and counseling aspects of treatment in this area. A good place to start is the World Professional Association for Transgender Health (WPATH, 2016), which provides ethical guidelines and standards of care for professionals working with transgender individuals (Davies et al., 2015).

The goal of treatment is to help the client identify and implement an effective speaking voice/style that is congruent with their gender identity. The broad goal encompasses a wide range of speech-language and communication areas:

- Vocal pitch
- Vocal resonance

- Vocal intonation

- Articulation

- Language usage

- Nonverbal communication (includes posture and body language)

The roles of SLPs working with transgender clients include a range of clinical responsibilities:

- Educating the client about the scope of treatment (see previous list) and the limitations of treatment

- Providing information about prevention of voice fatigue, strain, and potential vocal fold damage

- Teaching the client to observe/analyze their own communication style as well as other people

- Working directly with the client to modify six parameters of behavior as listed previously

- Providing a safe and supportive environment for the client to discuss emotions and concerns about using their target voice in the real world

Several aspects of voice production are generally considered to differ between males and females. Specifically, fundamental frequency range (particularly maximal fundamental frequency), average fundamental frequency, formant frequencies, and average intensity are considered important to listeners' perceptions of gender. Clients who have undergone transgender procedures have several options for altering their voice, if desired. Voice therapy can target alteration of pitch and/or register to more closely approximate the vocal attributes of the new gender. Biofeedback instruments can be beneficial in assisting clients to achieve a targeted pitch and register. Phonosurgical procedures also are available to alter the structural and mechanical components of the vocal tract. See the following sources for more information on vocal behaviors in this population: Fairchild and Stronach (2018), Davies (2017), Hirsch (2017), and Nolan et al. (2019).

The specific content of therapy sessions should be tailored to each client's needs and priorities. Best practices incorporate the following:

- Patient education about voice production and communication issues (e.g., explanation/demonstration of vocal fold anatomy and physiology)

- Vocal fold exercises for awareness

- Specific voice techniques for pitch, resonance, and intonation

- Consideration of other communication variables that affect perception of gender such as word choice, phrase structure and pausing, pragmatics, and nonverbal communication

Example Profiles

The following three profiles represent typical dysphonias of children and adults with different types of voice disorders. These examples have been designed to illustrate the selection of intervention targets as well as specific therapy activities and materials. Most of the chosen activities are easily implemented in either individual or group therapy settings.

PROFILE 1: CHILD—8-YEAR-OLD

Brian, an 8-year-old male, presents with a hoarse, low-pitched voice. Otolaryngological findings reveal prominent bilateral vocal nodules approximately 2 mm in size. Both vocal folds are swollen and irritated. Case history information obtained from his parents indicates that Brian is an extremely active child whose play activities are frequently accompanied by shouting and screaming. According to his mom, "Brian talks incessantly, from the moment he wakes up until it's time for bed." She also reported that Brian likes to make "sound effects," including car noises and monster voices. Brian shows no awareness of the dysphonic nature of his voice. Both Brian's parents and his classroom teacher noted that his voice quality deteriorates as the day progresses.

Selection of Therapy Targets. The overall communicative profile demonstrated by Brian is consistent with a dysphonia caused by vocal abuse/misuse. Based on his age and the pattern of hyperfunctional vocal behaviors, therapy will focus on the following areas: (a) identification of vocally abusive situations, (b) establishment of the target voice, and (c) elimination of the abusive behaviors. Most children with voice disorders do not recognize that a problem exists. Therefore, an important aspect of this approach is to facilitate an awareness in Brian, his parents, and his teacher of what constitutes abusive vocal behaviors as well as the situations in which these behaviors most frequently occur.

Sample Activities

Identify Situations Associated With Vocal Abuse

1. Observe Brian in home, play, and school settings for specified units of time (e.g., 15 min, recess period, and so on) to identify instances of hyperfunctional vocal behavior. Use this information to establish baselines regarding the type, context, and frequency of vocal abuse/misuse. These observations should be conducted on at least three occasions to ensure gathering of a representative sample of Brian's communicative behavior. Interviews with family members and others also can yield useful information regarding Brian's habitual vocal patterns. Develop a list of his most common types of vocal abuse/misuse and the situations in which they most frequently occur. Review this list with Brian and discuss how these behaviors have bothered his voice.

Establishing the Target Voice

2. Help Brian generate a list of 25 of his "likes" and "dislikes." Likes might include soccer, computer games, ping-pong, and playing with his best friend, Ian. Dislikes might include homework, broccoli, brushing his teeth, going shopping, and cleaning his room. Gather pictures or photographs depicting each item and tack the positive and negative items to separate walls. Model an excessively loud voice and a more desirable quiet voice until Brian can easily imitate each pattern. Explain to Brian that he will talk about the pictured items, alternately using his old loud voice and the new quieter voice. Instruct Brian to select one picture from the negative set and produce it along with the carrier phrase, "I don't like_____," using his old voice pattern. Then ask him to choose an item from the positive group and say the carrier phrase, "I do like_____," using the target voice. Encourage Brian

to pay attention to the differences in how these voices sound and feel. Continue to compare and contrast the desirable and undesirable loudness levels by repeating this alternating sequence until all items have been named.

Elimination of Abusive Vocal Behaviors

3. Provide Brian with a tally card or a simple behavioral response counter. Instruct Brian to record each time he catches himself yelling during a given time period. The clinician should specify time periods in which there will likely be at least 10 instances of the abusive behavior (e.g., recess). Have Brian tally the number of recorded behaviors at the end of each day and plot the number on a simple graph like the one shown in Form 10–1. As Brian's ability to accurately identify instances of vocal abuses improves, the specified time frame for self-monitoring can be progressively increased.

Form 10–1. VOCAL ABUSE CHART

Client's Name: _____ Setting: _____

PROFILE 2: ADULT—48-YEAR-OLD

Mr. Abdul, a 48-year-old professor of political science, reports a 2-year history of hoarseness and throat pain associated with teaching. He states that these symptoms are more severe during summer school because lecture periods are substantially longer than during the fall and spring semesters. A video of a typical lecture indicates that Mr. Abdul's speaking style in the classroom can be described as loud, forceful, and low pitched. In addition, Mr. Abdul is a member of a local repertory theater company and frequently performs in plays and musicals. A recent laryngoscopic examination reveals the presence of bilateral contact ulcers.

Selection of Therapy Targets. The aspects of voice production to be targeted are inappropriately low pitch, abrupt initiation of phonation, and excessive loudness. These features were selected because they constitute the primary symptoms of laryngeal hyperfunction in Mr. Abdul's profile.

Sample Activities

Adjusting Voice Pitch

1. Determine the client's optimal pitch through the procedure described in the section on treatment techniques for vocal hyperfunction. Devise a list of 25 sentences for a cloze task. Examples include the following:

> I'm going to the store and I'm going to buy some _____.
>
> I'm going on a trip and I'm packing _____.
>
> I'm going on a picnic and I'm taking _____.
>
> My favorite chili is made with _____.
>
> On our last vacation, we visited _____.
>
> If I win the lottery, I would buy _____.
>
> I'm sending a birthday card to _____.
>
> My favorite baseball player is _____.
>
> Last night for dinner I had _____.
>
> This old car needs new _____.

Explain that the clinician will read each sentence and present a cue or prompt (e.g., pitch pipe, piano note) representing the client's optimum pitch. Then the client completes the statement with a single word using the targeted pitch level. The difficulty level of this task can be increased by requiring the client to answer with a series of items rather than a single word.

Softening Glottal Attacks

2. The clinician models a soft glottal attack by yawning and producing single words that begin with /h/ or a vowel during the exhalation. Once the client can easily imitate this relaxed initiation of phonation, utterances can be progressively lengthened and may include initial phonemes other than /h/.

Explain to the client that the game of 20 Questions will be used to practice the yawn-sigh approach to phonation at the carrier-phrase level. Instruct the client to think of a person, place, or thing. The clinician then asks yes/no questions to determine the correct answer. Emphasize that the client should employ the yawn-sigh approach at the beginning of each response to the clinician's queries. For example:

Clinician: Are you thinking of a person?

Client: Yes, I'm thinking of a person.

Clinician: Is the person a female?

Client: No, the person is not a female.

Clinician: Is the person alive?

Client: Yes, the person is alive.

Task difficulty can be increased by reversing roles and instructing the client to spontaneously formulate the questions.

Reducing Loudness

3. Identify the optimal loudness level for the client as described in the section on vocal hyperfunction. Select listlike reading materials that can be easily divided into segments corresponding to single breath groups (e.g., directions to a destination such as a restaurant or movie theater, a recipe, instructions for assembling or operating a DVD player, and so on). Write each topic on an index card or sheet of paper and clearly delineate the utterance to be produced on each exhalation. Sample formats may include the following:

Directions
Turn left at the second traffic light./Pass the gas station on the right./Go two blocks and make your first left./The restaurant will be on your right.

Recipe
1) Combine flour and sugar in a bowl.
2) Add melted butter and one egg.
3) Mix thoroughly until batter is stiff.
4) Drop by the spoonful onto a cookie sheet.
5) Bake at 350° for 20 min.

Model reading each utterance aloud on a single exhalation. Instruct the client to imitate each production using the optimal loudness level identified previously.

PROFILE 3: VOCAL FOLD PARALYSIS—39-YEAR-OLD

Mrs. Simon, a 39-year-old female, was diagnosed with right unilateral adductor vocal fold paralysis 2 months ago. She sustained damage to the vagus nerve as a result of intubation during surgery. Mrs. Simon presents with an extremely quiet, weak, and breathy voice. Also evident are a hoarse vocal quality and low pitch with occasional pitch breaks. Decisions regarding surgical interventions such as phonosurgery are deferred for 6 months to allow for any spontaneous recovery of laryngeal function.

Selection of Therapy Targets. The vocal symptoms to be targeted are breathy, hoarse voice quality and reduced loudness level. These areas were chosen because they represent the primary characteristics of laryngeal hypofunction in Mrs. Simon's profile.

Sample Activities

Pushing/Pulling

1. Instruct the client to use one of the pushing/pulling techniques described in the section on laryngeal hypofunction to achieve firmer vocal fold approximation during phonation. Once closure has been achieved, emphasize the importance of an easy, relaxed pattern. Begin with prolongation of single vowels and progress hierarchically to the level of connected speech. At the connected speech level, the clinician poses simple questions, and the client responds while employing the pushing/pulling technique. Sample questions include the following:

   Where do you live?

   How long have you lived there?

   Do you have any brothers or sisters?

   What are their names?

   When is your birthday?

   Where do you work?

   What was your first job?

   What has been your favorite vacation?

   What did you do last weekend?

   What kind of car do you drive?

   What kind of car would you like to drive?

   What are your hobbies?

   What is your favorite movie?

   What do you like most about your job?

   What is your favorite holiday?

Increasing Loudness

2. Instruct the client to use the abdominal-diaphragmatic breathing pattern with phonation, as discussed in the section on vocal hypofunction, to achieve increased loudness. Stimuli may begin at the level of isolated vowels and advance systematically to the discourse level. At the discourse level, the clinician creates several written dialogues and provides two copies of each scenario. Assign the client one of the roles. Instruct her to place one hand on her abdomen to monitor the use of the target breathing pattern while reading her lines in the script. Following are sample scripts; additional dialogues can be found in Appendix 10–A on the companion website.

Calling Information

Operator: Hello. What city please?

Caller: College Park.

O: Yes?

C: I'd like the number for the post office on Route 1.

O: Thank you. That number is 800-555-2200.

Ordering a Pizza

Operator: Thank you for calling the pizzeria. Can you hold please?

Caller: Yes.

O: Thanks for holding. Can I take your order?

C: Yes, I'd like a large pepperoni pizza with extra cheese.

O: Any sodas with that?

C: I'll take two large sodas.

O: What's your address?

C: 1600 Pennsylvania Avenue.

O: And the phone number?

C: 203-4000.

O: OK. We'll be there in 30 minutes or less.

C: What's the total?

O: $14.50.

C: Thanks.

Helpful Hints

1. Clinicians may consider using speech-generating devices (e.g., tablet) for clients who cannot consistently generate sufficient voice production.

2. Clients with voice disorders that result from psychogenic factors, such as conversion dysphonias, may regain a completely normal voice within a single session.

3. Puppets can be very useful in negative practice activities for children who demonstrate dysphonias related to hyperfunction. For example, large or ugly puppets can adopt the abusive vocal pattern, while small or attractive puppets speak in the target voice.

4. With respect to the treatment of conversion disorders, the clinician must recognize that, although the voice is not actually lost, the loss of voice control is very real to the client.

5. Relatively loud masking or ambient noise can be useful for increasing loudness in some clients with weak, ineffective voices.

6. Irritating substances such as tobacco or alcohol can exacerbate the symptoms of an existing dysphonia.

7. Clinicians should be able to translate anatomical, physiological, and medical terminology used by other professionals (e.g., otolaryngologists) into clear and understandable explanations of a client's voice disorder.

8. Some aspects of voice production are difficult to explain verbally; use of visual imagery (such as a Nasometer II from PENTAX Medical Corporation) or computer display often helps clients grasp these concepts in a more concrete manner.

9. Despite the effectiveness of Botox injections, a client with long-standing spasmodic dysphonia may persist in the tendency to "push out" his or her voice. This type of individual may benefit from direct counseling/education to realize that his or her habit of effortful phonation is now unnecessary.

10. Therapy techniques that involve massage or other tactile stimulation may be inappropriate for clients who are hypersensitive or resistant to touch.

11. One strategy for promoting a positive therapeutic alliance with a transgender client is to actively seek their input on issues such as preferred pronoun usage and vocabulary.

Alaryngeal Speech

Alaryngeal speech refers to voice that emanates from a sound source other than the larynx. The surgical procedure known as **total laryngectomy** involves complete removal of the larynx due to malignant tumor or severe trauma. During total laryngectomy surgery, the larynx and its intrinsic muscles as well as the hyoid bone are removed. The trachea is then surgically attached to an opening (stoma) created in the neck just above the notch of the sternum. As a result, air from the lungs can no longer enter the vocal tract, and the voicing source has been removed, making normal phonation impossible. In addition to surgery, some individuals with laryngeal cancer may receive prior postoperative radiation and/or chemotherapy. Although concurrent chemoradiation is the widely used approach, a similar surgical approach is starting to gain attention. Near-total laryngectomy is a surgical procedure that preserves the voice by removing only certain parts of the laryngeal structures. Because only portions of the larynx are removed, near-total laryngectomy is only appropriate in patients with cancer localized to specific areas (D'Cruz et al., 2012).

A preoperative visit by the SLP plays an important role. The clinician can clearly explain the consequences of the surgical procedure on voice production and describe various methods of alaryngeal speech production. The visit also provides an ideal opportunity for assessment of the individual's habitual speaking patterns prior to surgery. Prater et al. (1999) suggest that the following factors be noted during the preoperative visit: (a) articulatory proficiency, (b) conversational speech rate, (c) dialectal patterns, and (d) degree of mouth opening used in conversation. Client and family counseling forms a major part of this preoperative visit and continues throughout the therapeutic process. Overall personal adjustment can facilitate successful long-term rehabilitation efforts (Schuster et al., 2003). The goal of therapy for individuals with laryngectomies is to establish an alternative mode of sound production that can be used for communication. Many factors may affect the prognosis for successful intervention:

- Extent of surgery (especially if significant portions of the tongue are also removed)

- Presence of significant hearing impairment (greatly reduces an individual's ability to acquire alaryngeal speech)

- Presence of excessive esophageal muscle tone

- Lengthy course of concurrent radiation treatment (may produce side effects that interfere with easy acquisition of alaryngeal speech)

- Limitations in cognitive, linguistic, or emotional status (may negatively affect an individual's ability to learn alaryngeal speech)

Treatment for Alaryngeal Clients

The search for an alternative method of sound production subsequent to laryngectomy is based on three general sources: external mechanical devices, functional use of the sphincterlike tissue at the junction of the **pharynx and esophagus (PE segment)** to produce esophageal speech, or the use of a prosthetic voice device inserted into a surgically created opening. The clinician should consult with the physician prior to and after surgery regarding the most appropriate form of alaryngeal speech for a given individual.

Mechanical Devices

Pneumatic Aids

These devices consist of a plastic housing that is held over the stoma connected to a small unit with a reed and a tube that is placed in the mouth. Air exhaled from the lungs through the stoma vibrates the reed, and the sound is carried to the oral cavity through the tubing. The speaker articulates this sound to produce speech.

Electronic Aids

Several types of electronic artificial larynges provide a battery-powered sound source, including the following: (Madhushankara et al., 2023; Rameau, 2020; Řepová et al., 2021):

- *Neck devices:* A handheld sound source (e.g., an electrolarynx) is placed against the neck. Sound is transmitted through the skin into the vocal tract. The clinician locates the most supple area on the client's neck and the aid is placed there, with the head of the aid in full contact with the skin. Typically, the best location is approximately 1 to 2 in. below the mandible near the midline of the neck. The client is instructed to hold the electrolarynx in his nondominant hand and turn it on while simultaneously shaping monosyllabic words containing bilabial consonants as clearly as possible. The client should be cautioned against the instinct to forcefully exhale, because this results in stoma noise that distracts the listener. As longer utterances are produced, the client must learn to turn the electrolarynx off during natural speech pauses and coordinate initiation of articulatory movement with finger movement for the "on" switch. The intelligibility of speech produced with an electrolarynx is greatly enhanced by the use of precise articulatory movements and reduced speaking rate. The feasibility of a hands-free electrolarynx is currently being explored. For example, one possible hands-free model utilizes oral movements, such as lingual movements, to active denture-based switches (Wan et al., 2012).

- *Oral devices:* These devices are similar to the pneumatic aid described previously, except the sound source is battery driven rather than arising from air exhaled through the stoma. Tubing should be placed in a corner of the mouth and angled up toward the hard palate to ensure that it is not occluded by the tongue or cheek. The client learns to articulate the sound carried to the oral cavity by the tubing. This type of aid is often used immediately after surgery because it does not interfere with sutures or swollen tissues. As with the neck version, training in the use of this device generally begins with monosyllabic words that contain bilabial consonants.

There are some disadvantages to the use of artificial larynges. The quality of the sound source is often judged as "unnatural," and these devices severely restrict the individual's ability to vary the pitch and loudness of his or her speech. However, there are also many positive aspects to the use of an artificial larynx. The device can be demonstrated prior to surgery and can be employed in the immediate postoperative period. The device also provides a means of communication that can be learned rapidly by most clients. Some laryngectomees will continue to use an electrolarynx as the primary method of communication; others will employ it as a temporary alternative until they master other forms of alaryngeal communication.

Esophageal Speech

This method of communication consists of using air passing through a narrow constriction in the esophagus as an alternative source of sound for speech (Doyle & Damrose, 2022; Graham, 2005). The quality of sound produced is perceived as more natural than that generated by an electrolarynx. The client's ability to rapidly intake and expel air from the esophagus and perform precise articulatory movements is the most critical aspect of effective esophageal speech. According to Casper and Colton (1998), at least one-third of laryngectomees will be unable to produce esophageal speech that is intelligible for daily communication purposes. Esophageal speech production operates on the principle that air of greater pressure in one location (mouth) will flow to a location of lesser pressure (esophagus) if the locations are connected (PE segment). The six main goals of intervention with esophageal speech as originally identified by Aronson in 1980 remain unchanged (Prater et al., 1999):

1. Easily and rapidly phonate on demand.
2. Use a rapid method of air intake.
3. Keep a short latency period between air intake and phonation.
4. Produce four to nine syllables per air charge.
5. Speak at a rate of 85 to 129 words per minute.
6. Speak with adequate intelligibility.

The basic sequence of training for esophageal speech includes the following steps:

Step 1: Establishing esophageal voice

Step 2: Gaining and maintaining control over production

Step 3: Increasing intelligibility of esophageal speech

Step 4: Increasing length of utterance production

Step 5: Mastering conversational nuances of pitch, loudness, and stress patterns

Esophageal speech training should begin as soon as possible after the client's discharge from the hospital. One rule of thumb states that an individual is ready to start learning esophageal speech when he or she can tolerate oral ingestion of food. A moderate pace of therapy is recommended. Some authors recommend incorporating highly proficient esophageal speakers into therapy programming to demonstrate techniques and provide performance feedback (Doyle & Finchmen, 2019). Verbal functionality of voice produced via esophageal/tracheoesophageal methods exerts an impact on the speaker's self-perceptions regarding quality of life (Allegra et al., 2019). Although many clients are extremely eager to master this procedure, therapy that proceeds too rapidly may result in unintelligible, forced speech with excessive stoma noise. (Table 10–3 provides basic guidelines for home practice of esophageal speech techniques.)

There are four main techniques for obtaining an esophageal air supply. From most to least efficient, they are consonant-injection, glossopharyngeal press, inhalation, and swallowing. Therefore, it is generally recommended that the clinician begin with the consonant-injection method. If the client is unsuccessful, proceed sequentially through the other methods until the client can consistently initiate phonation. At that point, the clinician may want to retry one of the more efficient methods.

Consonant-Injection Method

This method uses the intraoral air pressure that normally builds during production of high-pressure consonants, such as stops and fricatives, to inflate the esophagus. It has been described as the most efficient technique of esophageal air intake because air can be injected *simultaneously* with the production of a consonant rather than only during a pause or phrase interval. This results in minimal or no interruption in communication, unlike the other three methods.

Step 1: Client forces air into the esophagus by producing a whispered plosive bilabial consonant, such as /p/, repetitively four to five times. This repeated compression of air in the oral cavity should force some air into the esophagus.

Step 2: Client expels the air from the esophagus and attempts to phonate /pə/.

Step 3: Gradually introduce other voiceless plosives, fricatives, and affricates paired with /ə/ at the syllable level.

Step 4: Introduce monosyllabic words containing high-pressure consonants such as *pay, tap, toy, skate, stop, scotch.*

Step 5: Extend phonation to phrases that contain a preponderance of both voiced and voiceless high-pressure consonants such as "make it dark," "stop that cab," "cut the cake," and "take that skate."

Table 10–3
Homework Guidelines for Esophageal Speakers

1. Have reasonable expectations, especially during the initial period of treatment. It takes time to establish effective patterns of muscle control over esophageal speech production.
2. Practice for short, consistent periods (e.g., 10 min per hour) rather than for lengthy periods of time.
3. Exaggerated breathing patterns (either on inhalation or exhalation) do not make esophageal speech clearer or easier to understand.
4. Use of excessive muscular force does not make esophageal speech more intelligible; it only wears you out.

For some clients, this method may be less effective with stimulus items that consist mainly of vowels and low-pressure consonants. The relatively open-mouth articulatory configurations of these sounds may not allow the buildup of sufficient air pressure to insufflate the esophagus.

Glossopharyngeal Press Method

This method achieves esophageal air intake through tongue movements and is a useful alternative to consonant-injection for utterances loaded with low-pressure phonemes.

Step 1: Client closes lips and anchors the tongue tip against the alveolar ridge.

Step 2: The posterior portion of the tongue is moved backward along the hard and soft palates to pump air into the esophagus.

Step 3: The client expels air from esophagus and attempts to phonate vowels or mono-syllables. Extend length of utterance as the client's mastery of voluntary phonation improves.

Remind the client to refrain from actually completing a swallow when employing this technique.

Inhalation Method

In this method, air is supplied to the esophagus through relaxation of the PE segment during pulmonary inhalation. The expansion and contraction of chest muscles are used to direct air into the esophagus.

Step 1: The client inhales rapidly through the nose or covers the stoma midway through a quick inhalation.

Step 2: The client immediately expels the air and attempts production of /a/.

Step 3: Consonant-vowel (CV) syllables that contain stops are gradually introduced and content progresses to monosyllabic words.

Swallow Method

This method utilizes a controlled swallowing pattern to inject air into the esophagus. It is based on the fact that the PE segment tends to open spontaneously during a swallow because air is forced backward by the posterior movement of the tongue. This is the least efficient method of air injection and should be used only as a last resort. Primary disadvantages include (a) the extended latency between initiation of a swallow and the production of phonation; (b) the accumulation of air in the stomach as a result of repeated attempts at rapid swallowing; and (c) the inability to produce rapid, repetitive dry swallows as required for speech.

Step 1: The client swallows in a normal fashion by moving the tongue backward toward the pharynx.

Step 2: The client releases air and attempts to produce a CV syllable with an alveolar stop consonant such as "ta" and "da."

Tracheoesophageal (TEP) Speech

This method is an alternative to esophageal speech (Blom et al., 1998). A small device made of silicone is inserted into a surgically created opening between the trachea and esophagus to allow air from the lungs to reach the PE segment. This procedure can be performed during the primary laryngectomy surgery or at a later date. This technique, called **tracheoesophageal puncture (TEP)**, may be the quickest way for a client to regain near-normal speech after the larynx has been removed. Compared to users of artificial larynges, TE speakers report more positive long-term outcomes with regard to their communication abilities and their overall sense of well-being (Allegra et al., 2019). Patient selection for this procedure is often made by the surgeon. However, the clinician should be aware of some guidelines that are relevant to the selection of candidates for TEP. First, the client's overall health should be stable in all areas other than the laryngectomy. For example, an individual with poor respiratory function due to emphysema might not be able to generate enough pressure to move pulmonary air through the prosthesis to the PE segment.

Second, the client should possess the manual dexterity and cognitive skills required to use and care for the prosthesis on a daily basis. Ideally, the clinician should be involved in evaluating the suitability of a client for the TEP procedure; sizing the prosthesis; and training the client to insert, remove, and clean the prosthesis.

Once the fistula (punctured area) has healed sufficiently and the prosthesis has been inserted, the clinician may begin intervention according to this basic sequence of steps:

Step 1: Ask the client to inhale and then phonate on exhalation while the clinician uses a finger to occlude the stoma. It is important that the stoma be covered completely but with gentle pressure.

Step 2: The client digitally occludes the stoma during exhalation and attempts to phonate sustained sounds or words. Utterances should become longer and more effortless at a fairly rapid rate. (*Note:* Use of a tracheostoma valve can eliminate the need for manual occlusion of the stoma during speech production.)

For more information regarding this topic, consult the document published by the American Speech-Language-Hearing Association titled Communication After Total Laryngectomy.

Example Profile

The following profile illustrates characteristics typical of individuals who have undergone surgical removal of the larynx. Unlike other profiles throughout the book, the activities presented in this section are designed to illustrate a progression of intervention strategies that would be implemented over time with a single individual.

PROFILE 4: LARYNGECTOMY—62-YEAR-OLD

Mr. Evans, a 62-year-old male, underwent a total laryngectomy 3 months ago as a result of squamous cell carcinoma. Sutures have been removed, and he is currently able to take food by mouth. He received a postsurgical regimen of radiation treatment for 8 weeks. Currently, Mr. Evans communicates with an electrolarynx and by writing.

> **Selection of Therapy Targets.** The targets selected based on this profile illustrate the typical progression of esophageal speech programming and include (a) establishing phonation, (b) increasing duration of phonation, and (c) refining vocal pitch and intensity. One activity will address each of the target areas.

Sample Activities

Consonant-Injection Method

1. Instruct the client in the consonant-injection method of esophageal sound production as described in the section on esophageal speech. Once Mr. Evans can produce /pə/ rapidly in 10 consecutive trials, introduce CV syllables containing other voiceless plosives, fricatives, and affricates and then progress to monosyllabic words containing high-pressure consonants. Example stimuli include the following:

CV Syllables	CVC Words
/tə/	cup
/tɔ/	tub
/ti/	pat
/to/	cut
/kæ/	bag
/kɛ/	cheese
/ki/	church
/kʊ/	bit
/sə/	punch
/so/	cash
/sʊ/	bed
/si/	cat
/tʃʌ/	day
/tʃo/	date
/tʃə/	ghost

Increasing Duration of Phonation

2. Once esophageal speech has been reliably established at the level of monosyllabic CVC words, focus on increasing the duration of phonation. Write a list of three- to five-word phrases that are loaded with voiced and voiceless high-pressure consonants. Instruct the client to read these longer stimuli aloud while maintaining a consistent pattern of phonation. Sample stimuli include the following:

    Stop that cab
    Get the cup
    Buy the boot
    Touch the cat

Pull the tag

Call the cop

Go to bed

The time of day

Put it in the bank

A day at the beach

Teach the kids

Shut the door

Make it good

Coach the team

Get in the tub

Put on the cap

A lot of cash

Cash in the chips

Cut the tape

As the client progresses, the difficulty of this task can be increased. Write each phrase on separate index cards, shuffle the cards, and place the deck face down on the table. The client draws the top card from the pile without exposing its contents, reads it aloud, and the clinician attempts to imitate it. Emphasize that the clinician will be relying solely on the intelligibility of the client's esophageal speech to identify the entire phrase.

Refining Pitch and Intensity

3. The next phase of therapy focuses on refining communicative effectiveness by improving the client's ability to manipulate the pitch and loudness characteristics of esophageal speech (to the extent possible). Develop 10 groups of three-sentence sets. Each set should contain declarative, interrogative, and tag question versions of the same sentence (three to five words in length). Write each set on a single index card. Instruct the client to select a card and read each of the three sentences aloud using the appropriate alterations of pitch and increased loudness on the second and third versions. Encourage the client to try a variety of different head postures, which may facilitate increased pitch and loudness (e.g., slight head turning, chin lowering, head and chin extension). Examples include the following:

They know she's gone. They know she's gone?

They know she's gone, don't they?

There's no hot water.

There's no hot water?

There's no hot water, is there?

The office opens at 9 a.m.

The office opens at 9 a.m.?

The office opens at 9 a.m., doesn't it?

Mr. Smith is her dentist.

Mr. Smith is her dentist?

Mr. Smith is her dentist, isn't he?

They're going to the mall.

They're going to the mall?

They're going to the mall, aren't they?

The weather has improved.

The weather has improved?

The weather has improved, hasn't it?

It won't work for me.

It won't work for me?

It won't work for me, will it?

They shoot horses.

They shoot horses?

They shoot horses, don't they?

The budget was vetoed.

The budget was vetoed?

The budget was vetoed, wasn't it?

This is delicious soup.

This is delicious soup?

This is delicious soup, isn't it?

Helpful Hints

1. It is important for the client to avoid the use of excessive muscular tension during the production of esophageal speech. Overly rapid and effortful phonation is often accompanied by undesirable and distracting behaviors such as stoma noise, grimacing, and audible clunking during air injection.

2. A client can learn to self-monitor stoma noise using a microphone, stethoscope, or his or her hand held in front of the stoma.

3. The clinician may want to avoid the use of velar plosives such as /k/ in the early stages of esophageal speech training to prevent inadvertent production of pharyngeal speech (i.e., a Donald Duck voice).

4. The clinician needs to remember that esophageal speakers have much smaller reservoirs of air available for speech (i.e., less than 5 ml) than normal speakers (i.e., greater than 5 L). Therefore, they have a reduced capacity to generate lengthy utterances on a single injection of air.

5. Whenever possible, the clinician should arrange for the client to meet with a successful esophageal speaker either immediately prior to or following surgery. This visit can accomplish several goals at once. It serves as a motivator for the client; it demonstrates the communicative effectiveness of esophageal speech; and it allows the client and family to ask specific questions about the entire rehabilitation process.

6. A nonspeech communication system may need to be provided on an interim basis while the client is learning one of the alternative sound production methods.

7. Clinicians should be aware that clients may experience difficulty focusing on therapy goals due to preoccupation with global issues such as physical survival, economic pressures, and self-identity.

8. WebWhispers (https://webwhispers.org/) is an informational support site for individuals with laryngectomies and laryngeal cancer. The site includes several representative samples of laryngeal speech.

Conclusion

This chapter has presented basic information, protocols, and procedures for intervention with voice disorders at an *introductory* level. This information is intended only as a starting point in the reader's clinical education and training. For in-depth coverage of these areas, the following readings are recommended:

Boone, D. R., McFarlane, S. C., Von Berg, S., & Zraick, R. (2019). *The voice and voice therapy* (10th ed.). Pearson.

Ferrand, C. T. (2019). *Voice disorders: Scope of theory and practice* (2nd ed.). Pearson.

Kelchner, L. N., Baker Brehm, S., & Weinrich, B. D. (2014). *Pediatric voice: A modern collaborative approach to care*. Plural Publishing.

Sapienza, C., & Hoffman, B. (2021). *Voice disorders* (4th ed.). Plural Publishing.

Watts, C., & Awan, S. (2019). *Laryngeal function and voice disorders: Basic science to clinical practice*. Thieme.

Additional Resources

The Source for Children's Voice Disorders
This book provides information on assessing and treating voice disorders. It addresses vocal hyperfunction and abuse as well as other issues associated with the vocal tract (e.g., resonance). Includes a CD of reproducible forms as well as an informational PowerPoint presentation.

The Source for Voice Disorders: Adolescent and Adult
This book provides clinicians with assessment and treatment procedures. It discusses a variety of pathologies and how to address them through therapy. The book comes with a CD that contains handouts on evaluation procedures, therapy exercises, patient questionnaires, and educational resources.

Manual of Voice Therapy, Second Edition
This comprehensive reference includes information for pediatric through adult clients. It includes information about the various conditions that lead to voice disorders, the most recent developments in treatment methods and approaches, instrumentation, related medico-surgical management, counseling, and the challenges in management of voice disorders. This resource also contains a set of reproducible informational handouts for clients and families.

The Voice Diagnostic Protocol: A Practical Guide to the Diagnosis of Voice Disorders

This book serves to provide clinicians with information on how to assess voice disorders with a comprehensive approach. It has chapters that focus on the following topics: pitch, loudness, quality, respiratory control, dysphonias, and case studies. It also includes forms and materials for the evaluation process.

Clinical Management of Voice Disorders, Fourth Edition

This text addresses voice disorders, starting with anatomy and physiology and continuing to discuss a variety of evaluation procedures and tools, such as endoscopy and electroglottography. The book also includes information on a variety of voice disorders by category, including neurogenic disorders, psychogenic disorders, and laryngectomies.

Working With Voice Disorders: Theory and Practice, Third Edition

This text is meant to assist clinicians with the assessment and treatment of voice disorders. It contains sections on anatomy and physiology, disorders, and treatment approaches. The text is meant to encompass the entire rehabilitation process, starting with information for gathering a case history and progressing all the way through treatment sessions.

Martha Mouse and Baby Bear: Voice Adventures Card Deck

These cards contain illustrations of the characters Baby Bear and Martha Mouse. Different situations are presented on each card that the client has to identify as depicting positive or negative vocal behaviors. The cards are stored in a tin box and come in pairs for use in games.

Voice Treatment for Children and Adolescents

This book presents information on the practical assessment and treatment of voice disorders in children through a review of recent research and technological advancements in the area of voice. It also contains problem-solving and team intervention models appropriate for SLPs working in clinical, school, or medical settings.

Manual of Singing Voice Rehabilitation: A Practical Approach to Vocal Health and Wellness

This manual provides information for speech-language pathologists as well as singing teachers on how to treat singers with voice injuries. Written by an SLP, the manual presents information on voice pedagogy, voice pathology, and voice science in order to inform voice rehabilitation.

Client and Family Counseling

Counseling can be defined as an interpersonal relationship that is intended to alleviate emotional stress arising from or contributing to the primary communicative disorder. There are several theoretical schools of thought regarding the counseling process. Some of the most common include behavioral (Skinner, 1953), humanistic (Rogers, 1951), cognitive (Ellis, 1977), existential (Yalom, 1980), interpersonal (Sullivan, 1953), and wellness/positive psychology (Holland & Nelson, 2014) orientations. This chapter takes an eclectic approach to counseling and integrates the following underlying assumptions of several theoretical models (Flasher & Fogle, 2012; Shakespeare, 2006):

1. Human behavior can change or be changed.

2. Some behaviors (e.g., inadequate, dysfunctional, undesirable) warrant change.

3. Particular counseling techniques/interventions will effect change in client behavior.

4. Clients generally acknowledge the possibility that change will occur.

5. Clinicians expect clients to be actively involved in the therapeutic counseling process.

6. Clinicians should expand the scope of their counseling beyond the individual's behaviors to include a focus on relevant structural, environmental, and social barriers to change.

In speech-language intervention, counseling is an essential aspect of the therapeutic process. The American Speech-Language-Hearing Association's (ASHA, 2016) Scope of Practice emphasizes the importance of counseling in clinical work. Counseling fulfills several important functions:

- It allows the clinician to impart basic information to clients and their families.

- It provides opportunities for clients to verbalize feelings, fears, and uncertainties.

- It serves as an emotionally supportive milieu in which clients are comfortable making attitudinal and behavioral changes.

Although counseling is recognized as an integral part of treatment, clinicians often do not receive formal education or training in basic counseling skills (Beck, 2021; Beck & Verticchio, 2018; Doud, 2020). Many clinicians feel uncomfortable with this aspect of their professional role and are uncertain about the differences between psychotherapy and counseling. Psychotherapy involves the identification of unconscious patterns of behavior in a client in order to effect major personality changes. In contrast, counseling focuses on helping a client acknowledge feelings and engage in problem-solving to make personal adjustments (Luterman, 2020).

Counseling is the aspect of speech-language therapy that focuses on the person rather than the disorder. According to lore, Charles Van Riper often told his students, "It's not enough to know the kind of disorder a person has, one must know the kind of person who has the disorder." An effective therapeutic relationship must be built on mutual confidence, trust, respect, and consideration (Luterman, 2016; Rollin, 2000). Client and family perceptions of positive therapeutic/counseling relationships include the following characteristics:

- Sensitivity to and empathy for their feelings and circumstances

- Respect for them as individuals

- Honest, yet tactful, presentation of potentially unpleasant or emotionally charged information

- Motivation to actively participate in the therapy process

- Careful listening by the clinician that promotes effective communication and allows for the "venting" of feelings

Several variables can influence the counseling process. Both client and clinician bring their own needs, values, feelings, experiences, and expectations to the therapeutic relationship (Flasher & Fogle, 2012; Luterman, 2020). However, it is important for the clinician to practice selfless listening (e.g., to set aside his or her own personal views) in order to identify the client's concerns and to foster feelings of trust and security (Luterman, 2006). Both participants must recognize that the client's welfare is the central concern of the relationship and work together to improve the client's communicative status. It is important to understand that individual clients require varying amounts of time to form a bond of trust with another person. Therefore, clinicians need to be patient with clients who are slower to risk self-disclosure. In addition, clinicians must realize that, in most cases, a communicative disorder is a family problem rather than a problem of a single individual. Thus, counseling must address clients in the context of their overall life situations. Clinicians are encouraged to look beyond the observable aspects of client and family behavior and consider their internal emotional and affective states as well (Geller & Foley, 2009). In recent literature, the concept of "mindfulness" is discussed as a way to enhance a client's ability to actively focus on the present moment, adopt a nonjudgmental acceptance of their own thoughts and feelings, and develop self-compassion (Harley, 2018; Kinsella et al., 2020; Medina & Mead, 2021).

Counseling is an ongoing process and should not be viewed as a one-time event. It is incorporated into diagnostic as well as treatment sessions. In some cases, counseling may constitute the treatment process itself. For example, an intervention program for a person who stutters may consist entirely of counseling sessions that focus on reducing anxiety, boosting self-confidence, and modifying the environment to eliminate communicative stress. It is important for clinicians to realize that clients frequently receive services from multiple sources. Thus, collaboration among the professionals is crucial in communicating consistent counseling messages in order to minimize client/family misunderstanding and confusion.

Counseling is a relationship, and for any relationship to be successful, boundaries must be established (Flasher & Fogle, 2012; Stone & Olswang, 1989). This is a necessary first step, because boundaries define the function and role of each participant and clarify what will or will not be part of the therapeutic relationship. Setting specific parameters reduces anxiety for clients whose expectations about therapy may be confused or unclear. In the initial stage of intervention, the clinician is responsible for ensuring that boundaries are established and understood.

Clinicians also need to recognize the limits of their training/experience and realize when referrals need to be made to professionals with specialized counseling expertise (Flasher & Fogle, 2012; Luterman, 2020). Situations that are clearly beyond the scope of practice for a speech-language pathologist (SLP) may involve either the content or the style of the interaction. Content refers to the topic areas discussed within the therapeutic relationship. Topics that are generally considered inappropriate for discussion within the domain of speech-language pathology may include a client's marital problems, chronic depression, or unrelated health problems. Style involves the manner in which the clinician and client interact. Examples of inappropriate style include a client's unhealthy dependency on the clinician, unpredictable and repeated fluctuations of mood and temper, or undue anxiety on the part of the clinician before and after each therapy session.

Five Key Traits of an Effective Counselor

Many authors have discussed the interpersonal attributes of clinicians as counselors. Five key characteristics are presented here:

1. *Appropriate sharing:* Clinicians are often eager to establish a genuine connection with clients and their families. However, it is important for clinicians to recognize personal boundaries during these professional interactions. The type and amount of personal information that a clinician shares with clients should be carefully monitored, ensuring that the focus of counseling remains clearly on the clients and their needs. Clinicians should maintain objectivity regarding their personal relationship with clients (e.g., the difference between "being friendly" and "being a friend"; Shipley & Roseberry-McKibbin, 2006). An example of inappropriate sharing might be the following:

    > Client: I just can't seem to get members of my family to stop giving me advice about my stuttering.

    > Clinician: I know what you mean. My boyfriend is like that whenever I try to tell him about a problem I'm having.

2. *Nonjudgmental:* Counseling requires clinicians to provide support and encouragement to clients and families throughout the therapy process. Care should be taken to ensure that this feedback is not presented in terms of "good versus bad" or "right versus wrong." It is also important that clinicians refrain from imposing their own belief system/values onto their clients/families. An example of inappropriately judgmental behavior might be the following:

    > Client's wife: We really don't go to museums anymore because my husband has to use the wheelchair since his stroke.

    > Clinician: That shouldn't stop you! All museums these days have handicapped access and I'm sure your husband would enjoy visiting them.

3. *Tolerant of crying and emotional language:* There are points during the therapeutic process when clients may become emotional. These emotions can range from extreme happiness to hostility to self-pity. Beginning clinicians often feel the most uncomfortable with negative emotions such as crying or anger and seek to cut them off quickly. Yet effective counseling requires clinicians to recognize that allowing clients to express negative emotions can have

therapeutic value. An example of appropriate tolerance for emotional behavior might be the following:

> Client: (*crying and shouting*) It's just too hard—I'll never learn how to read!
>
> Clinician: (*waits until outburst is over*) It's OK to be upset—I know you're really frustrated today.

4. *Client- or family-centered:* The driving forces behind counseling are the needs and priorities of clients and their families. Effective counselors recognize that these needs may be in conflict with their own plan for intervention. The ability to adapt and accommodate clients' views while maintaining appropriate therapeutic focus is critical for successful counseling. An example of accommodating parental input might be the following:

> Client's parent: Benjamin isn't cooperating in therapy because he's bored. Can you use songs instead? He really likes singing.
>
> Clinician: Singing won't really help him learn to produce novel two- to three-word utterances. But we can use songs for our therapy goal on production of final consonants.

5. *Refrains from solving client issues:* Counseling is not designed to solve or prescribe solutions to client problems. Clients who discuss problems in therapy often just need someone to listen and are really not looking for specific advice. Effective counseling helps clients work toward identifying their own solutions for themselves and their families.

Another key aspect to being an effective counselor is continued dedication to professional literature and evidence-based practices (Holland & Nelson, 2018; Victorino & Hinkle, 2018). In addition to remaining updated on current practices, certain disorders and conditions will require SLPs to research other fields for a fuller understanding of their client's status. For example, a communication disorder associated with a degenerative disease would lead an SLP to obtain information on the medical characteristics and prognosis of the disease, including the projected timeline and expected trajectory of symptoms so as to inform treatment plans and to manage expectations (Holland & Nelson, 2018).

Stages of Counseling

Counseling is a dynamic process that continues throughout the course of a treatment program. As therapy progresses, the nature of counseling evolves through three main phases.

Establishing the Therapeutic Relationship

In this first phase, one of the clinician's primary responsibilities is to provide clients and their families with information. This information may pertain to the nature of the communicative disorder, possible treatment options, specific therapy techniques, the prognosis for improvement, and the level of commitment that therapy will require from the client and family. Clinicians must be sensitive to the amount of information that a client or family can handle at a given time. For example, the impact of an initial diagnosis of a communicative disorder may be devastating and preclude the processing of any other information presented at that time. Moreover, cognition becomes limited when emotions are elevated, making it difficult to process additional information (Luterman, 2006). When establishing a therapeutic relationship, the clinician functions in a directive role and assumes primary responsibility for setting the therapeutic agenda. The clinician determines the topics to be discussed, the activities to be performed, and the parameters of the client–clinician interpersonal relationship.

Implementing Counseling Intervention

This is the "work" stage of the client–clinician relationship. The focus of the counseling process shifts from an educational/informative mode to a problem-solving orientation. It is essential for clinicians to use their listening skills carefully in order to recognize the difference between "teaching moments" and "counseling moments." See the Helpful Hints section at the end of this chapter for books in the popular literature that provide insight into the lives of individuals with communication impairments. Therapy activities begin to focus directly on the client's deficits, and demands for behavioral change become more intense. Individual clients may demonstrate a variety of coping strategies or defense mechanisms such as avoidance, escape, humor, rationalization/intellectualization, and passive-aggression (Flasher & Fogle, 2012; Tanner, 2003). The client may begin to experience feelings of vulnerability, anxiety, and frustration, which may give rise to behaviors that are disruptive to the therapy process. Commonly seen manifestations may include (a) consistently arriving late for sessions, (b) chronically failing to complete homework assignments, (c) resisting therapy activities perceived as "too difficult," or (d) refusing/"forgetting" to attempt new communicative behaviors outside of the therapy setting. The clinician needs to recognize the feelings that motivate these behaviors in the client and focus counseling efforts on resolving these issues. Effective clinicians understand the need to recognize, accept, and work with—rather than against—a client's temperament. In this phase, the clinician begins to function in a more nondirective mode. The client is encouraged to assume more active responsibility for self-motivation and for determining the therapeutic agenda.

Terminating the Therapeutic Relationship

At this final stage, the clinician lays the groundwork for the closure of the relationship by preparing the client to become his or her own therapist (i.e., shifting the locus of control). Counseling efforts focus on validating accurate client perceptions and encouraging the client to assume full responsibility for maintaining the behavioral changes that have been accomplished in therapy. Counseling also should be directed toward ensuring that the client leaves therapy with a genuine conceptual understanding and healthy perspective regarding the nature of the communicative disorder. Clinicians should encourage clients to actively use self-advocacy skills in order to promote successful communicative outcomes once the therapeutic relationship has ended.

Client and Family Emotional Reactions to Communicative Disorders

Clients and their families often receive the diagnosis of a communicative impairment with a great sense of loss. This sense of loss can be manifested through a variety of strong emotional responses. Clinicians need to be aware of the range of possible emotions that clients or families may experience at different stages in the therapy process. The most common reactions that clinicians must recognize and be prepared to handle are the following:

- *Grief* is deep sorrow in response to a significant loss. There have been numerous attempts to identify the stages of the grieving process. Kübler-Ross (1969) discussed five stages, which include initial denial that a disorder exists, a bargaining phase in which "deals" are offered to ameliorate the severity or existence of the disorder (e.g., "If Billy stops stuttering, I'll never criticize him again"), and an acceptance stage in which the client and family adjust to the loss as a fact of life and begin focusing efforts toward rehabilitation. Alternatively, Luterman (2020) identified four stages of coping: denial, resistance, affirmation, and integration. See Tanner (2008) for a simple discussion of the acceptance of unwanted change following stroke.

- *Anger* is a strong feeling of displeasure characterized by resentment, hostility, or rage. With respect to a communicative disorder, anger is often an instinctive attempt at self-protection resulting from fear, powerlessness, and frustration. Sometimes, spouses or parents experience feelings of anger toward the family member with communicative impairment. However, they perceive this reaction as socially unacceptable; therefore, they may transfer their angry feelings toward the clinician.

- *Depression* is anger turned inward that results in passivity and feelings of helplessness. The client realizes that previous stages of anger and bargaining were ineffective and that the fact of the communication disorder must be faced. Depression is a relatively common emotion encountered in the counseling process. The clinician should be aware that this emotional state can become self-perpetuating and seriously impede a client's therapy progress.

- *Guilt* refers to self-blame and is frequently demonstrated by a client's immediate family members. These feelings tend to center on two types of issues: "Did I do something to cause (or contribute to) John's communicative disorder?" and "Am I getting the right type and amount of therapy for John?" Parents and family members may not necessarily verbalize these feelings but may act them out in the form of behavioral extremes, such as withdrawal from or overinvolvement in the therapeutic process. Clinicians need to be aware that some questions or comments routinely addressed to family members may inadvertently trigger feelings of guilt (e.g., "When did you first seek therapy for John's problem?" or "How do you deal with John's behavior at home?").

- *Shame* is an emotional state characterized by a negative evaluation of one's entire self and is accompanied by feelings of worthlessness and failure. It generates strong avoidance behaviors that may have a significant impact on a client's ability to participate effectively in counseling. Shame can be difficult to detect because there is no easily recognized facial expression or other overt manifestation, as in anger or depression.

- *Anxiety* refers to feelings of apprehension or distress that are generally not directly related to an immediate situation. This reaction may be present throughout the therapeutic process. During the initial stages of intervention, clients and their families are often uncertain about what to expect and also may question whether the clinician can truly help them. As therapy progresses, the focus of client anxiety may shift to the educational, vocational, or social repercussions of the communicative disorder.

- *Inadequacy* encompasses feelings of insufficiency or incompetence. Clients and their families frequently are overwhelmed by the diagnosis and implications of a communicative disorder. As a result, they rely heavily on the information and support provided by the clinician, especially in the initial stages of intervention. If feelings of confidence and self-esteem are not cultivated, this dependent relationship is likely to continue, and the clinician can become cast in the role of "rescuer" rather than a facilitator of change (Luterman, 2016).

- *Isolation* is a sense of personal detachment and remoteness from society. It can be self-imposed or result from others' rejection of the client. Isolation may arise from feelings, such as inadequacy and low self-esteem or from the perception that no one else can truly understand the client's situation. Strong feelings of isolation may exacerbate the intensity or duration of all the emotional reactions just discussed. The client's isolation from social interactions may severely impede the clinician's ability to establish an effective counseling relationship.

Clients rarely verbalize these emotions directly. Therefore, the clinician must be a keen observer of nonverbal and vocal behaviors that may be indicative of client distress. (See Forms 11–1 and 11–2 for checklists of client and clinician behaviors.)

Counseling Techniques for Communicative Disorders

One of the primary goals of counseling is to help clients and their families cope with the reality of the communicative disorder and foster the perspective that it constitutes only one aspect of the client's overall identity. The clinician's role is to assist clients in assuming responsibility for their own behavior and decisions. This goal is generally achieved through implementation of a variety of counseling techniques. Selection of specific procedures will depend on the personalities of the client and clinician as well as the constraints imposed by the communicative disorder. The following section briefly describes several of the counseling techniques most commonly used by SLPs.

- *Desensitization:* The client is guided through a hierarchy of situations from least to most anxiety provoking within the context of a safe and relaxed counseling environment. For example, a college student with a severe lisp can be gradually exposed to feared speaking situations that range from (a) an informal conversation with the clinician, (b) a formal presentation to the clinician, and (c) the same formal presentation to unfamiliar listeners in a classroom setting.

- *Relaxation:* Tension is reduced in muscle groups to alleviate a client's feelings of anxiety. For example, a client with a hyperfunctional voice disorder can be instructed to (a) alternately contract and release laryngeal muscles, (b) mentally visualize a peaceful setting, and (c) engage in deep diaphragmatic breathing.

- *Counterquestion:* A client may ask questions that appear to be requests for technical information but are actually intended to gain the clinician's confirmation or validation of a decision that has already been made. The clinician can respond to these types of remarks by posing a counterquestion that encourages the client to reveal the true intent of the original query. For example, a clinician may recognize that a mother who repeatedly inquires about the interpretation of her child's cognitive and language test scores may not truly be seeking technical information. The clinician can pose a counterquestion, such as, "Is there something in particular about these test scores that bothers you?" At this point, the mother may acknowledge that she recently refused to allow an Individualized Education Plan (IEP) team to label her child as "mentally retarded," and she is actually seeking support for this decision from the clinician.

- *Reframing:* A client or family is encouraged to modify views or attitudes toward a negative situation that cannot be changed. For example, a clinician may point out that family members have analyzed and improved their interpersonal relationships as a result of the client's stroke and subsequent aphasia. This technique should be introduced in the later stages of the therapeutic relationship only after the client or family has demonstrated a genuine acceptance of the communicative disorder.

- *Open-ended and indirect questions:* Questions are formulated in a manner that does not restrict the client or family's response to a simple one- or two-word utterance. This technique is used to elicit spontaneous and detailed responses that provide insight into the client's attitudes, knowledge, and feelings. One common example of an open-ended question is, "What are your major concerns about wearing a hearing aid?" A typical indirect question is, "I'd be interested in knowing your opinion of the new hearing aid."

- *Role-playing:* Problematic situations associated with the communicative disorder are identified, and structured opportunities are provided for a client to act out more appropriate behaviors in hypothetical contexts. For example, an adolescent who frequently misunderstands conversational messages may refuse to request clarification because "people will think I am stupid." Scripted scenarios can be developed and used to rehearse specific repair strategies for obtaining needed information without embarrassment.

- *Empathetic listening:* The clinician reflects back the content or emotions expressed by a client's message in a nonjudgmental manner. This is generally accomplished by merely repeating or rephrasing the client's comments in an objective fashion. Effective listening is characterized by consistent eye contact, attentive body language, and behaviors that encourage continued communication, such as head nods and "um hmm."

- *Paraphrasing content:* The clinician rephrases a client's message or statement in his or her own words. This "mirroring" allows the client to hear the message from another source and gives him or her the opportunity to amplify, clarify, correct, revise, or confirm the meaning.

- *Summarizing content:* This technique involves succinct, accurate paraphrasing of larger segments of client interaction (e.g., at least 10–15 min). The intent is for the clinician to capture the overall gist of the important elements of the preceding discourse.

In addition to overall strategies, Flasher and Fogle (2012) and Glade et al. (2018) provide counseling guidance with regard to specific communication disorders, including the following:

- Client age often factors into the counseling approach with individuals who stutter. For example, counseling may not be as direct with a preschool-aged individual as with an adult client.

- Voice disorders and associated changes in vocal characteristics can impact a person's self-identity as well as degree of social interactions. Intervention may need to target improving vocal quality while also addressing issues of vocal use with regard to daily activities.

- Dysphagia and swallowing protocols can cause a client to feel uncomfortable during meals, an activity of daily living that has a strong social component. Ongoing discussions with the client and his or her family are important to managing concerns that arise as the client adjusts to the current situation.

- For clients with hearing loss, the informational content of counseling changes as a function of a client's age or stage of development (e.g., school-age, adolescence, higher education, and transition to the workforce).

Form 11–1. CLIENT NONVERBAL AND VOCAL BEHAVIOR CHECKLIST

INSTRUCTIONS: Observe a live or recorded counseling session. Answer each of the following items by circling the letter in each set of three that corresponds to the most appropriate description of the client's nonverbal behaviors.

1. How is the client sitting?

   a. Rigidly   a. Very near the clinician   a. In constant motion

   b. Relaxed   b. At an average distance   b. In typical motion

   c. Slouched   c. Very far from the clinician   c. Motionless

2. How does the client look?

   a. Nervous   a. Happy   a. Well dressed   a. Friendly

   b. At ease   b. Concerned   b. Appropriately dressed   b. Business like

   c. Passive   c. Upset   c. Disheveled   c. Belligerent

3. How does the client communicate?

   a. Very quickly   a. Loudly   a. High-pitched voice

   b. At a normal rate   b. At normal intensity   b. Average voice

   c. Very slowly   c. Quietly   c. Low-pitched voice

   a. With appropriate affect and intonation   a. With many gestures

   b. With inappropriate affect and intonation   b. With some gestures

   c. With no affect or intonation   c. With no gestures

Source: Adapted from McDonald, P. A., & Haney, M. (1997). *Counseling the older adult: A training manual in clinical gerontology.* San Francisco, CA: Jossey-Bass.

Form 11–2. CLINICIAN/COUNSELOR BEHAVIOR CHECKLIST

INSTRUCTIONS: Observe a live or recorded counseling session. Respond to each statement with "Yes," "No," or "Not applicable" to describe the clinician's counseling behaviors.

(Note: Y = Yes; N = No; NA = Not applicable)

Nonverbal

_____ 1. The clinician maintained appropriate eye contact with the client.

_____ 2. The clinician was alert and responded with an animated facial expression.

_____ 3. The clinician refrained from nonverbally reinforcing the client's off-task or irrelevant remarks (i.e., head nods).

_____ 4. The clinician demonstrated relaxed body posture.

_____ 5. The clinician leaned forward as the client spoke.

_____ 6. The clinician used a variety of vocal intonation patterns.

_____ 7. The clinician's voice was sufficiently loud to be heard by the client.

_____ 8. The clinician used intermittent vocalization (e.g., mm-hmm) during the client's on-task, relevant remarks.

Verbal

_____ 1. The clinician's remarks usually addressed the most important aspects of each of the client's utterances.

_____ 2. The clinician encouraged the client to express feelings about the communicative disorder.

_____ 3. The clinician verbally identified and responded to the client's feelings.

_____ 4. Most of the clinician's questions were open-ended in nature and required more than a one- or two-word response from the client.

_____ 5. The clinician did not monopolize the available talk time in the session.

_____ 6. The clinician used purposeful silences to encourage the client to elaborate on responses.

_____ 7. The clinician made verbal responses that supported or reinforced some of the client's statements.

_____ 8. The clinician occasionally restated or clarified the client's remarks.

_____ 9. The clinician expressed a desire to understand the client's feelings and attitudes about the communication problem.

_____ 10. The clinician answered directly when the client asked for information or an opinion.

_____ 11. The clinician occasionally used counter-questions to respond to certain client queries.

_____ 12. The clinician occasionally offered an alternative and more positive perspective of some situation that the client has identified as distressing.

_____ 13. The clinician summarized key points of the session at appropriate junctures.

Source: Adapted from Cormier, L. S. & Hackney, H. (2008). _Counseling strategies and interventions_ (7th ed.). London, UK: Pearson Education.

Group Counseling

Some SLPs coordinate sessions that function as emotional support groups for clients and their families. Provision of therapy within a group setting can foster elements important to counseling, thus helping the group members to make progress (Erdman, 2009). Some of these factors include universality (i.e., the knowledge that an individual is not the only one experiencing a particular communication disorder), altruism (i.e., the feeling of self-importance and happiness that arises from providing support to other group members), and imitative behaviors (i.e., the development of compensatory strategies from watching other members; Erdman, 2009).

Clinicians need to be knowledgeable about group dynamics and be aware of the issues that tend to arise in this setting. Effective counseling skills enable the clinician to do the following:

- Determine appropriate composition and size of a group

- Set the procedures and norms for group interactions

- Promote an atmosphere of trust and unity among the group members

- Assume a less directive leadership role as the group matures

- Encourage a particular group member to risk self-disclosure

- Manage a dominant member who is monopolizing the group's time

- Manage confrontational interactions between or among group members

- Determine the hidden agendas of individual group members

- Extinguish comments and behaviors that detract from therapy goals

- Reinforce group members who make constructive comments to other group members

- Recognize an individual group member's need for more specialized counseling services and broach the topic skillfully

- Determine the appropriate juncture for terminating a group

(See Chapter 1 for a detailed discussion of the advantages and disadvantages of group sessions.)

Family Systems Counseling

Based on family systems theory, this approach acknowledges the central role that the family plays in a client's development and progress (Hunting Pompon et al., 2015). Key concepts of this theory are as follows: (a) change in one family member affects the entire family system, (b) the family unit is greater than the sum of its parts, and (c) families exist within the context of the larger society. In this view, families are dynamic units with specific communication and interaction patterns (Boyle & McDowell-Burns, 2015). Effective clinicians incorporate this family-centered perspective into their counseling efforts. It is noteworthy that such consideration is actually required by federal law under the provisions of the Individuals with Disabilities Education Act (2011).

An increasing variety of family structures are represented in clinical caseloads. Several societal factors contribute to this diversity, including differing cultural/ethnic backgrounds, poverty, and single-parent households, among a host of others. Accordingly, clinicians can expect a wide range of family involvement/participation in the intervention process. Therefore, the clinician's counseling efforts should be designed on a case-by-case basis to accommodate the needs of each family.

Helpful Hints

1. Clinicians can teach family members to employ empathetic listening techniques with clients to strengthen positive communication in the home environment.

2. The value of counseling is severely compromised if a clinician's personal feelings become a factor in the therapeutic relationship.

3. Important points can be emphasized by reiterating them in different ways at various stages of the counseling relationship.

4. The provision of a brief summary at the end of a counseling session may help the client focus on the most important points that were discussed. A written summary also may help the client to understand and remember terminology related to his or her communication disorder (e.g., dysarthria, anatomical terms).

5. The purpose of counseling is to provide a client with the information needed to manage and to treat the communication disorder; it is not intended to ameliorate problems in the client's personal life.

6. Reluctance, resentment, and opposition are predictable client reactions in the counseling process and should not evoke feelings of defensiveness on the part of the clinician.

7. A clinician's use of phrases such as "It is my impression . . ." or "I hear you saying . . ." are less likely to trigger defensive behaviors from a client than more direct statements such as "You are . . ." or "You can't . . ."

8. It is important for clinicians to realize that the overuse of positive remarks causes such reinforcers to become meaningless.

9. Counseling is more effective if it periodically acknowledges a client's strengths rather than focusing solely on weaknesses or limitations.

10. Clinicians should refrain from pressing a client for self-disclosure too early in the counseling relationship because it may actually increase a client's reluctance to confide in the clinician.

11. Sometimes, conflict within a group can be a sign that the group is working well as a unit. It frequently indicates that group members have developed a sense of trust and feel secure enough to disagree openly with each other.

12. Counseling that loses its focus or purpose becomes mere conversation and accomplishes little.

13. Clinicians can learn to identify "teaching" versus "counseling" moments. For example, some questions may be truly asked to request information (e.g., When did my child acquire this disorder?). However, sometimes the clinician may be able to discern that a question is meant more to address personal concerns (e.g., Did the parent have a role in the development of a communication disorder?).

14. The following books may help clinicians develop their empathetic listening skills and sharpen insights about living with communication disorders:

- Bauby, J.-D. (1997). *The diving bell and the butterfly: A memoir of life in death.* Knopf.

- Baxter, T. W. (2018). Relentless: How a massive stroke changed my life for the better. Greenleaf Book Group Press.

- Grandin, T. (2011). *The way I see it: A personal look at autism and Asperger's* (2nd ed.). Future Horizons.

- Haddon, M. (2003). *The curious incident of the dog in the night-time.* Doubleday.

- Hendrickson, J. (2023). *Life on delay: Making peace with a stutter.* Knopf Doubleday.

- Marks, L. (2018). *A stitch of time: The year a brain injury changed my language and life.* Simon & Schuster.

Conclusion

This chapter presented basic information, protocols, and procedures for counseling at an *introductory* level. This information is intended only as a starting point in the reader's clinical education and training. For more in-depth coverage of this area, the following readings are recommended:

Flasher, L. V., & Fogle, P. T. (2012). *Counseling skills for speech-language pathologists and audiologists* (2nd ed.). Cengage Learning.

Luterman, D. M. (2020). *Counseling persons with communication disorders and their families* (7th ed.). Pro-Ed.

Shipley, K. G., & Roseberry-McKibben, C. (2006). *Interviewing and counseling in communicative disorders: Principles and procedures* (3rd ed.). Pro-Ed.

Stein-Rubin, C., & Adler, B. (2016). *Counseling in Communication Disorders: Facilitating the Therapeutic Relationship.* SLACK Incorporated.

Additional Resources

Counseling in Speech-Language Pathology and Audiology: Reconstructing Personal Narratives, Second Edition
These authors illustrate how to integrate the concept of counseling into clinical practice. Replete with a variety of case studies, clinical guidelines, and actual transcripts of counseling interventions with clients and their families. This text offers a comprehensive, novel, and empirically informed approach to counseling.

Lifespan Perspectives on the Family and Disability, Second Edition
This resource examines how families cope, adapt, and grow through the challenge of living with a child with a disability. A family-centered focus is presented within a life span framework: infancy/early childhood, school years, transition from school to adult life, adult years.

Rehabilitation Counseling: Basics and Beyond, Fifth Edition (and E-Book)
This text provides clinicians with theoretical, research-based approaches to counseling as well as experience-driven practices. The authors frame counseling from the viewpoint of federal laws (e.g., Americans with Disabilities Act Amendments Act) as well as the issues that arise at different developmental stages (e.g., vocations/careers, sexual development).

Chapter 12

Multicultural Issues in Intervention/Diversity, Equity, Inclusion, and Accessibility (DEIA)

This topic is an evolving area of discussion that includes many important constructs, such as language, culture, ethnicity/race, geography, degree of acculturation, background, family type, values, belief systems, and gender identity. For the sake of simplicity and clarity, this chapter uses the term **cultural and linguistic diversity (CLD)** to represent this broad range of variables. The American Speech-Language-Hearing Association (ASHA) encourages speech-language pathologists (SLPs) to consider the impact of cultural factors as well as linguistic characteristics and unique values of individuals when designing and implementing intervention. **Culturally responsive** clinicians demonstrate respect for each individual's age, gender, ethnicity, and socioeconomic status among other factors. They readily acknowledge gaps regarding these variables in their own education and clinical experience. They recognize the importance of treating each client as an individual rather than imposing cultural stereotypes based on learned assumptions. Also, effective clinicians extend their culturally responsive focus beyond the therapy room to encompass their advocacy efforts with consideration of the health literacy, values, and preferences of specific communities. Several aspects of ASHA's Code of Ethics (2023) emphasize the responsibility to avoid discrimination and provide culturally and linguistically competent services (see Appendix A on the companion website). A more comprehensive discussion of cultural competence for SLPs is presented in the next section of this chapter. A recent paradigm shift identifies the impact of specific areas of multiculturalism: diversity, equity, inclusion, and accessibility (DEIA). These are a set of practices intended to mitigate discrimination and ensure that people from a broad set of backgrounds are represented and able to thrive. This terminology reflects current thinking in the field of speech-language pathology. It can encompass interpersonal communication, goal programming, types of reinforcement, and selection of therapy materials. For more comprehensive information on DEIA issues, readers are encouraged to explore example resources. The remainder of the chapter will focus on bilingualism as a method of highlighting the diversity of individuals with whom SLPs interact. There are a variety of terms used to describe individuals who are acquiring a second language. The most common include *dual-language learners, English learners*, and **English-language learners (ELLs)**. Again, for the sake of simplicity and clarity, this chapter uses the term *ELL* to represent these individuals. Similarly, the term *bilingual*, as used in this chapter, refers to individuals who speak two or more languages. L1 refers to an individual's native language, whereas L2 represents the second language.

In a related vein, dialects are variations within a single language and may encompass phonological, syntactic, semantic, and pragmatic components. Dialects may be associated with geographic, socioeconomic, or cultural/ethnic factors. Examples of dialects in English include African American English (AAE), Appalachian English, and Cajun English. Competent users of multiple languages or dialects often engage in **code-switching**, alternating use of each language/dialect depending on the context or listener needs.

The changing demographics of the United States have important implications for SLPs to consider. U.S. census (2015) data indicate that over 60 million Americans speak a language other than

English and that over 350 different languages are represented in that pool. The percentage of public school students in the United States who are ELLs is 10.4%, or 5.1 million students (National Center for Education Statistics [NCES], 2019). If communication disorders occur at the same prevalence rate as in the general U.S. population, then approximately 6.2 million CLD Americans currently have a communication disorder (Battle, 2012). The number of ELL students receiving speech-language services doubled between 1990 and 2000 and continues to rise. The majority of these students tend to be classified as demonstrating a learning disability (U.S. Department of Education, 2009). In the adult population, there is a steady increase in the number of CLD individuals receiving intervention for neurogenic communication disorders (Centeno, 2009).

At least 21.6% of individuals living in the United States speak a primary language other than English (U.S. Bureau of the Census, 2019). When individuals in this group demonstrate communication disorders, they may not be able to effectively participate in or derive maximal benefit from intervention. Unfortunately, only about 8.2% of certified ASHA members across the country can deliver clinical services in a language other than English, with 66% listing Spanish as the other language (ASHA, 2021). Each year, thousands of children from other countries are adopted by American families. However, there has been a sharp decline in international adoptions. In 2004, Americans adopted a record high of 22,989 children from overseas; in 2021, 1,785 children were adopted from abroad by American citizens (U.S. Department of State, 2021). These **international adoptees**, increasingly from China and Eastern Europe, sometimes spend their earliest years in settings characterized by inadequate nutrition, lack of stimulation, and lack of interpersonal/social interaction (Hwa-Froelich & Matsuo, 2019). As a result, they show evidence of a fundamental attachment disorder and demonstrate significant developmental impairments, especially in cognitive, linguistic, and behavioral skills. Due to the increasing rate of referral for assessment and treatment for this population, SLPs need to be aware that the age of adoption appears to be the most critical factor in eventual language outcome. Glennen's (2015) study indicated that children adopted before 2 years catch up to their chronological peers within 15 months of adoption. Two years of exposure to the new language is required for children adopted at age 3 to reach age-level expectations, while children adopted at 4 years require 3 years of exposure to achieve the language skills of chronological-aged peers (Glennen, 2014, 2015). Still, some internationally adopted children will demonstrate language acquisition skills in the normal range, but generally below their native English-speaking peers. A study comparing language acquisition in individuals adopted from China and Canadian-born children acquiring French found that certain aspects of language may be more difficult for children to acquire as they learn their second "first" language. Among their difficulties were receptive syntax and morphology and expressive vocabulary (Gauthier & Genesee, 2011).

Cultural Competence

Cultural competence has been defined as the "ability to think, feel, and act in ways that acknowledge, respect and build upon ethnic, cultural, and linguistic diversity" (Lynch & Hanson, 2011). Cultural competence is a clinician's ability to adjust his or her views and behavior in relation to another culture's norms. Culturally competent clinicians demonstrate understanding of the impact of cultural differences on individual behavior. Within the clinical setting, flexibility is important in adapting and reacting to CLD variables. However, it is important for clinicians to recognize that individual differences exist even within specific cultural groups. To avoid stereotyping, clinicians should view clients as individuals first and members of particular ethnicities or cultures second (Battle, 2012;

Hamilton et al., 2018; Hopf et al., 2021; Roseberry-McKibbin, 2007). Clinicians may use a DEIA paradigm in the development of their therapeutic programming. In 2021, ASHA developed a series of cultural competency checklists to support clinicians' growth in this area:

- The "self-reflection" checklist is designed to heighten clinicians' awareness of their own views regarding the influence of cultural variables in areas such as child-rearing practices and social communication.

- A second checklist reviews clinicians' understanding of the impact of cultural variables on the current policies/procedures within their employment setting.

- A third checklist provides an opportunity for clinicians to consider the impact of cultural variables on their provision of therapy services.

Members of various cultures have widely differing views regarding the nature and appropriate treatment of communication disorders. Use of professional terminology varies widely from country to country and may affect clinician–client communication during the intervention process. For example, the term *dyslexia* in Russia is confined to those with reading problems only. However, in Italy, the same term refers to writing difficulties as well (Smythe & Everatt, 2002). Even issues as fundamental as whether a disability exists or should be treated are subject to cultural interpretation (Adler, n.d.). Battle (1997) highlights this point by contrasting the belief systems of Native American and Chinese cultures. Native Americans embrace a philosophy that life should be in harmony with nature. Thus, a communication disorder may be considered a part of life that should be accepted rather than changed. In contrast, Chinese cultural tradition regards a disability as an irreversible punishment for the transgressions of ancestors. Members of either culture, therefore, may be reluctant to engage in the therapeutic process. Other consequences of cultural differences may become obvious when parental expectations of a child differ from school expectations. Thus, the child receives "mixed messages" and has to find a way to resolve the conflict between the two sets of expectations.

Numerous other culture-specific factors may have an influence on the clinician's approach to clients with communication disorders and their families. Battle (2012) provides the following illustrations:

- Islamic tradition does not permit a female client to receive therapy services from a male clinician. Extended family members may expect to participate in therapy sessions and might be offended if they are excluded.

- Hinduism allows no photographs or videotapes of female clients.

- Japanese mothers tend to use less verbal (and more nonverbal) communication behaviors than middle-class American mothers when interacting with their young children.

- Hispanic families may experience difficulty acknowledging disabilities that have no visible physical manifestations (e.g., language or articulation disorder, dyslexia, and so on).

- Asian cultures often view social skills as a critical component of intelligence, whereas Western European cultures' model of intelligence involves innate cognitive skills.

There are several broad categories of CLD variables to consider in delivery of intervention services. The following sections illustrate them with three examples.

Cultural/Ethnic Background

Prior to initiating the intervention process, clinicians should engage in self-reflection to identify core aspects of their own values and belief systems. Roseberry-McKibbin (2007) identified several assumptions that are common to clinicians reared in mainstream American culture. Examples include the following:

- Punctuality is an indicator of mutual respect in a therapeutic relationship.

- In meetings, value is placed on "getting to the point" quickly and directly.

- The age and gender of the clinician relative to the client are much less important than the clinician's level of competence.

- Written documentation is an integral component of all interactions with clients/families.

- Treatment is warranted even for individuals with no observable physical disability.

- The ultimate goal of intervention is independent functioning.

These beliefs may be in substantial contrast to those held by individuals from CLD backgrounds. Some examples of these differences are discussed here in an attempt to illustrate the scope of knowledge required to develop multicultural competence.

Socioeconomic Status (SES)

Socioeconomic status (SES) is a way of ranking relative position in a society based on class, status, and power. It is frequently represented by financial resources/wealth, level of education, and occupation.

Clients of lower SES may be primarily concerned with practical issues of daily living that revolve around making ends meet, both financially and personally. Their priority in therapy may be to seek immediate solutions and concrete, observable behavioral changes. An intervention approach that focuses on increasing self-awareness and insight into the personal dynamics associated with a communication disorder may not be highly valued. Recommendations and referrals that may arise from the intervention process should be made with full consideration of each client's financial and personal situation. Huang et al. (2023) suggest that SES may be a strong predictor of cognitive communicative behaviors than other factors such as racial-ethnic background. In addition, maternal education level has been found to positively correlate with children's vocabulary knowledge (Bruce et al., 2022).

SLP educational and clinical training programs increasingly are incorporating information on CLD issues. In addition to the traditional focus on the characteristics of CLD individuals, some programs emphasize the knowledge and skills that clinicians must master to demonstrate cultural competence. Quach and Tsai (2017) identified several competencies from which the following are adapted:

- Clinician establishes a clinical environment that values diversity

- Clinician utilizes client's experiences and culture to inform clinical programming

- Clinician adapts assessment methods to meet the needs of CLD clients and use the data to develop culturally sensitive programming

- Clinician works collaboratively with families and significant others from culturally diverse communities

Linguistic Differences

In addition to SES and cultural/ethnic factors, the intervention process may be affected by language differences with clients from diverse backgrounds (Huang & Kan, 2019; Hyter & Salas-Provance, 2021). These differences involve nonverbal, paralinguistic, and verbal aspects of communication. With respect to nonverbal behaviors, beginning clinicians may assume that certain communication behaviors have universal meanings. In fact, tremendous variation exists in the interpretation of these expressions. Three examples that are particularly relevant to therapy provided by SLPs are eye contact, smiling, and seating arrangement. Caucasian Americans exhibit a much greater degree of eye contact as listeners than as speakers, while African Americans tend to demonstrate the opposite pattern (i.e., greater eye contact when speaking than listening), see Hudley et al. (2018). Moreover, Asians/Pacific Islanders often perceive eye contact as an expression of hostility, whereas Native Americans tend to interpret direct eye contact as a sign of disrespect. Similar variation exists with respect to smiling: Western cultures assign positive meaning to this facial expression; the Japanese culture associates smiling with shyness or embarrassment; and other Asian cultures may interpret smiling as a sign of weakness or superficiality. Finally, Westerners seem to prefer a seating arrangement in which the client and clinician face each other across a table. Native Americans may be most comfortable with a side-by-side arrangement (Sue & Sue, 2012).

In the United States, native speakers of tonal languages continue to increase; nearly 3 million residents speak Chinese, such as Mandarin and Cantonese (U.S. Bureau of the Census, 2021). Chinese is considered a tonal language, in which pitch is used to discriminate between the meanings of individual words (e.g., /ma/ can have at least three meanings depending on the lexical tone used by the speaker). These lexical tones vary within a speaker's pitch range and change over time. The ability to perceive lexical tones is correlated with activity in the language-dominant left hemisphere of the brain for native speakers of tonal languages. In contrast, lexical tones presented to native speakers of nontonal languages tend to activate the right hemisphere of the brain, because the tones carry no linguistic relevance for them.

Many English sounds are not used in other languages. Clinicians treating communication disorders in individuals from CLD backgrounds should keep in mind these speech sound repertoire differences (Kress, 2009). Table 12–1 provides examples. Clearly, verbal language differences are

Table 12–1
Sounds from English Not Used in Other Languages

Language	Sounds
Spanish	/dʒ/ /j/ /ʃ/ /θ/ /z/
Chinese	/b/ /tʃ/ /d/ /dʒ/ /g/ /oa/ /ʃ/ /θ/ /ð/ /v/ /z/
French	/tʃ/ /i/ /j/ /ŋ/ /u/ /θ/ /ð/
Italian	/a/ /ð/ /ɑr/ /e/ /dʒ/ /h/ /ŋ/ /θ/

Source: Adapted from *English Language Learners: Differentiating Between Language Acquisition and Learning Disabilities* (p. 17), by J. Klingner and A. Eppolito, 2014. Copyright 2014 Council for Exceptional Children. All rights reserved.

culturally determined and may influence semantic, phonologic, syntactic, and morphologic behaviors. Moreover, pragmatic language issues such as appropriate topics of conversation, turn-taking rules, and the effects of social status between communication partners are culturally bound. For specific information regarding nonverbal and verbal characteristics of three main cultural groups—African American, Hispanic, and Asian—refer to Tables 12–2 through 12–10.

Table 12–2
Consonant Sound Production Characteristics of African American English (AAE)

Phoneme	Description
/n/	Replaced by nasalized vowel in the final position (e.g., bin → /bĩ/)
/w, d/	Omitted in initial position for specific words (e.g., was → /əz/; don't → /ont/)
/ŋ/	Replaced by /n/ especially in final position (e.g., going → /goɪn/)
/l, r/	Omitted in medial and final positions (e.g., poor → /po/) Replaced occasionally by /ə/ in final position (e.g., pill → /pɪə/; here /hiə/)
/θ/	Replaced by /t/ or /f/ in initial, medial, and final positions (e.g., author → /ɔfə/; math → /mæf/)
/ð/	Replaced by /d/ in initial position and /d/ or /v/ in medial and final positions (e.g., this → /dɪs/; mother → /mʌvɚ/)
/z/	Omitted or replaced by /d/ before nasal sounds (e.g., isn't /ɪdnt/)
Blends	
/str/	Replaced by /skr/ (e.g., street → /skrit/)
/ʃr/	Replaced by /str/ (e.g., shrill → /strɪl/)
/θr/	Replaced by /θ/ (e.g., throw → /θo/)
/pr, br, gr, kr/	Omission of /r/ (e.g., apron → /epən/; agriculture → /ægɪkəltʃɚ/)
Consonant Clusters	
/sk, nd, sp, ft, ld, dʒd, st, sd, nt/	Deletion of second consonant in final word position (e.g., left → /lɛf/; cold → /kol/; desk → /dɛs/)

Sources: Adapted from "Some Aspects of African-American Vernacular English Phonology," by G. Bailey and E. Thomas, 1998, in *African-American English: History and Use* (pp. 85–109), by S. Mufwene, J. Rickford, G. Bailey, and J. Baugh (Eds.), London: Routledge; *Cultural and Linguistic Diversity Resource Guide for Speech-Language Pathologists*, by B. Goldstein, 2000, Clifton Park, NY: Cengage Learning; *Language Development: An Introduction* (8th ed.), by R. E. Owens, 2011, Needham Heights, MA: Allyn & Bacon; "Some Linguistic Features of Negro Dialect," by R. Fasold and W. Wolfram, 1970, in *Teaching Standard English in the Inner City* (pp. 41–86), by R. Fasold and R. Shuy (Eds.), Washington, DC: Center for Applied Linguistics; *Social Dialects: Differences vs. Disorders*, by R. Williams and W. Wolfram, 1977, Washington, DC: American Speech-Language-Hearing-Association.

Table 12–3
Morphologic and Syntactic Characteristics of African American English (AAE)

Structure	Description
Verbs	
Regular past -ed	Not obligatory and frequently omitted (e.g., I **talk** to him last week)
Irregular past	May remain uninflected or regularized with "-ed" (e.g., He **begin** work yesterday; She **knowed** all about it)
Regular present third-person singular	Not obligatory and frequently omitted (e.g., John **sleep** too much)
Irregular present third-person singular	Not obligatory and frequently omitted (e.g., He always **do** silly things)
Future tense	"Will" is replaced by "gonna"; "will" is omitted preceding the verb "be" (e.g., The dog **gonna** bite you; I **be** back tomorrow)
Copula and auxiliary	Not obligatory and may be omitted if contractible (e.g., He **ready**; They **eating**)
Perfect tense	"Been" is used to signify action in the distant past (e.g., He died long ago → He **been** dead)
Habitual state	Ongoing or general states are marked by uninflected "be" (e.g., She **be** funny)
Modals	Double modals are permissible with forms such as *might*, *could*, and *should* (e.g., They **might could** come)
Noun Phrases	
Regular plural -s	Not obligatory and frequently omitted when quantifiers are present (e.g., I see three **book** over there)
Irregular plural	May be doubly inflected (e.g., Help me find the **childrens**)
Possessive -'s	Not obligatory and frequently omitted when word order indicates possession (e.g., **Debbie** bike got wet)
Pronouns	
Apposition	Pronoun immediately follows the referent noun (e.g., My brother **he** bigger than you)
Relative pronouns	Not obligatory and frequently omitted (e.g., There's the **dog bit** me)
Reflexive pronouns	Reflexive -*self* form can be extended to possessive pronouns (e.g., **hisself; theirself**)
Demonstratives	Certain demonstrative/pronominal phrases are permissible (e.g., **These here** apples; **Them there** toys)

continues

Table 12–3
continued

Structure	Description
Adverbs and Adjectives	
Comparatives and superlatives	The forms *-er* and *-est* can be extended to many adjectives (e.g., **worser, horriblest**)
	The modifiers *more* and *most* can be added to comparative and superlative forms (e.g., **more taller; most oldest**)
Intensifiers	Certain modifiers can be added to adverbs or adjectives for emphasis (e.g., **right** quick; **plumb** crazy)
Negation	
Ain't	"Ain't" is a permissible negative form (e.g., I **ain't** got any money)
Multiple negation	Double and triple negative markers are permissible (e.g., **Nobody don't** like me; **Nobody don't never** talk to him)
Interrogatives	
Indirect questions	The inverted form may be used for indirect questions (e.g., I wonder what **was he** singing)
	The uninverted form may be used for direct questions (e.g., What **he was** eating?)
	The conditional conjunction *if* is replaced by *do* (e.g., I wonder **do** you hear me?)

Sources: Adapted from "Some Linguistic Features of Negro Dialect," by R. Fasold and W. Wolfram, 1970, in *Teaching Standard English in the Inner City* (pp. 41–86), by R. Fasold and R. Shuy (Eds.), Washington, DC: Center for Applied Linguistics; *Cultural and Linguistic Diversity Resource Guide for Speech-Language Pathologists*, by B. Goldstein, 2000, Clifton Park, NY: Delmar Cengage Learning; *Language Development: An Introduction* (8th ed.), by R. E. Owens, 2011, Needham Heights, MA: Allyn & Bacon; *Multicultural Students With Special Language Needs* (3rd ed.), by C. Roseberry-McKibbin, 2008, Oceanside, CA: Academic Communication Associates; "Dialect Forms During Discourse of Poor, Urban African-American Preschoolers," by J. Washington and H. Craig, 1994, *Journal of Speech and Hearing Research, 37*, 816–823; *Social Dialects: Differences vs. Disorders*, by R. Williams and W. Wolfram, 1977, Washington, DC: American Speech-Language-Hearing-Association.

Clinical Considerations for Children

Provision of effective intervention for children from CLD backgrounds requires basic knowledge of second-language acquisition in childhood. This knowledge base includes important terminology, patterns of L2 acquisition, and models of bilingual education.

Terminology

There are three main types of bilingualism:

- **Ambilingual:** Speaks both languages with the proficiency of a native speaker
- **Equilingual:** Communicates effectively in both languages
- **Semilingual:** Demonstrates poor mastery of both L1 and L2

Table 12–4
Pragmatic Characteristics of African American English (AAE)

- Direct eye contact is used in the speaker role, whereas indirect eye contact is associated with the listener role. Speakers of other dialects may interpret this indirect eye contact as inattentiveness or disrespect.

- Interruptions during conversation are permissible, and the role of speaker is yielded to the most assertive conversational partner. This interaction pattern may be interpreted by non-AAE speakers as impolite or rude.

- Silence is used as a communication strategy in unfamiliar situations or to refute a speaker's statement. In other dialects, this silence may be interpreted as lack of knowledge or acceptance of the speaker's statement.

- Questions about personal matters such as family, health, and education are considered rude and discourteous when addressed to a new acquaintance.

- Humor and sarcasm are highly valued aspects of communicative interactions and are often expressed in ritualized exchanges of insults and comebacks. These interactions may be misinterpreted by non-AAE speakers as instances of negative and hostile behavior.

- Conversations are considered to be private; verbal contributions from individuals outside the immediate conversational group are perceived as impolite eavesdropping behavior (even if the comments were intended to be helpful).

- Intense and demonstrative speech behavior is permissible in public conversational interactions. Speakers of other dialects may interpret this emotional display as irresponsible or in bad taste.

Sources: Adapted from *Communication Development and Disorders in African-American Children*, by A. Kamhi, K. Pollock, and J. Harris, 1996, Baltimore, MD: Paul H. Brookes; *Language Disorders From Infancy to Adolescence: Assessment and Intervention*, by R. Paul, 2007, Boston, MA: Mosby.

Mastery of a language can be described in two major ways:

- **Proficiency:** Competence in or mastery of a given language; may change over time

- **Dominance:** Preference for or comfort with a specific language in a particular context

Acquisition of L2 can be described according to two major functions (Butler, 2013; Godfroid & Hopp, 2022):

- **Basic interpersonal communication skills (BICS):** Use of language for social purposes (e.g., conversation, play, requesting, greetings). It is often supported by contextual cues, gestures, or facial expressions and takes 2 to 3 years to develop fully.

- **Cognitive-academic language proficiency skills (CALPS):** Use of language effectively for academic learning purposes (e.g., make inferences, compare and contrast, synthesize). Contextual cues and other supports are usually not available, so the individual must primarily rely on the linguistic code itself to derive meaning. This set of language skills generally takes about 5 to 7 years to develop fully.

Table 12-5
Speech Sound Production Characteristics of Spanish-Influenced English (SIE)

Phoneme	Description
/ɪ, æ/	Do not exist in Spanish and are replaced by other vowels (e.g., mister → /mistɚ/)
/d/	Dentalized in medial position
/ŋ/	Replaced by /n/ in the final position (e.g., song → /sɔn/)
/j/	Replaced by /dʒ/ in initial position (e.g., you → /dʒu/)
/ʃ/	Replaced by /tʃ/ in all positions (e.g., sheet → /tʃit/; washer → /wɔtʃɚ/)
/tʃ/	Replaced by /ʃ/ in all positions (e.g., chain → /ʃen/; teacher → /tiʃɚ/)
/dʒ/	Replaced by /j/ in initial and medial positions (e.g., major → /mejɚ/)
/θ/	Replaced by /t/ in initial and final positions and omitted in medial position (e.g., think → /tɪnk/; baths → /bæs/)
/v/	Replaced by /b/ in all positions (e.g., vowel → /baul/; oven → /ʌbɛn/)
/z/	Replaced by /s/ in all positions (e.g., zero → /siro/; blizzard → /blɪsɚd/)
/ð/	Replaced by /d/ in initial and final positions; replaced by /d/, /v/, or /θ/ in medial position (e.g., they → /de/; brother → /brʌθɚ/)
	Consonants in the final position are usually devoiced (e.g., cab → /kæp/; bug → /bʌk/)
	A schwa or /ɛ/ is often added before consonant blends beginning with /s/ (e.g., speech → /əspitʃ/; slow → /ɛslo/)

Sources: Adapted from *Communication Disorders in Multicultural and International Populations* (4th ed.), by D. E. Battle, 2012, St. Louis, MO: Mosby; *Cultural and Linguistic Diversity Resource Guide for Speech-Language Pathologists*, by B. Goldstein, 2000, Clifton Park, NY: Delmar Cengage Learning; *Language Development: An Introduction* (8th ed.), by R. E. Owens, 2011, Needham Heights, MA: Allyn & Bacon; *Language Disorders from Infancy to Adolescence: Assessment and Intervention*, by R. Paul, 2007, Boston, MA: Mosby.

L1 and L2 can influence one another in the following reciprocal ways:

- **Language interference/transfer:** The grammar, vocabulary, phonology, or pragmatics of L1 may have an impact on the production of utterances in L2. These effects are frequently perceived as errors.

- **Language loss:** Previously mastered skills in L1 can be negatively affected by the introduction of L2. If usage of L1 decreases significantly, the child will likely lose some degree of proficiency in that language.

Table 12-6
Morphologic and Syntactic Characteristics of Spanish-Influenced English (SIE)

Structure	Description
Verbs	
Regular past -ed	Not obligatory and frequently omitted (e.g., I **talk** to him last week)
Regular present third-person singular	Not obligatory and frequently omitted (e.g., John **sleep** too much)
Future	Use of *go* + *to* with omission of the verb *to be* as well as the progressive marker *-ing* (e.g., I **go to** store)
Copula	Occasional use of *have* instead of *be* in certain instances (e.g., I **have** 14 years)
Noun Phrases	
Regular plural -s	Not obligatory and frequently omitted (e.g., I see three **book** over there)
Possessive -'s	Replaced by prepositional phrase following the noun (e.g., This is the shirt **of my brother**)
Articles	Not obligatory and frequently omitted (e.g., They went **to movie**)
Pronouns	
Possessive pronouns	Replaced with article in reference to body parts (e.g., I broke **the** leg)
Subject pronouns	May be omitted when subject is specified in the preceding utterance (e.g., Maria is pretty. **Got** a new dress)
Adjectives	
Comparative -er	Replaced by modifier *more* (e.g., That table is **more** long)
Negation	
No	*No* replaces "auxiliary + *not*" before a verb (e.g., He **no** drink milk)
	No replaces *don't* in imperative forms (e.g., **No** touch that)
Interrogatives	
Inversion	Not obligatory and replaced by rising intonation (e.g., **Mama is** gone?)
Do insertion	Not obligatory and frequently omitted (e.g., **You want** more soup?)

Sources: Adapted from *Communication Disorders in Multicultural and International Populations* (4th ed.), by D. E. Battle, 2012, St. Louis, MO: Mosby; *Cultural and Linguistic Diversity Resource Guide for Speech-Language Pathologists*, by B. Goldstein, 2000, Clifton Park, NY: Delmar Cengage Learning; *Language Development: An Introduction* (8th ed.), by R. E. Owens, 2011, Needham Heights, MA: Allyn & Bacon; *Language Disorders From Infancy to Adolescence: Assessment and Intervention*, by R. Paul, 2007, Boston, MA: Mosby.

Table 12–7
Pragmatic Characteristics of Spanish-Influenced English (SIE)

- Indirect eye contact is used in conversation to convey attentiveness or respect. Speakers of other dialects may interpret this behavior in the opposite manner.

- Distance between speakers during conversation is relatively close.

- Touching one's communication partner is common during conversations. This contact may be perceived as offensive by speakers of other cultural orientations.

- Interruptions during conversation are permissible. This pattern of interaction may be interpreted by non-SIE speakers as impolite or rude.

- Formal or business conversations are opened with personal questions and remarks, which can be extensive. Speakers of other dialects may interpret this style of conversational initiation as intrusive, a sign of procrastination, or as "a waste of time."

Sources: Adapted from *Assessment and Intervention Resource for Hispanic Children*, by H. Kayser, 1998, San Diego, CA: Singular Publishing; *Language Disorders From Infancy to Adolescence: Assessment and Intervention*, by R. Paul, 2007, Boston, MA: Mosby.

Table 12–8
Speech Sound Production Characteristics of Asian-Influenced English (AIE)

- Speakers of AIE may shorten, lengthen, or otherwise distort English vowels. For example native speakers of Mandarin may produce *bead* as /bId/ or *fit* as /fit/.

- AIE speakers tend to omit or distort final consonants because the rule systems of many Asian languages highly restrict or eliminate consonant sounds in the final position (e.g., *did* → /dɪ/).

- In many Asian languages, /r/ and /l/ are not categorized as distinctly separate phonemes. As a result, these sounds may be used interchangeably in English (e.g., *rice* → /lais/).

- Consonant blends are uncommon in many Asian languages. AIE speakers tend to simplify clusters either by inserting a /ə/ into the blend (e.g., speakers of Chinese and Japanese) or by omitting the entire cluster (e.g., speakers of Vietnamese).

- Several Asian languages are predominantly monosyllabic in nature. AIE speakers may shorten or misplace stress on multisyllabic words (e.g., sepa'rately).

- Asian languages such as Chinese, Vietnamese, or Laotian use changes in "tone" (prosody) to signify changes in word meaning. In contrast, tonal changes in English are used to differentiate declarative from interrogative utterances and to convey communicative intent (e.g., sarcasm, humor, protest). AIE speakers may experience difficulty acquiring English intonation patterns, and their messages may frequently be misinterpreted.

Sources: Adapted from *Assessing Asian Language Performance: Guidelines for Assessing Limited-English-Proficient Students*, by L. L. Cheng, 1987a, Gaithersburg, MD: Aspen; "Cross-Cultural and Linguistic Considerations in Working With Asian Populations," by L. L. Cheng, 1987b, *ASHA, 29*, 33–38; *Language Development: An Introduction* (8th ed.), by R. E. Owens, 2011, Needham Heights, MA: Allyn & Bacon.

Table 12–9
Morphologic and Syntactic Characteristics of Asian-Influenced English (AIE)

Structure	Description
Verbs	
Regular past -ed	Not obligatory and frequently omitted (e.g., He **walk** home yesterday)
Irregular past	May be regularized with *–ed* or doubly inflected, even in the perfect tense (e.g., He **sleeped** in the bed; He **didn't ran** home; He **had wented**)
Singular present	Not obligatory and frequently omitted in third person; overly inflected in second person (e.g., He usually **walk** to school; You **talks** too loud)
Auxiliary	*Be* and *do* may be omitted or remain uninflected (e.g., He **eating** dinner now; He **do** not know her)
Perfect tense	Marker *-en* is not obligatory and frequently omitted (e.g., I **have speak** to her)
Noun Phrases	
Regular plural -s	Not obligatory and frequently omitted when quantifiers are present (e.g., I have **three shirt**)
Irregular plural	May be doubly inflected and overregularized (e.g., She brushed her **teeths**)
Possessive -'s	Not obligatory and frequently omitted (e.g., That my **mom** hat)
Pronouns	
Possessive	Pronoun usage may be confused (e.g., I see **she** car)
Case	Subject and object pronouns may be confused (e.g., **Him** coming soon)
Gender	Male and female pronouns may be confused (e.g., I meet **her** wife)
Demonstratives	Singular and plural pronouns may be confused (e.g., He own **that** cars)
Adjectives	
Comparatives	The form *-er* may be extended to many adjectives (e.g., **gooder, honester**)
	The modifier *more* may be added to comparative forms (e.g., She is **more shorter** than me)
Negation	
Multiple negation	Double negative markers are permissible (e.g., He **didn't** have **none**)
No	*No* replaces "auxiliary + *not*" (e.g., He **no** live here)
Interrogatives	
Inversion	Not obligatory and replaced by rising intonation (e.g., **You are** coming home?)
Do insertion	Not obligatory and frequently omitted (e.g., **You see** her today?)

continues

Table 12–9
continued

Structure	Description
Prepositions	May be omitted or confused (e.g., I put **it drawer**; I am **at kitchen**)
Conjunctions	Not obligatory and frequently omitted (e.g., **Brother sister** went home)
Articles	May be omitted or overused (e.g., I saw **boy**; I go to **the school**)
Word Order	Changes in word order frequently occur (e.g., I have **car new**; **Book mine** got lost; He put **down it**)

Sources: Adapted from "Cross-Cultural and Linguistic Considerations in Working With Asian Populations," by L. L. Cheng, 1987b, *ASHA, 29*, 33–38; *Language Development: An Introduction* (8th ed.), by R. E. Owens, 2011, Needham Heights, MA: Allyn & Bacon.

Table 12–10
Pragmatic Characteristics of Asian-Influenced English (AIE)

- Direct eye contact is avoided; indirect eye contact is used in conversation to convey respect. Speakers of other dialects may interpret this behavior unfavorably.

- Interruptions during conversations are considered impolite. Children who ask questions or interrupt teachers during classroom lectures are considered disobedient. Western cultures may perceive this behavior (i.e., not asking questions during lecture) as passive and nonparticipatory.

- Third-party introductions are preferred to informal self-introductions, especially when interacting with individuals of high status. Non-AIE speakers may regard this preference for formal introductions as unfriendly or aloof behavior.

- Questions about age, marital status, or employment are considered appropriate, even of new acquaintances in order to establish proper social distance between or among the speakers. Western cultures may regard such queries as inappropriate or nosy, especially in initial conversations.

- Professionals are automatically treated with respect and are regarded as authorities.

- Kinship terms may be used with elders who are not family members as an indication of respect.

- Embarrassment is a common reaction to praise; humility is emphasized and highly valued.

- Feelings are not openly exhibited; public affection is not displayed. The facial expressions of AIE speakers may remain impassive even when being provoked or reprimanded. Western speakers may perceive this affect as indifference or insensitivity.

- Giggling may reflect shyness or embarrassment rather than amusement.

- Direct and open disagreement is infrequent, particularly with individuals regarded as high-status professionals or authorities. Speakers in Western cultures may misinterpret this behavior as an indication of agreement.

Sources: Adapted from *Assessing Asian Language Performance: Guidelines for Assessing Limited-English-Proficient Students,* by L. L. Cheng, 1987a, Gaithersburg, MD: Aspen; Cross-Cultural and Linguistic Considerations in Working With Asian Populations, by L. L. Cheng, 1987b, *ASHA, 29*, 33–38; *Collaborating With Interpreters and Translators,* by H. W. Langdon and L. R. Cheng, 2002, Eau Claire, WI: Thinking Publications.

Patterns of Second-Language Acquisition

There are two major patterns of L2 acquisition:

- **Simultaneous** (Bialystok, 2018; Dale et al., 2018a; Preston et al., 2022): The child is exposed to and acquires L1 and L2 from birth. In this ideal, although rare scenario, the child develops BICS in both languages with relatively equivalent levels of proficiency.

- **Sequential/successive** (Bialystok, 2018; Dale et al., 2018b; Preston et al., 2022): L2 is introduced later in childhood, usually after 3 years of age, when a significant portion of BICS in L1 is already in place.

The age or stage at which L2 is introduced strongly influences the degree of bilingualism that a child will demonstrate (Marian & Hayakawa, 2021; Montanari et al., 2018). For example, if L2 is introduced in the early primary grades, then the child will tend to present as *equilingual* (i.e., able to communicate effectively in either language). Children who are exposed to L2 at later ages or grade levels will generally present in a manner that more closely resembles *semilingual* (i.e., does not demonstrate native proficiency in either language). In addition to the age of exposure, the relative amounts that each language is used as well as the contexts in which each are used also affect the degree of bilingualism.

Educational Models

Various educational approaches exist for children from CLD backgrounds:

- **Immersion:** L1 is deemphasized, and all instruction is conducted in L2.

- **Transitional:** L1 is used to teach L2 until students can acquire the classroom curriculum effectively in L2 (at which point L1 is faded out).

- **Maintenance:** Both L1 and L2 continue to be used in instructional settings to varying degrees, with the goal of maintaining some level of proficiency in the child's native language.

Clinical Considerations for Adult Populations

Very little information is available to guide clinicians in the treatment of adults from CLD backgrounds. Following is a compilation of clinically relevant information that SLPs can incorporate into the development and delivery of intervention (Babatsouli, 2021; Larkman et al., 2022; Vicente et al., 2019):

- Language disorders often exist in both languages. Thus, assessments in each language are necessary to determine the types of linguistic difficulties in each language.

- For bilingual speakers, the same type and severity of aphasia may be present in both languages, or severity may be greater in one language (even after adjusting for premorbid proficiency levels).

- An effective approach for enhancing recovery from aphasia in bilingual speakers includes an emphasis on cross-linguistic generalization from a treated to an untreated language.

- Word retrieval can be improved in bilingual aphasia by selecting training stimuli that are similar in both meaning and phonetic form across L1 and L2 (e.g., *plate/plato* rather than *apple/manzana*). This clinical concept also applies to emphasizing the underlying processes that are common to both languages (e.g., attention, categorization, problem-solving strategies).

- Repeated presentation of therapy stimuli may improve the ability to gain or regain cognitive skills in L1 or L2.

- Therapy provided only in L2 results in positive outcomes even with bilingual speakers with chronic aphasia (Larkman et al., 2022). Direct treatment in L2 alone does not harm L1 unless it is accompanied by a recommendation to avoid use of L1 outside the clinic setting. However, complete inattention to one language in the clinical setting combined with a recommendation to avoid using it outside the clinic may result in a persistent and greater impairment in that language.

- Speech-language intervention most often is conducted in the language that is common to both the clinician and the client. For this reason, programming should incorporate stimulation/facilitation strategies for the nontreated language in environments outside of the clinical setting.

For dysarthric speakers of tonal languages (i.e., when single-word meanings are conveyed by tones), therapy that targets pitch variation at the single-word level may be the most effective approach for improving a client's ability to accurately produce the tones. Therapy can be structured to emphasize functional communication that involves longer utterances accompanied by more contextual cues for the listener. This strategy will decrease dependence on single-word production, which is highly reliant on tone variation to signal meaning.

Clinical Considerations for Multilingual Populations With Language Disorders

As in typically developing individuals, there are many factors that influence the effects of multilingualism on individuals with developmental disorders. Goral and Conner's (2013) literature review provides guidance for treating multilingual individuals with language disorders. Although the literature is currently limited in this area, there are several findings that can inform intervention as well as provide information for multilingual and multicultural families:

- When possible, a bilingual approach to therapy with individuals with specific language impairment (SLI) can result in benefits to both languages (Kohnert et al. 2020; Law et al., 2019). Furthermore, L2 gains from bilingual treatment were comparable to L2 treatment alone.

- For SLI, treatment in L1 has been found to benefit L2 abilities, although the opposite scenario of treatment in L2 has not been found to provide much benefit to L1.

- No evidence supports the notion that exposing individuals with autism spectrum disorders to multiple languages will negatively impact their abilities to learn and use multiple languages.

- Although individuals with Down syndrome can learn to effectively communicate in multiple languages, strategies such as repetition and highly structured language interventions may be necessary to facilitate multiple language learning.

In addition to cultural and linguistic diversity, SLPs also face a diverse variety of disorders within their scope of practice. Factors and strategies to consider with regard to specific disorders and conditions among CLD populations include the following:

- Individuals with brain injury (e.g., traumatic brain injury [TBI], aphasia) may feel socially isolated depending on cultural views on neurogenic disorders. Participation in rehabilitation also may differ based on a culture's view of possible treatments and outcomes (Qualls, 2012).

- Dysphagia intervention in CLD populations requires consideration of factors such as the role of food and meals within the culture, nutrition and health issues related to dietary preferences of a culture, and culture-specific dietary restrictions (Ambrocio & Shune, 2022; Qualls, 2012).

- The linguistic properties of a language can impact the manner in which motor speech disorders manifest. For example, intervention for an individual with dysarthria who speaks a tonal language may require a greater emphasis on targeting suprasegmental aspects than intervention for an individual who speaks a nontonal language (Qualls, 2012).

- Some cultures may have theories as to the cause of certain disorders, such as stuttering, that are not based in scientific evidence (Medina et al., 2023; Robinson, 2012; Souza Mumy, 2023; Üstün-Yavuz et al., 2021). Patient and caregiver counseling can help promote greater understanding of communication disorders and the role of intervention.

- Voice and the vocal characteristics that are considered normal vary from culture to culture (Procter & Joshi, 2022). Thus, an individual may not perceive his or her voice as disordered in a new cultural context (e.g., nasality). Conversely, an SLP may not perceive certain vocal qualities as disordered (e.g., vocal volume). Pretreatment interviews and assessments can help an SLP to ascertain the client's motives for seeking intervention (Behlau & Murry, 2012).

Helpful Hints

1. Children from Spanish-speaking and African American backgrounds tend to learn vocabulary words more effectively in tasks that involve descriptions and functions of target words rather than in tasks that emphasize labeling.

2. Some vocabulary words are differentially harder for specific CLD groups of children because of reduced exposure to certain words and/or prior experiences. In the selection of vocabulary targets, clinicians need to consider a child's prior knowledge and experiences rather than using curriculum as the sole source of material.

3. Use formal titles and full names when addressing adult clients. First names or nicknames may be considered condescending or offensive.

4. Clinicians should make every effort to learn the correct pronunciation of clients' and family members' names.

5. There may be cultural inhibitions about sharing personal information. Clinicians should carefully explain the meaning and parameters of confidentiality in the clinical process.

6. When intervention requires information gathering about family members or personal issues, the clinician should review standardized questionnaires and omit or modify items as appropriate given a client's specific background.

7. Clients from CLD backgrounds may require additional support in developing mainstream cultural knowledge (e.g., history, arts, news events) to facilitate their acquisition of reading and writing skills.

8. Use of dialects such as AAE should not be assumed for any particular individual. Use of AAE may be influenced by factors such as age, SES, and geographic region.

9. A speaker's use of code-switching should not be interpreted as an indicator of poor linguistic mastery. In fact, a speaker of multiple languages or dialects should be encouraged to code-switch strategically to maximize communication success in different environments with different listeners.

10. The role of the family varies in different cultures. This aspect may impact factors such as the point of contact for a family as well as the family's view on completing homework assignments in the home environment.

11. Although it is important to be aware of CLD factors when planning intervention, it is also important to note that individual variation occurs within cultures. Thus, a client's cultural and linguistic preferences are best identified through interactions that will either confirm or alter expected CLD norms.

12. Interpreters may be needed to discuss intervention progress with family members. In addition, ASHA provides resources (e.g., informational brochures) that are written in other languages to help provide information to linguistically diverse clients.

13. In-service trainings on CLD, especially the aspects specific to the cultures and languages present in one's work environment, can provide beneficial information for staff members (e.g., teachers, other therapists) to use when interacting with clients from diverse backgrounds.

14. Clinicians can increase awareness of their sensitivity regarding clients/patients from CLD backgrounds. ASHA provides a "Personal Reflection Checklist" that can be used for this purpose (ASHA, 2010).

Conclusion

This chapter has presented basic information and considerations for multicultural issues in intervention at an *introductory* level. This information is intended only as a starting point in the reader's clinical education and training. For in-depth coverage of this area, the following readings are recommended:

Battle, D. E. (2012). *Communication disorders in multicultural and international populations* (4th ed.). Mosby.

Grosjean, F., & Byers-Heinlein K. (2018). *The listening bilingual: Speech perception, comprehension, and bilingualism.* Wiley & Sons.

Hyter, Y., & Salas-Provance, M. (2022). *Culturally responsive practices in speech, language, and hearing sciences* (2nd ed.). Plural Publishing.

Li, S., Hiver, P., & Papi, M. (Eds.). (2022). *The Routledge handbook of second language acquisition and individual differences.* Taylor & Francis.

Paul, R., Norbury, C., & Gosse, C. (2018). *Language disorders from infancy through adolescence: Listening, speaking, reading, writing, and communicating* (5th ed.). Elsevier.

Additional Resources

Bilingual Language, Speech, and Special Education Dictionary

This resource is for English and Spanish speakers and provides definitions for terms commonly used by speech-language pathologists, audiologists, and special educators. It also includes terminology related to Individualized Education Program (IEP) objectives and clinician–family interactions.

Working With Interpreters and Translators: A Guide for Speech-Language Pathologists and Audiologists

This text provides the SLP with information on how to conduct interviews, assessments, and conferences with individuals with limited English proficiency. It covers areas such as cultural considerations, training suggestions for interpreters and translators, and best practice recommendations for conducting assessments with and without materials in a given language.

Chapter 13

Contemporary Issues

The field of speech-language pathology is characterized by a foundation of solid knowledge in the area of communication disorders. There also are a multitude of emerging areas of interest that are relevant on a profession-wide scale. Of these evolving topics, the authors chose four areas for introductory-level discussion in this chapter: critical thinking, telepractice, clinical simulation training, and billing/coding issues. The dynamic nature of growth and change in these areas will require effective clinicians to continue their learning throughout their careers.

Critical Thinking

As defined in Chapter 1, critical thinking is the objective analysis and evaluation of an issue to form a reasoned judgment that goes beyond memorization/recall of information and is free from feelings or personal biases. Critical thinking is practiced intentionally. It requires evaluating claims of others and judging the acceptability/reliability of an argument. Many resources identify critical thinking as an important skill for both clinicians and students but often fail to provide an accompanying rationale. Based on our collective years of experience, the authors of this text believe that in most situations, including professional ones, individuals tend to rely heavily on familiar beliefs, which may lead to unintentionally biased thinking and poor decision-making. Therefore, mindful engagement in and application of the critical-thinking process can significantly minimize the impact of cognitive bias on clinical work. For more detailed information, see the scoping literature review by Berg et al. (2023).

Components of Critical Thinking

In 2015, the American Speech-Language-Hearing Association (ASHA) identified critical thinking and evidence-based problem-solving as fundamental to clinical practice and suggested that it underlies all treatment decisions. The description of critical thinking outlined by Finn et al. (2016) is a useful tool for "thinking about thinking." Following is a list of the major components of their rubric, which is then followed by a brief discussion of each facet:

1. Argument analysis

    Stage A: interpretation

    Stage B: evaluation

    Stage C: metacognition

2. Thinking disposition

3. Knowledge of cognitive biases

Argument Analysis

This is a fundamental component of the critical-thinking process. *Interpretation* as the initial stage requires the clinician to recognize when uncertainty exists in a given situation and deliberately weigh the need for critical thinking to counterbalance that perceived uncertainty. The clinician must decide how much he or she knows about the relevant point/topic and clarify what further information is necessary to achieve reasonably effective decisions. *Evaluation* is the next stage in argument analysis and examines the relevancy or plausibility of reasons for supporting a particular decision. The quality and amount of evidence are important aspects to be considered during this phase of the process. For instance, personal experience/anecdotes may not be weighted as heavily as data from a randomly controlled trial. In turn, a reason that seems more substantive may, upon reflection, be judged as relevant to only a narrowly restricted population of clients. *Metacognition* is the final stage of the argument analysis component of critical thinking. It obligates the clinician to actively engage in attempts to objectively monitor his or her use of critical-thinking skills. Mindful application and monitoring of success of critical-thinking strategies can help facilitate solid decision-making in nearly all clinical situations.

Thinking Disposition

Thinking dispositions consist of various attitudes toward forming/modifying beliefs and making decisions, and they are often considered essential complements to critical thinking. In more familiar terms, these can be considered as "values" or "intellectual traits." The most useful example of this concept is "open-mindedness." This refers to the degree to which an individual is willing to consider alternative viewpoints rather than relying on a reflexive belief that a familiar or previously favored approach is the best. Thinking dispositions that favor a balanced and relatively objective attitude toward evaluating competing sources of knowledge are key to the implementation of successful decision-making and problem-solving.

Knowledge of Cognitive Biases

Implicit biases are well-documented "thinking errors." These tendencies influence the unintentional development of erroneous beliefs and act as lenses that have the power to distort objective evaluation of facts and other information (i.e., cognitive dissonance). Much discussion in the literature is devoted to a particular form of skewed thinking known as "confirmation bias," which can significantly impact clinical work. This proposition assumes that humans are predisposed toward evidence that supports their existing beliefs and that we ignore, downplay, or distort evidence that questions these biases (Nickerson, 1998). Reactions to the cognitive dissonance created by new information can range from, "Well, this must be right since it fits neatly with what I already know about the topic" versus the opposite end of the comfort spectrum: "Well, this point of view is nonsense since it is completely at odds with what I already know about the topic." Clinicians are encouraged to actively consider the possibility that confirmation bias is operating at least occasionally in their clinical decision-making process and seek out ways to recognize/mitigate this implicit influence on their thinking.

Strategies/Techniques for Promoting Critical Thinking

In the literature from many fields, there are rubrics/guidelines that encourage critical thinking (Dwyer, 2017). Rubrics with easily depicted visual representations can serve as examples of critical-thinking approaches that are applicable to the education and clinical work of speech-language pathologists (SLPs). Three approaches are depicted:

- **Bloom's cognitive taxonomy** (Figure 13–1)

- **Argument mapping** (Figure 13–2): The purpose of mapping is to (a) uncover the logical structure of arguments, (b) identify unstated assumptions, (c) evaluate the support an argument offers for a conclusion, and (d) aid in understanding of debates. Argument maps often are designed to visually support deliberation of issues and/or ideas (van Gelder, 2015; Yilmaz-Na, & Sönmez, 2023).

- **Reflective thinking** (Figure 13–3): One long-standing and effective framework for encouraging thoughtful decision-making and problem-solving is the What—So What—Now What process.

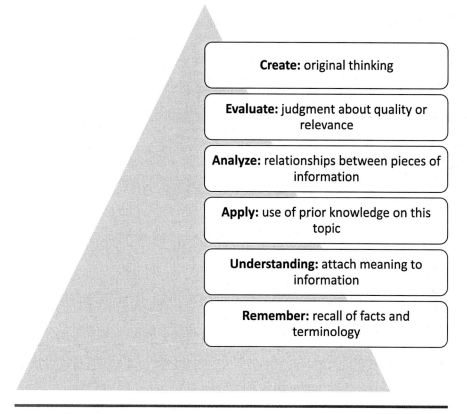

Figure 13–1
Bloom's taxonomy. Adapted from Knowledge Pyramid (2001).

Figure 13–2
Argument map.

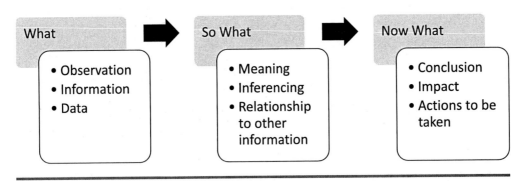

Figure 13–3
What—So What—Now What.

When uncertainty arises in clinical work, the following list of reflective questions (adapted from Browne & Keely, 2015) can be useful in guiding clinicians through the critical-thinking process:

- What are the issues?

- What are the reasons?

- What words or phrases are ambiguous?

- What are the assumptions?

- Are there fallacies in the reasoning?

- How good is the evidence?

- Are there rival causes?

- Are the statistics deceptive?

- What significant information is missing?

- What reasonable conclusions are possible?

Repeated learning opportunities with the application of critical thinking are necessary for this thinking orientation to become a routine clinical practice. Student clinicians, in particular, can benefit from a combined approach to instruction that is taught (a) as the content of a course on critical thinking and (b) as part of speech-language pathology course/clinical material (Cook et al., 2019; Grillo et al., 2015; McCurtin et al., 2019; Morris et al., 2018). Clinicians must design their selected instructional strategies based on client need and the existing evidence base. An important part of strategy development is being prepared to incorporate critical thinking while engaged in treatment planning and implementation. Interprofessional collaboration will be an important part of clinical practice throughout a clinician's career, and critical thinking is recognized as a core competency for engaging in that process (Interprofessional Education Collaborative Expert Panel, 2011).

Telepractice

Telepractice (and its educational counterpart, telesupervision) is a clinical model that is used for the provision of services to clients or groups of clients and can serve as a clinical educational model. It involves the use of telecommunications to deliver clinical services at a distance. SLPs use telepractice to treat clients who cannot participate in face-to-face therapy because of distance, mobility issues, or unavailability of SLPs in underserved regions or to provide access to SLPs in specialized areas of expertise (ASHA, n.d.-a). In addition, telepractice can be used for other important professional responsibilities, such as participating in or leading Individualized Education Program (IEP) meetings. From the perspective of clinical education, telesupervision, or e-supervision, refers to the use of video-/audioconferencing technologies or electronic messaging (such as email) to provide clinical supervision to students at a distant site.

When used appropriately, telepractice models may help address the following:

- Persistent and growing shortages of SLPs by increasing the number of qualified SLPs from communication science disorders (CSD) programs

- Issues of limited clinical capacity while ensuring a high-quality supervisory experience

- The persistent issue of available extern practicum sites by increasing the number and variety of potential clinical practicum placements and experiences for students

- The needs of some students whose geographic locations require long-distance clinical supervision

Two common descriptors of these service/education models are synchronous and asynchronous. Synchronous telepractice occurs between a client and clinician in real time using video- or audioconferencing and simulates traditional face-to-face therapy sessions. In synchronous telesupervision, the student and supervisor communicate in real time using web-conferencing technologies. This provides live supervision of student clinicians in off-campus clinical placements. In asynchronous models of telepractice and telesupervision (also called "store and forward"), images or data are captured and transmitted for later viewing, reviewing, or interpretation by a professional (e.g., voice clips, session segments). Sometimes, these two models are used in combination with one another and are referred to as hybrid applications. Telepractice/telesupervision can be implemented in any setting as long as the services comply with national, state, institutional, and professional regulations or policies. These settings include schools, medical centers, rehabilitation hospitals, community health centers, outpatient clinics, universities, homes, residential health care facilities, and childcare centers. The onset of the pandemic resulted in a dramatic shift in service delivery for adults and children from traditional in-person treatment to remote telepractice services using Zoom or other synchronous videoconferencing technologies (Jakubowitz & Edwards-Gaither, 2023). Campbell and Goldstein (2021) put forth the term "telepractitioners" to describe this new role of speech-language clinicians in an online treatment environment.

Evidence Base for Telepractice

The literature regarding the efficacy of telepractice has increased since the onset of the pandemic. In general, most systematic reviews found significant support for the use of telepractice in speech-language therapy as well as other health care fields (deNocker & Toolan, 2023; Kichloo et al., 2020). Many of the treatment-efficacy articles focus on particular disorders (e.g., apraxia, aphasia, autism, etc.). The next two paragraphs will present an overview of selected articles that address efficacy in adult and pediatric populations.

Available evidence indicates that telepractice/teletherapy is an appropriate and effective treatment model for adults. Weidner and Lowman's (2021) systematic review showed that telepractice was most successful for patients with chronic aphasia, Parkinson's disease, and dysphagia. Chaudhary et al. (2021) reported similar positive findings for adults with fluency, voice, swallowing and neurogenic disorders. Future research efforts using well-designed studies will contribute to a fuller understanding of the effects and challenges of speech-language telepractice with adults.

The evidence base for telepractice with children includes many studies that focus on speech sound production and autism. Preliminary evidence suggests that school-age children with speech sound disorders (Coufal et al., 2018) and childhood apraxia of speech (Bahar et al., 2022) achieve meaningful improvement in their therapeutic programs when delivered remotely via telepractice. For children with autism, Christopolou et al. (2022) and Sutherland et al. (2018) found significant evidence regarding the equivalency of remote versus in-person service delivery. Parents and students rate telepractice efficacy as high but report that "distant" treatment is less effective than an on-site mode of service delivery (Lam et al., 2021).

Privacy and Regulatory Issues

Patient privacy concerns should be considered carefully when telepractice is chosen as a service delivery mechanism. Some current videoconferencing systems may meet data security requirements for the Health Insurance Portability and Accountability Act (HIPAA), especially through formal business associate agreements. It is the clinician's responsibility to ensure that the platform being used to deliver therapeutic services is sufficiently secure. The website for the U.S. Department of Health and Human Services provides detailed guidance regarding patient privacy. It is equally important that clinicians who use social media (e.g., to ask advice about a case) carefully consider patient confidentiality. Simply omitting patient names from your postings is insufficient to protect their identity. Even information on clinicians' social media profiles (e.g., where they live or work) can contribute to unintentional breaches of patient confidentiality. SLPs can consult the ASHA Code of Ethics (2023) for further guidance (see Appendix A on the companion website).

In addition to federal regulations prescribed by HIPAA, state and/or local regulations applicable to telepractice must also be considered. Currently, best practices suggest that the SLPs should hold valid licensure in the home state as well as the state in which the services are received. The state-by-state section of ASHA's website clearly describes regulatory information relevant to telepractice for all 50 states. This is a rapidly evolving area of clinical practice, and SLPs need to stay abreast of regulatory changes.

Basic Clinician Competencies With Technology

Beyond knowledge of therapy content, clinicians need to demonstrate additional mastery of fundamental technology skills in order to successfully engage in telepractice (Curtis, 2014):

- Identify basic equipment needed to complete telepractice session
- Enter a meeting via a click
- Start audio
- Start video
- Adjust audio and video settings
- End or leave a meeting

The specifics of these skills will vary with the equipment and meeting platform being used.

Candidates for Telepractice Services

Selection

Many factors affect the success of intervention delivered via telepractice. One of the most important tasks for clinicians is to identify appropriate clients as candidates. There are several areas that SLPs should consider during the selection process (adapted from ASHA, n.d.-a). These include the following:

- Physical/sensory characteristics (e.g., hearing, vision, manual dexterity)
- Cognitive ability (e.g., problem-solving, memory, executive function)
- Behavioral characteristics (e.g., on-task focus, attention span, hyperactivity)
- Communication abilities (e.g., language comprehension, speech intelligibility, literacy skills)
- Access to technology (e.g., adequate equipment, reliable internet connections, tech support availability)
- Environment (e.g., minimal visual distractions, quiet setting, sufficient lighting)

Matching Session Design With Client Traits

As noted in Chapter 1, session design must be tailored to the needs and characteristics of individual clients. This same principle applies for a telepractice model of intervention. Based on the work of Curtis (2014), some examples for calibrating general client traits with session techniques are presented and can be applied to pediatric or adult cases:

Inattentive or Behavioral Issues

- Emphasize turn-taking tasks and preferred activities
- Balance client-directed and SLP-directed tasks

- Engage an "assistant" (e.g., spouse; classroom aide) within the client's physical environment to familiarize a client with a visual schedule of therapy activities prior to the therapy session

- Limit tasks to 10 items/trials

Difficulties With Transitions

- Keep stimulus format as consistent as possible throughout a session (e.g., cartoon figures versus photographs versus word lists)

- Closely monitor rate and volume variations of stimulus presentation

- Be prepared to "mute" or control the client's mouse during periods of persistent off-task behavior

The use of technology is expanding the ability of SLPs to deliver intervention into more remote geographic regions (e.g., rural communities) and to less familiar populations (e.g., prison inmates). Telepractitioners may fail to recognize cultural needs or barriers associated with a specific case as a result of the absence of in-person contact with the client. Self-monitoring for implicit or linguistic bias can help SLPs establish stronger and more effective therapeutic alliances with their clients. Therefore, clinicians must develop basic attitudes and interpersonal skills that value diversity (Edwards-Gaither, 2018).

Simulation Technologies

Simulations are student-centered instructional approaches and are increasingly being used in CSD educational programs to provide valuable clinical training experiences for future SLPs. Use of this teaching approach can be particularly valuable within the context of interprofessional education (IPE) in which students from multiple disciplines collaborate on the same training case. Simulation methods are used to enrich/enhance student learning delivered by traditional teaching methods. Simulated learning experiences also promote critical-thinking skills, such as self-reflection, problem-solving, self-confidence, and improved interpersonal skills. Simulations provide students with a representation of a real-world event with a primary focus on the patient's profile. There are various forms of simulation technologies, and the two most commonly used methods in the clinical preparation of SLPs are standardized patients and computer-based simulations.

Standardized Patients (SPs)

A standardized patient (SP) is an individual who is trained to act as an actual patient in a realistic, consistent, and repeatable way. The simulation includes body language, physical findings, and emotional and personality traits (Picou & Tharpe, 2015; Stead et al., 2023). SPs are trained to exhibit specific patterns of behaviors and responses during clinician–client interactions (Baylor et al., 2017; Carter, 2019) and provide every student with a similar experience. As discussed by Carter (2019), SPs do well portraying overt symptoms (e.g., stuttering, vocal tremors, speech sound errors, etc.) but do less well portraying covert symptoms, such as reduced language comprehension. This limitation becomes significant for clinical training in critical areas such as developmental language disorders. In addition, the authors currently are unaware of any studies in speech-language pathology in which children are trained as standardized patients.

Computer-Based Learning Experiences (CBLEs)

Computer-based simulations are powerful tools for learning. In CBLEs, the simulation is presented on a computer screen and is often based on technology that is used in gaming technologies (Dudding & Nottingham, 2018). Most often, these simulated learning environments use a case-based learning model. This approach provides multimodal input (video, audio, text) that is compatible with a broad range of student clinician learning styles. Students can control the pace and sequencing of information presentation, including repetition, as needed. Computer simulation programs often provide consistent feedback to learners, which allows them to monitor their progress through the case material. Van der Kleij et al. (2015) found that students' ability to monitor their own progress based on feedback facilitated increased understanding of complex material. As an example, SimuCase is a computer-based program designed for speech-language pathology training programs. The training cases are created by experienced SLPs, cover a broad range of disorders/ages, and incorporate a strong focus on formative feedback.

Implementation

Research indicates that there are three components of best practice in simulations, regardless of the platform chosen (Dudding & Ingram, 2018), as discussed in the following sections.

Prebrief

Students meet with their instructor prior to the simulation activity to become familiar with the technology and to be introduced to the specific case. The student and instructor discuss and agree on the learning objectives for the activity.

Case Work (Scenario)

Students engage in the simulation activity with the guidance of an experienced instructor. The activity involves decision-making about a wide range of issues, such as pre-session planning, client interactions, implementation of relevant clinical work, and final summary/recommendations. Students will benefit from strong instruction during this portion of the simulated learning experience. Clarification and reinforcement of key teaching points are integral parts of this component.

Debrief

Significant student learning occurs in this component of the simulation experience (Dudding et al., 2019). Discussion generally focuses on the details of the case as well as the student's ability to integrate the clinical knowledge presented. One of the most important aspects of the debrief phase is the student's engagement in self-reflection and generalization.

Coding and Reimbursement

Reimbursement is an important and complex issue in health care. New developments in this area occur frequently and rapidly. Therefore, a comprehensive discussion of reimbursement issues is beyond the scope of this book. However, a brief introduction to several important concepts is provided in this section. Clinicians should be aware that insurers require the use of sets of alphanumeric codes to identify important information about patients. These include Current Procedural Terminology (CPT) codes and International Classification of Diseases, Tenth Revision (ICD-10) codes. Descriptions of a client's diagnosis or condition must be assigned an appropriate ICD-10 code, whereas descriptions of services provided/procedures performed need to be identified with CPT codes. The use of these in documentation may vary according to the setting in which intervention is provided.

CPT Codes

CPT codes were first developed in 1966 for the medical profession and are updated on an annual basis. In the early 1990s, these codes were expanded to include other health care professionals. The basic codes have five digits, and each code represents a specific type of service or procedure (e.g., evaluation, screening treatment). These codes are used for insurance coverage/payment and data analysis. There is a differential value assigned to each code based on factors such as level of expertise required, time/equipment required, and level of patient risk.

ICD-10 Codes

Developed by the World Health Organization to standardize disease classification across settings and providers, SLPs use these codes to identify specific disorders, such as cleft palate hearing loss, language impairment, and aphasia. Given the complexity of the ICD-10 coding system, clinicians must familiarize themselves with the correct application of subcodes and subclassifications related to their caseload and work setting.

Documentation

Accurate documentation describes the care provided and supports the codes used for billing/payment. Insurance companies or other agencies analyze documentation to determine payment in a process called *utilization review*. Documentation serves as the official record of frequency and types of services delivered. Types of documentation for SLPs include evaluation report, treatment plan/plan of care, progress notes, and discharge summaries. Goals and progress should be written in measurable terms.

Finally, several websites provide detailed information about appropriate use of these code sets. Clinicians can refer to the Centers for Medicare and Medicaid, the American Medical Association, and ASHA for more information. In particular, the ASHA website contains several resources including a model superbill (a comprehensive list of possible CPT codes for clinicians working with a variety of patient populations), FAQs, and informational modules on coding. In addition, this website provides information on Medicaid, Medicare, and private insurance. Coding, documentation, and reimbursement are complex aspects of professional practice; SLPs are encouraged to remember the acronym "ACUTE" (accurate, code-able, understandable, timely, error free).

Helpful Hints

1. Clinicians can use client case studies to promote active learning and clinical problem solving, as important components of critical thinking.

2. Technology often fails when least expected; clinicians should prepare back-up plans that can be used immediately when glitches occur in audio/visual systems or internet connections.

3. Students who struggle with grasping/using simulation technology may benefit from repeated exposures (three or more times) to the same videotaped simulation session within a short amount of time.

Conclusion

This chapter presented basic information on several topics of emerging importance to our profession. It is intended only as a starting point in the reader's clinical education and training. For in-depth coverage of these areas, the following readings are recommended.

Critical Thinking

Abrami, P. C., Bernard, R. M., Borokhovski, E., Waddington, D. I., Wade, C. A., & Persson, T. (2015). Strategies for teaching students to think critically: A meta-analysis. *Review of Educational Research, 85*(2), 275–314.

Browne, M. N., & Keeley, S. M. (2015). *Asking the right questions: A guide to critical thinking* (11th ed.). Prentice Hall.

Dwyer, C. P. (2017). *Critical thinking: Conceptual perspectives and practical guidelines.* Cambridge University Press.

Telepractice

Biggs, E. E., Therrien, M. C., Snodgrass, M. R., & Douglas, S. N. (2022). Voices from the field: Strategies for effective telepractice for children with autism who use augmentative and alternative communication. *Perspectives of the ASHA Special Interest Groups, 7*(2), 324–337.

Cutchin, G. M., Shelly, S., Petty, B., van Leer, E., Tripp, R. M., Klein, A. M., & Gillespie, A. I. (2023). A comparison of voice therapy attendance rates between in-person and telepractice. *American Journal of Speech-Language Pathology, 32*(3),1154–1164.

Edwards-Gaither, L. (2018). Cultural considerations for telepractice: An introduction for speech-language pathologists. *Perspectives of the ASHA Special Interest Groups, 3*(18), 13–20.

Jacobs, M., Briley, P. M., Fang, X., & Ellis, C. (2021). Telepractice treatment for aphasia: Association between clinical outcomes and client satisfaction. *Telemedicine Reports, 2*(1), 118–124.

Luxton, D. D., Nelson, E. L., & Maheu, M. M. (2016). *A practitioner's guide to telemental health: How to conduct legal, ethical, and evidence-based telepractice.* American Psychological Association.

Stone, J. (2019). *Integrating technology into modern therapies: A clinician's guide to developments and interventions.* Routledge.

Simulations

 Dudding, C., Brown, D., Estis, J., Szymanski, C., Zraick, R., & Mormer, E. (2019). *Best practices in healthcare simulations.* https://growthzonesitesprod.azureedge.net/wp-content/uploads/sites/1023/2020/03/Best-Practices-in-CSD.pdf

Dudding, C., & Ingram, S. (2018). *Health care simulation in clinical education.* https://academy.pubs
.asha.org/2018/08/health-care-simulation-in-clinical-education/

Hill, A. E., Ward, E., Heard, R., McAllister, S., McCabe, P., Penman, A., ... Walters, J. (2021). Simulation can replace part of speech-language pathology placement time: A randomised controlled
trial. *International Journal of Speech-Language Pathology, 23*(1), 92–102.

Nagdee, N., Sebothoma, B., Madahana, M., Khoza-Shangase, K., & Moroe, N. (2022). Simulations
as a mode of clinical training in healthcare professions: A scoping review to guide planning in
speech-language pathology and audiology during the COVID-19 pandemic and beyond. *South
African Journal of Communication Disorders, 69*(2), 905.

Riley, R. H. (Ed.). (2008). *Manual of simulation in healthcare.* Oxford University Press, USA.

Weir-Mayta, P., Green, S., Abbott, S., & Urbina, S. (2020). Incorporating IPE and simulation experiences into graduate speech-language pathology training. *Cogent Medicine, 7*(1), 1847415.

Coding and Reimbursement

Nikjeh, D. A. (2019). Ethical decision making: Coding and compliance dilemmas for speech-language
pathologists. *Perspectives of the ASHA Special Interest Groups, 4*(6), 1289–1297.

Schwartz, S. A. (2020). Frequent billing misconceptions and potential related dilemmas faced by
speech-language pathologists. *Perspectives of the ASHA Special Interest Groups, 5*(1), 97–101.

Swigert, N. B. (2018). *Documentation and reimbursement for speech-language pathologists: Principles and
practice.* Slack.

References

Adler, R. (n. d.). *Multicultural issues.* SpeechPathology.com. http://www.speechpathology.com/ask-the-experts/multicultural-issues-932

Adlof, S. M., & Hogan, T. P. (2019). If we don't look, we won't see: Measuring language development to inform literacy instruction. *Policy Insights from the Behavioral and Brain Sciences, 6*(2), 210–217.

Ahn, H. N., & Wampold, B. E. (2001). Where oh where are the specific ingredients? A meta-analysis of component studies in counseling and psychotherapy. *Journal of Counseling Psychology, 48*(3), 251.

Alamer, A., Melese, H., & Nigussie, F. (2020). Effectiveness of neuromuscular electrical stimulation on post-stroke dysphagia: A systematic review of randomized controlled trials. *Clinical Interventions in Aging, 15*(2020), 1521–1531.

Albert, M., Sparks, R., & Helm, N. (1973). Melodic intonation therapy for aphasia. *Archives of Neurology, 29*, 130–131.

Alegria, R., Vaz Freitas, S., & Manso, M. C. (2020). Effectiveness of voice therapy in patients with vocal fold nodules: A systematic search and narrative review. *European Archives of Oto-Rhino-Laryngology, 277*, 2951–2966.

Alhinti, L., Christensen, H., & Cunningham, S. (2020). An exploratory survey questionnaire to understand what emotions are important and difficult to communicate for people with dysarthria and their methodology of communicating. *International Journal of Psychological and Behavioral Sciences, 14*(7), 187–191.

Allghlerl, C., Bettens, K., Bruneel, L., D'haeseleer, E., Van Gaever, E., & Van Lierde, K. (2020). Effectiveness of speech intervention in patients with a cleft palate: Comparison of motor-phonetic versus linguistic-phonological speech approaches. *Journal of Speech, Language, and Hearing Research, 63*(12), 3909–3933.

Alighieri, C., Van Lierde, K., De Caesemaeker, A. S., Demuynck, K., Bruneel, L., D'haeseleer, E., & Bettens, K. (2021). Is high-intensity speech intervention better? A comparison of high-intensity intervention versus low-intensity intervention in children with a cleft palate. *Journal of Speech, Language, and Hearing Research, 64*(9), 3398–3415.

Allegra, E., La Mantia, I., Bianco, M. R., Drago, G. D., Le Fosse, M. C., Azzolina, A., . . . Saita, V. (2019). Verbal performance of total laryngectomized patients rehabilitated with esophageal speech and tracheo-esophageal speech: Impacts on patient quality of life. *Psychology Research and Behavior Management, 12*(2019), 675–681.

Allison, K. M., Cordella, C., Iuzzini-Seigel, J., & Green, J. R. (2020). Differential diagnosis of apraxia of speech in children and adults: A scoping review. *Journal of Speech, Language, and Hearing Research, 63*(9), 2952–2994.

Ambrocio, K. R., & Shune, S. E. (2022). Using backward design in dysphagia management: A paradigm shift toward more culturally responsive care. *Perspectives of the ASHA Special Interest Groups, 7*(6), 1998–2011.

American Psychiatric Association. (2013). *Diagnostic and statistical manual of mental disorders* (5th ed.).

American Speech-Language-Hearing Association (n.d.-a). *Telepractice* [Practice portal]. https://www.asha.org/Practice-Portal/Professional-Issues/Telepractice/

American Speech-Language Hearing Association (n.d.-b). *Communication after total laryngectomy* [Practice portal]. https://www.asha.org/practice-portal/clinical-topics/head-and-neck-cancer/communication-after-total-laryngectomy/

American Speech-Language-Hearing Association. (2000). *Roles and responsibilities of speech-language pathologists with respect to reading and writing in children and adolescents: Position statement, technical report, and guidelines.* https://www.asha.org/policy/ps2001-00104/

American Speech-Language-Hearing Association. (2007a). *Childhood apraxia of speech: Position statement.* https://www.asha.org/policy/ps2007-00277/

American Speech-Language-Hearing Association. (2007b). *Scope of practice in speech-language pathology.* http://www.asha.org/policy

American Speech-Language-Hearing Association. (2008). *Roles and responsibilities of speech-language pathologists in early intervention: Position statement, technical report, and guidelines.* https://www.asha.org/uploadedFiles/Demographic-Profile-Bilingual-Spanish-Service-Members.pdf

American Speech-Language-Hearing Association. (2015). *Practice portal: Spoken language.* https://www.asha.org/practice-portal/clinical-topics/spoken-language-disorders/

American Speech-Language-Hearing Association. (2016). *Scope of practice in speech-language pathology.* https://www.asha.org/policy/sp2016-00343/

American Speech-Language-Hearing Association. (2021). *2021 Demographic Profile of ASHA Members Providing Multilingual Services.* https://www.asha.org/siteassets/surveys/demographic-profile-bilingual-spanish-service-members.pdf

American Speech-Language-Hearing Association. (2023). *Code of ethics.* http://www.asha.org/policy/

Americans with Disabilities Amendments Act. (2008). https://www.eeoc.gov/statutes/ada-amendments-act-2008

Anderson, J., Wagovich, S., & Hall, N. (2006). Nonword repetition skills in young children who do and do not stutter. *Journal of Fluency Disorders, 31,* 177–199.

Anderson, J. D., & Conture, E. G. (2004). Sentence structure priming in young children who do and do not stutter. *Journal of Speech, Language, and Hearing Research, 47,* 552–571.

Anderson, K. L., & Goldstein, H. (2004). Speech perception benefits of FM and infrared devices to children with hearing aids in a typical classroom. *Language, Speech, and Hearing Services in Schools, 35,* 169–184.

Andrews, C., O'Brian, S., Onslow, M., Harrison, E., Packman, A., & Menzies, R. (2012). Syllable-timed speech treatment for school age children who stutter: A Phase I trial. *Language, Speech, and Hearing Services in Schools, 43,* 359–369.

Andrews, G., & Harris, M. (1964). The syndrome of stuttering. *Clinics in Developmental Medicine, 17.* Heinemann Medical Books.

Angadi, V., Croake, D., & Stemple, J. (2019). Effects of vocal function exercises: A systematic review. *Journal of Voice, 33*(1), 124.e13–124.e34.

Arciuli, J., Stevens, K., Trembath, D., & Simpson, I. (2013). The relationship between parent report of adaptive behavior and direct assessment of reading ability in children with autism spectrum disorders. *Journal of Speech, Language, and Hearing Research, 56*(6), 1837–1844.

Arnott, S., Onslow, M., O'Brian, S., Packman, A., Jones, M., & Block, S. (2014). Group Lidcombe Program treatment for early stuttering: A randomized controlled trial. *Journal of Speech, Language, and Hearing Research, 57*(5), 1606–1618.

Aronson, A. E., & Bless, D. (2009). *Clinical voice disorders* (4th ed.). Thieme Medical.

Asperger, H. (1944). Die "Autistischen Psychopathen" im Kindesalter. *European Archives of Psychiatry and Clinical Neuroscience, 117*(1), 76–136.

Association on Higher Education and Disability. (2008). [AHEAD is the leading professional membership association for individuals committed to equity for persons with disabilities in higher education.]. https://www.ahead.org/

Aulisio, M. C., Han, D. Y., & Glueck, A. C. (2020). Virtual reality gaming as a neurorehabilitation tool for brain injuries in adults: A systematic review. *Brain Injury, 34*(10), 1322–1330.

Avramovic, Rietdijk, R., Attard, M., Kenny, B., Power, E., & Togher, L. (2023). Cognitive and behavioral digital health interventions for people with traumatic brain injury and their caregivers: A systematic review. *Journal of Neurotrauma, 40*(3–4), 159–194.

Babatsouli, E. (2021). Diversity considerations in speech and language disorders: A focus on training. In J. S. Damico, N. Müller, & M. J. Ball (Eds.), *The handbook of language and speech disorders* (2nd ed., pp. 33–52). Wiley Blackwell.

Baddeley, A. D. (2007). *Working memory, thought, and action.* Oxford University Press.

Badian, N. A. (1999). Reading disability defined as a discrepancy between listening and reading comprehension. *Journal of Learning Disabilities, 32,* 138–148.

Bahar, N., Namasivayam, A. K., & van Lieshout, P. (2022). Telehealth intervention and childhood apraxia of speech: A scoping review. *Speech, Language and Hearing, 25*(4), 450–462.

Bahia, M. M., & Lowell, S. Y. (2020). A systematic review of the physiological effects of the effortful swallow maneuver in adults with normal and disordered swallowing. *American Journal of Speech-Language Pathology, 29*(3), 1655–1673.

Bailey, G., & Thomas, E. (1998). Some aspects of African-American vernacular English phonology. In S. Mufwene, J. Rickford, G. Bailey, & J. Baugh (Eds.), *African-American English: History and use* (pp. 85–109). Routledge.

Baker, E. (2012). Optimal intervention intensity. *International Journal of Speech-Language Pathology, 14*(5), 401–409.

Baker, E., & McLeod, S. (2011). Evidence-based practice for children with speech sound disorders: Part 1 narrative review. *Language, Speech, and Hearing Services in Schools, 42*(2), 102–139.

Baker, E., Williams, A. L., McLeod, S., & McCauley, R. (2018). Elements of phonological interventions for children with speech sound disorders: The development of a taxonomy. *American Journal of Speech-Language Pathology, 27*(3), 906–935.

Baker, S. K., Simmons, D. C., & Kameenui, E. J. (1998). Vocabulary acquisition: Reading bases. In D. C. Simmons & E. J. Kameenui (Eds.), *What reading research tells us about children with diverse learning needs: Bases and basics* (pp. 183–217). Lawrence Erlbaum.

Bakker, M., Beijer, L., & Rietveld, T. (2019). Considerations on effective feedback in computerized speech training for dysarthric speakers. *Telemedicine and e-Health, 25*(5), 351–358.

Ball, M. J. (2016). *Principles of clinical phonology.* Psychology Press.

Ballard, K. J. (2001). Response generalization in apraxia of speech treatments: Taking another look. *Journal of Communication Disorders, 34,* 3–20.

Ballard, K. J., Robin, D. A., McCabe, P., & McDonald, J. (2010). A treatment for dysprosody in childhood apraxia of speech. *Journal of Speech, Language, and Hearing Research, 53*(5), 1227–1245.

Balou, M., Herzberg, E. G., Kamelhar, D., & Molfenter, S. M. (2019). An intensive swallowing exercise protocol for improving swallowing physiology in older adults with radiographically confirmed dysphagia. *Clinical Interventions in Aging, 14,* 283–288.

Balthazar, C. H., & Scott, C. M. (2018). Targeting complex sentences in older children with specific language impairment: Results from an early-phase treatment study. *Journal of Speech, Language, and Hearing Research, 61(3),* 713–728.

Bambara, L. M., Cole, C. L., Kunsch, C., Tsai, S. C., & Ayad, E., (2016). A peer-mediated intervention to improve the conversational skills of high school students with autism spectrum disorder. *Research in Autism Spectrum Disorders, 27,* 29–43.

Bane, M., Angadi, V., Dressler, E., Andreatta, R., & Stemple, J. (2019). Vocal function exercises for normal voice: The effects of varying dosage. *International Journal of Speech-Language Pathology, 21*(1), 37–45.

Banerjee, R., & Luckner, J. (2014). Training needs of early childhood professionals who work with children and families who are culturally and linguistically diverse. *Infants and Young Children, 27*(1), 43–59.

Barkley, R. A. (1996). Linkages between attention and executive functions. In G. R. Lyon & N. A. Krasnegor (Eds.), *Attention, memory, and executive function* (pp. 307–325). Brookes.

Barkley, R. A. (1997). *ADHD and the nature of self-control.* Guilford Press.

Barlow, J. A., & Gierut, J. A. (2002). Minimal pair approaches to phonological remediation. *Seminars in Speech and Language, 23*(1), 57–68). Thieme Medical Publishers.

Baron-Cohen S., Leslie, A. M., & Frith, U. (1985). Does the autistic child have a "theory of mind"? *Cognition, 21,* 37–46.

Barwood, C. H. S., & Murdoch, B. E. (2013). rTMS as a treatment for neurogenic communication and swallowing disorders. *Acta Neurologica Scandinavica, 127*(2), 77–91.

Barwood, C. H. S., Murdoch, B. E., Whelan, B. M., Lloyd, D., Riek, S., O'Sullivan, J. D., . . . Wong, A. (2012). Improved receptive and expressive language abilities in nonfluent aphasic stroke patients after application of rTMS: An open protocol case series. *Brain Stimulation, 5,* 274–286.

Basso, A. (2018). Spontaneous recovery and language rehabilitation. In X. Seron & G. Deloche (Eds.), *Cognitive approaches in neuropsychological rehabilitation* (pp. 17–38). Routledge.

Basso, A., & Macis, M. (2011). Therapy efficacy in chronic aphasia. *Behavioral Neurology, 24,* 317–325.

Bates, C., Baxter, P., Bonney, H., Bremner, F., Bunn, L., Carrillo Perez-Tome, M., . . . Ealing, J. (2016). *Management of the ataxias towards best clinical practice.* Ataxia UK. https://www.ataxia.org.uk/Handlers/Download.ashx?IDMF=ed02c727a034-4c99-b2fb-4623479d5c88

Bates, E., Camaioni, L., & Volterra, V. (1975). The acquisition of performatives prior to speech. *Merrill-Palmer Quarterly, 21,* 205–224

Bates, E., & MacWhinney, B. (1987). Competition, variation, and language learning. In B. MacWhinney (Ed.), *Mechanisms of language learning* (pp. 157–194). Lawrence Erlbaum.

Battle, D. E. (1997). Multicultural considerations in counseling communicatively disordered persons and their families. In T. A. Crowe (Ed.), *Applications of counseling in speech-language pathology and audiology* (pp. 118–141). Williams & Wilkins.

Battle, D. E. (2012). *Communication disorders in multicultural and international populations* (4th ed.). Mosby.

Bauman-Waengler, J. (2011). *Articulatory and phonological impairments: A clinical focus* (4th ed.). Pearson.

Baxter, S., Johnson, M., Blank, L., Cantrell, A., Brumfitt, S., Enderby, P., & Goyder, E. (2016). Non-pharmacological treatments for stuttering in children and adults: A systematic review and evaluation of clinical effectiveness, and exploration of barriers to successful outcomes. *Health Technology Assessment, 20*(2), 1–302.

Baxter, T. W. (2018). *Relentless: How A massive stroke changed my life for the better.* Greenleaf Book Group Press.

Baylor, C., Burns, M. I., Struijk, J., Herron, L., Mach, H., & Yorkston, K. (2017). Assessing the believability of standardized patients trained to portray communication disorders. *American Journal of Speech-Language Pathology, 26*(3), 791–805.

Bear, D., & Templeton, S. (1998). Explorations in spelling: Foundations for learning and teaching phonics, spelling, and vocabulary. *The Reading Teacher, 52,* 222–242.

Beck, A. M., Kjaersgaard, A., Hansen, T., & Poulsen, I. (2018). Systematic review and evidence-based recommendations on texture modified foods and thickened liquids for adults (above 17 years) with oropharyngeal dysphagia—An updated clinical guideline. *Clinical Nutrition, 37*(6), 1980–1991.

Beck, A. R. (2021). A review of mindfulness and communication sciences and disorders students. *Perspectives of the ASHA Special Interest Groups, 6*(4), 795–805.

Beck, A. R., & Verticchio, H. (2018). Effectiveness of a method for teaching self-compassion to communication sciences and disorders graduate students. *American Journal of Speech-Language Pathology, 27*(1), 192–206.

Beck, A. T., Rush, A., Shaw, B., & Emery, G. (1979). *Cognitive therapy of depression.* Guilford Press.

Beck, I. L., McKeown, M. G., & Kucan, L. (2013). *Bringing words to life: Robust vocabulary instruction.* Guilford Press.

Behlau, M., & Murry, T. (2012). International and intercultural aspects of voice and voice disorders. In D. E. Battle (Ed.), *Communication disorders in multicultural and international populations* (4th ed., pp. 174–207). Mosby.

Behn, N., Francis, J., Togher, L., Hatch, E., Moss, B., & Hilari, K. (2021). Description and effectiveness of communication partner training in TBI: A systematic review. *Journal of Head Trauma Rehabilitation, 36*(1), 56–71.

Belanger, H. G., Kretzmer, T., Yoash-Gantz, R., Picket, T., & Tupler, L. A. (2009). Cognitive sequelae of blast-related versus other mechanisms of brain trauma. *Journal of the International Neuropsychological Society, 15*, 1–8.

Bellini, S., & Akullian, J. (2007). A meta-analysis of video modeling and video self-modeling interventions for children and adolescents with autism spectrum disorders. *Exceptional Children, 73*(3), 264–287.

Bellon-Harn, M. L. (2012). Dose frequency: Comparison of language outcomes in preschool children with language impairment. *Child Language Teaching and Therapy, 28*(2), 225–240.

Bellugi, U. (1967). *The acquisition of negation* [Unpublished doctoral dissertation]. Harvard University.

Benedict, H. (1979). Early lexical development: Comprehension and production. *Journal of Child Language, 6*, 183–200.

Bennett, T. A., Szatmari, P., Bryson, S., Duku, E., Vaccarella, L., & Tuff, L. (2013). Theory of mind, language and adaptive functioning in ASD: A neuroconstructivist perspective. *Journal of the Canadian Academy of Child and Adolescent Psychiatry, 22*, 13–19.

Berg, C., Philipp, R., & Taff, S. D. (2023). Scoping review of critical thinking literature in healthcare education. *Occupational Therapy in Health Care, 37*(1), 18–39.

Berndt, R. S., Mitchum, C. C., & Wayland, S. (1997). Patterns of sentence comprehension in aphasia: A consideration of three hypotheses. *Brain and Language, 60*, 197–221.

Bernthal, J. E., Bankson, N. W., & Flipsen, P. (2009). *Articulation and phonological disorders: Speech sound disorders in children.* Pearson.

Berthier, M. L. (2021). Ten key reasons for continuing research on pharmacotherapy for post-stroke aphasia. *Aphasiology, 35*(6), 824–858.

Berthier, M. L., Pulvermuller, F., Davila, G., Casares, N. G., & Gutierrez, A. (2011). Drug therapy of post-stroke aphasia: A review of current evidence. *Neuropsychology Review 21*, 302–317.

Betts, S., Feichter, L., Kleinig, Z., Connell-Debais, A., Thai, H., Wong, C., & Kumar, S. (2018). Telerehabilitation versus standard care for improving cognitive function and quality of life for adults with traumatic brain injury: A systematic review. *Internet Journal of Allied Health Sciences & Practice, 16*(3), 1–16.

Bialystok, E. (2018). Bilingual education for young children: Review of the effects and consequences. *International Journal of Bilingual Education and Bilingualism, 21*(6), 666–679.

Biggs, E. E., Therrien, M. C., Snodgrass, M. R., & Douglas, S. N. (2022). Voices from the field: Strategies for effective telepractice for children with autism who use augmentative and alternative communication. *Perspectives of the ASHA Special Interest Groups, 7*(2), 324–337.

Bislick, L. (2020). A phonomotor approach to apraxia of speech treatment. *American Journal of Speech-Language Pathology, 29*(4), 2109–2130.

Blache, S. (1989). A distinctive feature approach. In N. Creaghead, P. Newman, & W. Secord (Eds.), *Assessment and remediation of articulatory and phonological disorders* (pp. 361–382). Charles E. Merrill.

Black, L. I., Vahratian, A., & Hoffman, H. J. (2015). *Communication disorders and use of intervention services among children aged 3–17 years: United States, 2012.* U.S. Department of Health and Human Services, Centers for Disease Control and Prevention, National Center for Health Statistics.

Block, S., Ingham, R., & Bench, R. (1996). The effects of the Edinburgh Masker on stuttering. *Australian Journal of Human Communication Disorders, 24*, 11–18.

Blom, E. D., Singer, M. I., & Hamaker, R. C. (1998). *Tracheoesophageal voice restoration following total laryngectomy.* Singular Publishing.

Blood, G. W. (1995). POWER2: Relapse management with adolescents who stutter. *Language, Speech, and Hearing Services in Schools, 26*, 169–179.

Blood, G. W., & Conture, E. G. (1998). Outcomes measurement issues in fluency disorders. In C. M. Frattali (Ed.), *Measuring outcomes in speech-language pathology* (pp. 387–405). Thieme.

Bloodstein, O. (1960). The development of stuttering: II. Development phases. *Journal of Speech and Hearing Disorders, 25*, 366–376.

Bloodstein, O. (1987). *A handbook on stuttering.* National Easter Seals Society.

Bloodstein, O. (1975). Stuttering as tension and fragmentation. In *Stuttering: A second symposium*. Harper & Row.

Bloodstein, O., & Ratner, N. (2008). *A handbook on stuttering* (6th ed.). Delmar Cengage Learning.

Bloodstein, O., Ratner, N. B., & Brundage, S. B. (2021). *A handbook on stuttering* (7th ed.). Plural Publishing.

Bloom, L. (1973). *One word at a time: The use of single-word utterances before syntax*. The Hague Mouton.

Bloom, P. (2000). *How children learn the meanings of words*. MIT Press.

Bloom, B. S., Airasian, P., Cruikshank, K., Mayer, R., Pintrich, P., Raths, J., & Wittrock, M. (2001). *A taxonomy for learning, teaching, and assessing: A revision of Bloom's taxonomy of educational objectives*. Pearson.

Blosser, J., & Neidecker, E. A. (2002). *School programs in speech-language pathology: Organization and service delivery* (4th ed.). Allyn & Bacon.

Bondy, A. S., & Frost, L. A. (1994). The picture exchange communication system. *Focus on Autism and Other Developmental Disabilities, 9*(3), 1–19.

Boone, D. R., McFarlane, S. C., Von Berg, S., & Zraick, R. (2019). *The voice and voice therapy* (10th ed.). Pearson.

Bothe, A. K., Davidow, J. H., Bramlett, R. E., & Ingham, R. J. (2006). Stuttering treatment research 1970–2005: I. Systematic review incorporating trial quality assessment of behavioral, cognitive, and related approaches. *American Journal of Speech-Language Pathology, 15*, 321–341.

Boutsen, F., Park, E., Dvorak, J., & Cid, C. (2018). Prosodic improvement in persons with Parkinson disease receiving SPEAK OUT!® voice therapy. *Folia Phoniatrica Et Logopaedica, 70*, 51–58.

Boyd, B. A., Odom, S. L., Humphreys, B. P., & Sam, A. M. (2010). Infants and toddlers with ASD: Early identification and early intervention. *Journal of Early Intervention, 32*, 75–98.

Boyle, R., & McDowell-Burns, M. (2015). Modalities of marriage and family therapy supervision. In K. Jordan (Ed.), *Couple, marriage, and family therapy supervision* (pp. 51–70). Springer.

Boyle, S. A., McNaughton, D., & Chapin, S. E. (2019). Effects of shared reading on the early language and literacy skills of children with autism spectrum disorders: A systematic review. *Focus on Autism and Other Developmental Disabilities, 34*(4), 205–214.

Braden, C., Hawley, L., Newman, J., Morey, C., Gerber, D., & Harrison-Felix, C. (2010). Social communication skills group treatment: A feasibility study for persons with traumatic brain injury and comorbid conditions. *Brain Injury, 24*(11), 1298–1310.

Brady, M. C., Ali, M., VandenBerg, K., Williams, L. J., Williams, L. R., Abo, M. ... & Harris Wright, H. (2022). Precision rehabilitation for aphasia by patient age, sex, aphasia severity, and time since stroke? A prespecified, systematic review-based, individual participant data, network, subgroup meta-analysis. *International Journal of Stroke, 17*(10), 1067–1077.

Brady, M. C., Kelly, H., Godwin, J., & Enderby, P. (2012). Speech and language therapy for aphasia following stroke. *Cochrane Database of Systematic Reviews, 2012*(5), CD000425.

Brady, M. C., Kelly, H., Godwin, J., Enderby, P., & Campbell, P. (2016). Speech and language therapy for aphasia following stroke. *Cochrane Database of Systematic Reviews, 2016*(6), CD000425.

Brady, N. C., Marquis, J., Fleming, K., & McLean, L. (2004). Prelinguistic predictors of language growth in children with developmental disabilities. *Journal of Speech, Language, and Hearing Research, 47*, 663–677.

Breit-Smith, A., Justice, L. M., McGinty, A. S., & Kaderavek, J. (2009). How often and how much? Intensity of print referencing intervention. *Topics in Language Disorders, 29*, 360–369.

Brennan-Jones, C. G., White, J., Rush, R. W., & Law, J. (2014). Auditory-verbal therapy for promoting spoken language development in children with permanent hearing impairments. *Cochrane Database of Systematic Reviews, 2014*(3), CD010100.

Brent, G., & Yairi, E. (2012). Disfluency patterns and phonological skills near stuttering onset. *Journal of Communication Disorders, 45*, 426–438.

Brignell, A., Chenausky, K. V., Song, H., Zhu, J., Suo, C., & Morgan, A. T. (2018). Communication interventions for autism spectrum disorder in minimally verbal children. *Cochrane Database of Systematic Reviews, 2018*(11), CD012324.

Brignell, A., Krahe, M., Downes, M., Kefalianos, E., Reilly, S., & Morgan, A. (2021). Interventions for children and adolescents who stutter: A systematic review, meta-analysis, and evidence map. *Journal of Fluency Disorders, 70*, 105843.

Brock, K. L. (2016). Which AAC interface design facilitates communicative interactions for persons with nonfluent aphasia? *EBP Briefs, 11*(1), 1–15.

Brown, R. (1968). *Words and things*. The Free Press.

Brown, R. (1973). *A first language*. Harvard University Press.

Browne, M. N., & Keeley, S. M. (2015). *Asking the right questions: A guide to critical thinking* (11th ed.). Prentice Hall.

Bruce, M., Miyazaki, Y., & Bell, M. A. (2022). Infant attention and maternal education are associated with childhood receptive vocabulary development. *Developmental Psychology, 58*(7), 1207–1220.

Brundage, S. B., & Bernstein Ratner, N. (2022). Linguistic aspects of stuttering: Research updates on the language–fluency interface. *Topics in Language Disorders, 42*(1), 5–23.

Bruner, J. (1974). The organization of early skilled action. In M. P. M. Richards (Ed.), *The integration of a child into a social world* (pp. 167–184). Cambridge University Press.

Bruner, J. (1977). Early social interaction and language acquisition. In H. R. Schaffer (Ed.), *Studies in mother-infant interaction* (pp. 271–289). Academic Press.

Bruner, J. (1983). *Child's talk: Learning to use language* (pp. 67–88). W. W. Norton.

Bruner, J. S. (1960). *The process of education: A searching discussion of school education opening new paths to learning and teaching.* Vintage Books.

Brutten, E., & Shoemaker, D. (1967). *The modification of stuttering.* Prentice Hall.

Bryans, L. A., Palmer, A. D., Anderson, S., Schindler, J., & Graville, D. J. (2021). The impact of Lee Silverman Voice Treatment (LSVT LOUD®) on voice, communication, and participation: Findings from a prospective, longitudinal study. *Journal of Communication Disorders, 89,* 106031.

Bucur, M., & Papagno, C. (2019). Are transcranial brain stimulation effects long-lasting in post-stroke aphasia? A comparative systematic review and meta-analysis on naming performance. *Neuroscience & Biobehavioral Reviews, 102,* 264–289.

Bulow, M., Speyer, R., Baijens, L., Woisard, V., & Ekberg, O. (2008). Neuromuscular electrical stimulation (NMES) in stroke patients with oral and pharyngeal dysfunction. *Dysphagia, 23*(3), 302–309.

Bunton, K. (2008). Speech vs. nonspeech: Different tasks, different neural organizations. *Seminars in Speech and Language, 29,* 267–275.

Burns, S. M., Griffin, P., & Snow, C. E. (1999). *Starting out right: A guide to promoting children's reading success.* National Academy Press.

Butler, Y. G. (2013). Bilingualism/multilingualism and second-language acquisition. In T. K. Bhatia & W. C. Ritchie (Eds.), *The handbook of bilingualism and multilingualism* (pp. 109–136). Wiley Blackwell.

Cabbage, K. L., & DeVeney, S. L. (2020). Treatment approach considerations for children with speech sound disorders in school-based settings. *Topics in Language Disorders, 40*(4), 312–325.

Cabbage, K. L., & Hitchcock, E. R. (2022). Clinical considerations for speech perception in school-age children with speech sound disorders: A review of the current literature. *Language, Speech, and Hearing Services in Schools, 53*(3), 768–785.

Cable, A. L., & Domsch, C. (2010). Systematic review of the literature on the treatment of children with late language emergence. *International Journal of Language & Communication Disorders, 46,* 1–17.

Caesar, L. G. (2013). Providing early intervention services to diverse populations: Are speech-language pathologists prepared? *Infants & Young Children, 26*(2), 126–146.

Cahana-Amitay, D., Albert, M. L., & Oveis, A. (2013). Psycholinguistics of aphasia pharmacotherapy: Asking the right questions. *Aphasiology, 27,* 1–22.

Calandrella, A. M., & Wilcox, M. J. (2000). Predicting language outcomes for pre-linguistic children with developmental delay. *Journal of Speech, Language, and Hearing, 43,* 1061–1071.

Campbell, D. R., & Goldstein, H. (2021). Genesis of a new generation of telepractitioners: The COVID-19 pandemic and pediatric speech-language pathology services. *American Journal of Speech-Language Pathology, 30*(5), 2143–2154.

Carlisle, J. F., & Goodwin, A. P. (2014). Morphemes matter: How morphological knowledge contributes to reading and writing. In C. A. Stone, E. R. Silliman, B. J. Ehren, & G. P. Wallach (Eds.), *Handbook of language and literacy: Development and disorders* (pp. 265–282). Guilford Press.

Carnaby, G. D., LaGorio, L., Silliman, S., & Crary, M. (2020). Exercise-based swallowing intervention (McNeill Dysphagia Therapy) with adjunctive NMES to treat dysphagia post-stroke: A double-blind placebo-controlled trial. *Journal of Oral Rehabilitation, 47*(4), 501–510.

Carroll, J. M., Holliman, A. J., Weir, F., & Baroody, A. E. (2019). Literacy interest, home literacy environment and emergent literacy skills in preschoolers. *Journal of Research in Reading, 42*(1), 150–161.

Carson, L., Baker, E., & Munro, N. (2022). A systematic review of interventions for late talkers: Intervention approaches, elements, and vocabulary outcomes. *American Journal of Speech-Language Pathology, 31*(6), 2861–2874.

Carter, A. S., Messinger, D. S., Stone, W. L., Celimli, S., Nahmias, A. S., & Yoder, P. (2011). A randomized controlled trial of Hanen's "More Than Words" in toddlers with early autism symptoms. *Journal of Child Psychology and Psychiatry, 52*(7), 741–752.

Carter, M. D. (2019). The effects of computer-based simulations on speech-language pathology student performance. *Journal of Communication Disorders, 77,* 44–55.

Caselli, M. C., Rinaldi, P., Stefanini, S., & Volterra, V. (2012). Early action and gesture "vocabulary" and its relation with word comprehension and production. *Child Development, 83*(2), 526–542.

Casper, J. (2000). Treatment approaches and measurement of vocal function: Confidential voice. In J. C. Stemple (Ed.), *Voice therapy: Clinical studies* (2nd ed., pp. 128–139). Thomson Delmar Learning.

Casper, J. K., & Colton, R. H. (1998). *Clinical manual for laryngectomy and head/neck cancer rehabilitation* (2nd ed.). Delmar Cengage Learning.

Catts, H. W., Hogan, T. P., & Adlof, S. M. (2005). Developing changes in reading and reading disabilities. In H. W. Catts & A. G. Kamhi (Eds.), *The connections between language and reading disabilities* (pp. 50–71). Lawrence Erlbaum.

Caute, A., Pring, T., Cocks, N., Cruice, M., Best, W., & Marshall, J. (2013). Enhancing communication through gesture and naming therapy. *Journal of Speech, Language, and Hearing Research, 56*(1), 337–351.

Centeno, J. G. (2009). Issues and principles in service delivery to communicatively impaired-minority bilingual adults in neurorehabilitation. *Seminars in Speech and Language, 30*(3), 139–152.

Centers for Disease Control and Prevention. (2013). *Traumatic brain injury in the United States: Fact sheet.* http://www.cdc.gov/traumaticbraininjury/get_the_facts.html

Centers for Disease Control and Prevention. (2018). *Autism spectrum disorder (ASD).* https://www.cdc.gov/ncbddd/autism/index.html

Cepeda, N. J., Pashler, H., Vul, E., Wixted, J. T., & Rohrer, D. (2006). Distributed practice in verbal recall tasks: A review and quantitative synthesis. *Psychological Bulletin, 132*(3), 354.

Chang, S. E., Horwitz, B., Ostuni, J., Reynolds, R., & Ludlow, C. (2011). Evidence of left frontal inferior premotor structural and functional connectivity deficits in adults who stutter. *Cerebral Cortex, 21,* 2507–2518.

Chapey, R. (2008). *Language intervention strategies in aphasia and related neurogenic communication disorders* (5th ed.). Lippincott Williams & Wilkins.

Charlop, M. H., Lang, R., & Rispoli, M. (2018). *Play and social skills for children with autism spectrum disorder.* Springer International Publishing.

Chaudhary, T., Kanodia, A., Verma, H., Singh, C. A., Mishra, A. K., & Sikka, K. (2021). A pilot study comparing teletherapy with the conventional face-to-face therapy for speech-language disorders. *Indian Journal of Otolaryngology and Head & Neck Surgery, 73*(3), 366–370.

Chen, Z., & Kuo, L. J. (2017). Language and literacy development among children with autism spectrum disorder. *Journal of Childhood & Developmental Disorders, 3*(3), 1–4.

Cheng, I., Sasegbon, A., & Hamdy, S. (2022). A systematic review and meta-analysis of the effects of intraoral treatments for neurogenic oropharyngeal dysphagia. *Journal of Oral Rehabilitation, 49*(1), 92–102.

Cheng, L. L. (1987a). *Assessing Asian language performance: Guidelines for assessing limited-English-proficient students.* Aspen.

Cheng, L. L. (1987b). Cross-cultural and linguistic considerations in working with Asian populations. *ASHA, 29,* 33–38.

Cherney, L. R., Gardner, P., Logemann, J. A., Newman, L. A., O'Neil-Pirozzi, T., Roth, C. R., & Solomon, N. P. (2010). The role of speech-language pathology and audiology in the optimal management of the service member returning from Iraq or Afghanistan with a blast-related head injury: Position of the Communication Sciences and Disorders Clinical Trials Research Group. *Journal of Head Trauma Rehabilitation, 25*(3), 219–224.

Cherney, L. R., Patterson, J. P., Raymer, A., Frymark, T., & Schooling, T. (2008). Evidence-based systematic review: Effects of intensity of treatment and constraint-induced language therapy for individuals with stroke-induced aphasia. *Journal of Speech, Language, and Hearing Research, 51,* 1282–1299.

Chin, S. B., Tsai, P. L., & Gao, S. (2003). Connected speech intelligibility of children with cochlear implants and children with normal hearing. *American Journal of Speech-Language Pathology, 12,* 440–451.

Chiou, H. S., & Yu, V. Y. (2018). Measuring life participation, communicative confidence, language, and cognition in people with aphasia. *Perspectives of the ASHA Interest Groups, 3*(2), 4–12.

Chomsky, N. (1965). *Aspects of a theory of syntax.* MIT Press.

Chomsky, N., & Halle, M. (1968). *The sound pattern of English.* Harper & Row.

Christopoulou, M., Drosos, K., & Petinou, K. (2022). Recent advances of telepractice for autism spectrum disorders in speech and language pathology. *Neuropsychiatric Disease and Treatment, 18,* 2379–2389.

Chrysikou, E. G., & Hamilton, R. H. (2011). Noninvasive brain stimulation in the treatment of aphasia: Exploring interhemispheric relationships and their implications for neurorehabilitation. *Restorative Neurology and Neuroscience 29*(6), 375–394.

Chumpelik, D. (1984). The PROMPT system of therapy: Theoretical framework and applications for developmental apraxia of speech. *Seminars in Speech and Language, 5,* 139–155.

Cirrin, F. M., Schooling, T. L., Nelson, N. W., Diehl, S. F., Flynn, P. F., Staskowski, M., . . . Adamczyk, D. F. (2010). Evidence-based systematic review: Effects of different service delivery models on communication outcomes for elementary school-age children. *Language, Speech, and Hearing Services in Schools, 41*(3), 233–264.

Clark, H. (2003). Neuromuscular treatments for speech and swallowing: A tutorial. *American Journal of Speech Language Pathology, 12,* 400–415.

Clark, H., Lazarus, C., Arvedson, J., Schooling, T., & Frymark, T. (2009). Evidence-based systematic review: Effects of neuromuscular electrical stimulation on swallowing and neural activation. *American Journal of Speech-Language Pathology, 18,* 361–375.

Clark, J. G. (1981). Uses and abuses of hearing loss classification. *ASHA, 23*, 493–500.

Cleave, P. L., Becker, S. D., Curran, M. K., Horne, A. J. O. V., & Fey, M. E. (2015). The efficacy of recasts in language intervention: A systematic review and meta-analysis. *American Journal of Speech-Language Pathology, 24*(2), 237–255.

Coelho, C., Lê, K., Mozeiko, J., Hamilton, M., Tyler, E., Krueger, F., & Grafman, J. (2013). Characterizing discourse deficits following penetrating head injury: A preliminary model. *American Journal of Speech Language Pathology, 22*(2), S438–S448.

Coelho, C. A., Sinotte, M. P., & Duffy, J. R. (2008). Schuell's stimulation approach to rehabilitation. In R. Chapey (Ed.), *Language intervention strategies in aphasia and related neurogenic communication disorders* (pp. 403–449). Lippincott Williams & Wilkins.

Cohan, S. L., Chavira, D. A., & Stein, M. B. (2006). Practitioner review: Psychosocial interventions for children with selective mutism: A critical evaluation of the literature from 1990–2005. *Journal of Child Psychology and Psychiatry, 47*(11), 1085–1097.

Cohen, S. M., Kim, J., Roy, N., Asche, C., & Courey, M. (2012). Prevalence and causes of dysphonia in a large treatment-seeking population. *Laryngoscope, 122*(2), 343–348.

Coleman, C. (2013, November 21). *Community-centered stuttering intervention: Widening the treatment circle* [Seminar presentation]. Annual Convention of the American Speech-Language-Hearing Association, Chicago, IL.

Coleman, C., & Yaruss, J. S. (2014). A comprehensive view of stuttering: Implications for assessment and treatment. *Perspectives on School-Based Issues, 15*(2), 75–80.

Coleman, M. R., Roth, F. P., & West, T. (2009). *Road-Map to PreK RTI: Applying response to intervention in preschool settings.* National Center for Learning Disabilities.

Conture, E. G. (1996). Treatment efficacy: Stuttering. *Journal of Speech and Hearing Research, 39*, S18–S26.

Cook, K., Tillard, G., Wyles, C., Gerhard, D., Ormond, T., & McAuliffe, M. (2019). Assessing and developing the written reflective practice skills of speech-language pathology students. *International Journal of Speech-Language Pathology, 21*(1), 46–55.

Cooper, E., & Cooper, C. (2003). *Cooper personalized fluency control therapy for adolescents and adults: Clinician's manual.* Pro-Ed.

Cornett, R. O. (1967). Cued speech. *American Annals of the Deaf, 112*, 3–13.

Coufal, K., Parham, D., Jakubowitz, M., Howell, C., & Reyes, J. (2018). Comparing traditional service delivery and telepractice for speech sound production using a functional outcome measure. *American Journal of Speech-Language Pathology, 27*(1), 82–90.

Cowan, N. (2008). What are the differences between long-term, short-term, and working memory? *Progress in Brain Research, 169*, 323–338.

Creaghe, N., & Kidd, E. (2022). Symbolic play as a zone of proximal development: An analysis of informational exchange. *Social Development, 31*(4), 1138–1156.

Creaghe, N., Quinn, S., & Kidd, E. (2021). Symbolic play provides a fertile context for language development. *Infancy, 26*(6), 980–1010.

Croot, K. (2002). Diagnosis of AOS: Definition and criteria. *Seminars in Speech and Language, 23*, 267–279.

Cuadrado, E. M., & Weber-Fox, C. M. (2003). Atypical syntactic processing in individuals who stutter: Evidence from event-related brain potentials and behavioral measures. *Journal of Speech, Language, and Hearing Research, 46*, 960–976.

Curtis, T. R. (2014). Case studies for telepractice in AAC. *Perspectives on Augmentative and Alternative Communication, 23*(1), 42–54.

Dahlberg, C., Hawley, L., Morey, C., Newman, J., Cusick, C. P., & Harrison-Felix, C. (2006). Social communication skills in persons with post-acute traumatic brain injury: Three perspectives. *Brain Injury, 20*(4), 425–435.

Dale, P., & Hayden, D. (2013) Treating speech subsystems in CAS with tactual input: The PROMPT approach. *American Journal of Speech-Language Pathology, 22*, 644–661.

Dale, P. S. (1980). Is early pragmatic development measurable? *Journal of Child Language, 8*, 1–12.

Daliri, A., Wieland, E. A., Cai, S., Guenther, F. H., & Chang, S. E. (2018). Auditory-motor adaptation is reduced in adults who stutter but not in children who stutter. *Developmental Science, 21*(2), e12521.

Dalton, B., Pisha, B., Eagleton, M., Coyne, P., & Deysher, S. (2002). *Engaging in the text: Final report to the U.S. Department of Education.* CAST.

Darley, F. L., Aronson, A. E., & Brown, J. R. (1969a). Clusters of deviant speech dimensions in the dysarthrias. *Journal of Speech and Hearing Research, 12*, 462–496.

Darley, F. L., Aronson, A. E., & Brown, J. R. (1969b). Differential diagnostic patterns of dysarthria. *Journal of Speech and Hearing Research, 12*, 246–269.

Darley, F. L., Aronson, A. E., & Brown, J. R. (1975). *Motor speech disorders.* Saunders.

Darling-White, M., & Huber, J. E. (2017). The impact of expiratory muscle strength training on speech breathing in individuals with Parkinson's disease: A preliminary study. *American Journal of Speech-Language Pathology, 26*(4), 1159–1166.

Davies, S. (2017). The evidence behind the practice: A review of WPATH suggested guidelines in transgender voice and communication. *Perspectives of the ASHA Special Interest Groups, 2*(10), 64–73.

Davies, S., Papp, V. G., & Antoni, C. (2015). Voice and communication change for gender nonconforming individuals: Giving voice to the person inside. *International Journal of Transgenderism, 16*(3), 117–159.

Davis, G. A. (2007). Cognitive pragmatics of language disorders in adults. *Seminars in Speech and Language, 28*, 111–121.

David, G. A. (1993). *A survey of adult aphasia and related language disorders* (2nd ed.). Prentice-Hall.

Davis, G. A., & Wilcox, M. J. (1981). Incorporating parameters of natural conversation in aphasia treatment. In R. Chapey (Ed.), *Language intervention strategies in adult aphasia* (pp. 169–193). Williams & Wilkins.

Dawson, G., & Bernier, R. (2013). A quarter century of progress on the early detection and treatment of autism spectrum disorder. *Development and Psychopathology, 25*, 1455–1472.

Dawson, G., Rogers, S., Munson, J., Smith, M., Winter, J., Greenson, J., . . . Varley, J. (2010). Randomized, controlled trial of an intervention for toddlers with autism: The early start Denver model. *Pediatrics, 125*(1), e17–e23.

D'Cruz, A. K., Sharma, S., & Pai, P. S. (2012). Current status of near-total laryngectomy: Review. *Journal of Laryngology and Otology, 126*, 556–562.

de Araújo Pernambuco, L., Espelt, A., Balata, P. M. M., & de Lima, K. C. (2015). Prevalence of voice disorders in the elderly: A systematic review of population-based studies. *European Archives of Otorhino-Laryngology, 272*(10), 2601–2609.

De Nil, L. F., & Kroll, R. M. (2001). Searching for the neural basis of stuttering treatment outcome: Recent neuroimaging studies. *Clinical Linguistics and Phonetics, 15*(1–2), 163–168.

de Nocker, Y. L., & Toolan, C. K. (2023). Using telehealth to provide interventions for children with ASD: A systematic review. *Review Journal of Autism and Developmental Disorders, 10*(1), 82–112.

Denton, C. A., Cirino, P. T., Barth, A. E., Romain, M., Vaughn, S., Wexler, J., . . . Fletcher, J. M. (2011). An experimental study of scheduling and duration of "Tier 2" first-grade reading intervention. *Journal of Research on Educational Effectiveness, 4*(3), 208–230.

Deshmukh, R. S., Pentimonti, J. M., Zucker, T. A., & Curry, B. (2022). Teachers' use of scaffolds within conversations during shared book reading. *Language, Speech, and Hearing Services in Schools, 53*(1), 150–166.

Desjardins, M., Halstead, L., Cooke, M., & Bonilha, H. S. (2017). A systematic review of voice therapy: What "effectiveness" really implies. *Journal of Voice, 31*(3), 392.e13–393.e32.

DeThorne, L. S., & Gerlach-Houck, H. (2023). Resisting ableism in school-based speech-language therapy: An invitation to change. *Language, Speech, and Hearing Services in Schools, 54*(1), 1–7.

DeThorne, L. S., & Searsmith, K. (2021). Autism and neurodiversity: Addressing concerns and offering implications for the school-based speech-language pathologist. *Perspectives of the ASHA Special Interest Groups, 6*(1), 184–190.

DeVeney, S. L., & Peterkin, K. (2022). Facing a clinical challenge: Limited empirical support for toddler speech sound production intervention approaches. *Language, Speech, and Hearing Services in Schools, 53*(3), 659–674.

DeVilliers, P. A., & DeVilliers, J. G. (1979). *Early language (the developing child).* Harvard University Press.

de Wit, E., Visser-Bochane, M. I., Steenbergen, B., van Dijk, P., van der Schans, C. P., & Luinge, M. R. (2016). Characteristics of auditory processing disorders: A systematic review. *Journal of Speech, Language, and Hearing Research, 59*(2), 384–413.

Diamond, K. E., Justice, L. M., Siegler, R. S., & Snyder, P. A. (2013). *Synthesis of IES research on early intervention and early childhood education.* National Center for Special Education Research, Institute of Education Sciences, U.S. Department of Education.

DiLollo, A., & Neimeyer, R. A. (2020). *Counseling in speech-language pathology and audiology: Reconstructing personal narratives.* Plural Publishing.

Dipper, L., Marshall, J., Boyle, M., Botting, N., Hersh, D., Pritchard, M., & Cruice, M. (2021). Treatment for improving discourse in aphasia: A systematic review and synthesis of the evidence base. *Aphasiology, 35*(9), 1125–1167.

Dockrell, J. J. (2014). Developmental variations in the production of written text: Challenges for students who struggle with writing. In C. A. Stone, E. R. Silliman, B. J. Heren, & G. P. Wallach (Eds.), *Handbook of language and literacy: Development and disorders.* (2nd ed., pp. 505–523). Guilford Press.

Dodd, B., & Bradford, A. (2000). A comparison of the three therapy methods for children with different types of developmental phonological disorder. *International Journal of Language and Communication Disorders, 35*, 189–209.

Dodd, B., Holm, A., Crosbie, S., & McIntosh, B. (2010). Core vocabulary intervention for inconsistent speech disorder. In L. Williams, S. McLeod, & R. McCauley (Eds.), *Interventions for speech sound disorders in children* (pp. 117–136). Brookes.

Doogan, C., Dignam, J., Copland, D., & Leff, A. (2018). Aphasia recovery: When, how and who to treat? *Current Neurology and Neuroscience Reports*, *18*(12), 1–7.

Dore, J. (1974). A pragmatic description of early language development. *Journal of Psycholinguistic Research*, *3*, 343–350.

Doud, A. K., Hoepner, J. K., & Holland, A. L. (2020). A survey of counseling curricula among accredited communication sciences and disorders graduate student programs. *American Journal of Speech-Language Pathology*, *29*(2), 789–803.

Douglas, J. M., Bracy, C. A., & Snow, P. C. (2016). Return to work and social communication ability following severe traumatic brain injury. *Journal of Speech, Language, and Hearing Research*, *59*(3), 511–520.

Dowdall, N., Melendez-Torres, G. J., Murray, L., Gardner, F., Hartford, L., & Cooper, P. J. (2020). Shared picture book reading interventions for child language development: A systematic review and meta-analysis. *Child Development*, *91*(2), e383–e399.

Doyle, P. C., & Damrose, E. J. (2022). Has esophageal speech returned as an increasingly viable postlaryngectomy voice and speech rehabilitation option? *Journal of Speech, Language, and Hearing Research*, *65*(12), 4714–4723.

Doyle, P. C., & Finchem, E. A. (2019). Teaching esophageal speech: A process of collaborative instruction. In P. C. Doyle (Ed.), *Clinical care and rehabilitation in head and neck cancer* (pp. 145–161). Springer International Publishing.

Druker, K., Mazzucchelli, T., Hennessey, N., & Beilby, J. (2020). An evaluation of an integrated stuttering and parent-administered self-regulation program for early developmental stuttering disorders. *Journal of Speech, Language, and Hearing Research*, *63*(9), 2894–2912.

Druker, K. C., Mazzucchelli, T. G., & Beilby, J. M. (2019). An evaluation of an integrated fluency and resilience program for early developmental stuttering disorders. *Journal of Communication Disorders*, *78*, 69–83.

Dudding, C., Brown, D., Estis, J., Szymanski, C., Zraick, R., & Mormer, E. (2019). *Best practices in healthcare simulations. Council of Academic Programs in Communication Sciences and Disorders (CAPCSD).* https://growthzonesitesprod.azureedge.net

Dudding, C. C., & Ingram, S. (2018). *Healthcare simulation in clinical education.* ASHA Access Academics and Research Newsletter. https://www.asha.org/Articles/Health-Care-Simulation-in-ClinicalEducation/

Dudding, C. C., & Nottingham, E. E. (2018). A national survey of simulation use in university programs in communication sciences and disorders. *American Journal of Speech-Language Pathology*, *27*(1), 71–81.

Duffy, J. R. (2020). *Motor speech disorders: Substrates, differential diagnosis, and management* (4th ed.). Elsevier/Mosby.

Duhon, G. J., Mesmer, E. M., Atkins, M. E., Greguson, L. A., & Olinger, E. S. (2009). Quantifying intervention intensity: A systematic approach to evaluating student responses to increasing intervention frequency. *Journal of Behavioral Education*, *18*, 101–118.

Duke, N. K., & Bennett-Armistead, V. S. (2003). *Reading & writing informational text in the primary grades.* Scholastic Teaching Resources.

Dunn, C. C., Walker, E. A., Oleson, J., Kenworthy, M., Van Voorst, T., Tomblin, J. B., . . . Gantz, B. J. (2014). Longitudinal speech perception and language performance in pediatric cochlear implant users: The effect of age at implantation. *Ear and Hearing*, *35*(2), 148–160.

Durand, M. (1990). *Severe behavior problems: A functional communication training approach.* Guilford Press.

Dworkin, J. P. (1991). *Motor speech disorders: A treatment guide.* Mosby Year Book.

Dwyer, C. P. (2017). *Critical thinking: Conceptual perspectives and guidelines.* Cambridge University Press.

Dykens, E. M., & Lense, M. (2011). Intellectual disabilities and autism spectrum disorder: A cautionary note. In Amaral, D., Geschwind, D., & Dawson, G. (Eds.), *Autism spectrum disorders*, (pp. 261–269). Oxford Academic.

Ebbers, S. M., & Denton, C. A. (2008). A root awakening: Vocabulary instruction for older students with reading difficulties. *Learning Disabilities Research and Practice*, *23*(2), 90–102.

Edeal, D., & Gildersleeve-Neumann, C. (2011). The importance of production frequency in therapy for childhood apraxia of speech. *American Journal of Speech-Language Pathology*, *20*, 95–110.

Edgar, J. D. (2003). Respiration and swallowing in healthy adults and infants. *Perspectives on Swallowing and Swallowing Disorders*, *12*, 2–6.

Edwards-Gaither, L. (2018). Cultural considerations for telepractice: An introduction for speech-language pathologists. *Perspectives of the ASHA Special Interest Groups*, *3*(18), 13–20.

Efstratiadou, E. A., Papathanasiou, I., Holland, R., Archonti, A., & Hilari, K. (2018). A systematic review of semantic feature analysis therapy studies for aphasia. *Journal of Speech, Language, and Hearing Research*, *61*(5), 1261–1278.

Eisenberg, S. (2014). What works in therapy: Further thoughts on improving clinical practice for children with language disorders. *Language, Speech, and Hearing Services in Schools*, *45*(2), 117–126.

Ellis, A. (1977). The basic clinical theory of rationalemotive therapy. In A. Ellis & R. Grieger (Eds.), *Handbook of rational-emotive therapy* (pp. 3–34). Springer.

Ellis, C., & Urban, S. (2016). Age and aphasia: A review of presence, type, recovery and clinical outcomes. *Topics in Stroke Rehabilitation*, *23*, 430–439.

Elman, R. J. (2007). The importance of aphasia group treatment for rebuilding community and health. *Topics in Language Disorders, 27*, 300–308.

Elman, R. J., & Bernstein-Ellis, E. (1999). The efficacy of group communication treatment in adults with chronic aphasia. *Journal of Speech, Language, and Hearing Research, 42*, 411–419.

Elsabbagh, M., & Johnson, M. H. (2010). Getting answers from babies about autism. *Trends in Cognitive Sciences, 14*(2), 81–87.

Erdman, S. A. (2009). Therapeutic factors in group counseling: Implications for audiologic rehabilitation. *SIG 7 Perspectives on Aural Rehabilitation and Its Instrumentation, 16*(1), 15–28.

Erikson, E. H. (1968). *Identity: Youth and crisis.* W. W. Norton.

Erickson, K. A., (2017). Comprehensive literacy instruction, interprofessional collaborative practice, and students with severe disabilities. *American Journal of Speech-Language Pathology, 26*(2), 193–205.

Ertmer, D., & Goffman, L. (2011). Speech production accuracy and variability in young cochlear implant recipients: Comparisons with typically developing age peers. *Journal of Speech, Language, and Hearing Research, 54*, 177–189.

Ertmer, D. J. (2005). *The source for children with cochlear implants.* LinguiSystems.

Escalona, S. (1973). Basic modes of social interaction: Their emergence and patterning during the first two years of life. *Merrill-Palmer Quarterly, 19*, 205–232.

Faham, M., Ahmadi, A., Silverman, E., Harouni, G. G., & Dabirmoghaddam, P. (2021). Quality of life after botulinum toxin injection in patients with adductor spasmodic dysphonia; a systematic review and meta-analysis. *Journal of Voice, 35*(2), 271–283.

Fairchild, M., & Stronach, S. (2018). Holistic voice therapy for the whole person: University of Minnesota faculty and students learn about—and provide—transgender voice treatment. *ASHA Leader, 23*(8), 38–39.

Farquharson, K., Tambyraja, S. R., & Justice, L. M. (2020). Contributions to gain in speech sound production accuracy for children with speech sound disorders: Exploring child and therapy factors. *Language, Speech, and Hearing Services in Schools, 51*(2), 457–468.

Fasold, R., & Wolfram, W. (1970). Some linguistic features of Negro dialect. In R. Fasold & R. Shuy (Eds.), *Teaching standard English in the inner city* (pp. 41–86). Center for Applied Linguistics.

Ferrier, L. J. (1978). Some observations of errors in context. In N. Waterson & C. Snow (Eds.), *The development of communication* (pp. 301–309). Wiley.

Fey, M. (1985). *Language intervention with young children.* Allyn & Bacon.

Fey, M. E. (1986). *Language intervention with young children.* College Hill Press.

Fey, M. E., Yoder, P. J., Warren, S. F., & Bredin-Oja, S. L. (2013). Is more better? Milieu communication teaching in toddlers with intellectual disabilities. *Journal of Speech, Language, and Hearing Research, 56*(2), 679–693.

Finch, E., Rumbach, A. F., & Park, S. (2018). Speech pathology management of non-progressive dysarthria: A systematic review of the literature. *Disability and Rehabilitation, 42*(3), 296–306. https://doi.org/10.1080/09638288.2018.1497714

Finn, P. (2003). Evidence-based treatment of stuttering: I. Clinical significance of behavioral stuttering treatments. *Journal of Fluency Disorders, 28*, 209–218.

Finn, P., Brundage, S. B., & DiLollo, A. (2016). Preparing our future helping professionals to become critical thinkers: A tutorial. *Perspectives of the ASHA Special Interest Groups, 1*(10), 43–68.

First Words Project. (2021). *A longitudinal research investigation to identify early signs of communication disorders in children from 9 to 24 months of age.* https://firstwordsproject.com

Flasher, L. V., & Fogle, P. T. (2012). *Counseling skills for speech-language pathologists and audiologists* (2nd ed.). Delmar Cengage Learning.

Fodor, J. A. (1975). *The language of thought* (Vol. 5). Harvard University Press.

Forrest, K. (2002). Are oral-motor exercises useful in the treatment of phonological/articulatory disorders? *Seminars in Speech and Language, 23*, 15–26.

Foundas, A. L., Mock, J. R., Corey, D. M., Golob, E. J., & Conture, E. G. (2013). The SpeechEasy device in stuttering and nonstuttering adults: Fluency effects while speaking and reading. *Brain and Language, 126*(2), 141–150.

Fox, C., Ebersbach, G., Ramig, L., & Sapir, S. (2012). LSVT LOUD and LSVT BIG: Behavioral treatment programs for speech and body movement in Parkinson disease. *Parkinsons Disease, 2012*, 1–12. https://doi.org/10.1155/2012/391946

Franzone, E. (2009). *Steps for implementation: Functional communication training.* The National Professional Development Center on Autism Spectrum Disorders. Waisman Center, University of Wisconsin.

Frattali, C. M., Thompson, C. K., Holland, A. I., Wohl, C. B., & Ferketic, M. M. (2003). *Functional Assessment of Communication Skills for Adults (FACS).* American Speech-Language-Hearing Association.

Fredman, T. (2017). Altering the prosodic features of motherese to promote joint attention in language delayed children. *EBP Briefs, 12*(1), 1–10.

Freed, D. (2012). *Motor speech disorders: Diagnosis and treatment* (2nd ed.). Delmar Cengage Learning.

Froeschels, E. (1952). Chewing method as therapy. *Archives of Otolaryngology*, *56*, 427–434.

Froeschels, E., Kastein, S., & Weiss, D. A. (1955). A method of therapy for paralytic conditions of the mechanisms of phonation, respiration and glutination. *Journal of Speech and Hearing Disorders*, *20*, 365–370.

Fuchs, D., & Fuchs, L. S. (2006). Introduction to response to intervention: What, why, and how valid is it? *Reading Research Quarterly*, *41*, 92–99.

Fuchs, D., & Fuchs, L. S. (2017). Critique of the national evaluation of response to intervention: A case for simpler frameworks. *Exceptional Children*, *83*(3), 255–268.

Fuchs, L. S. (2002). Best practices in defining student goals and outcomes. In A. Thomas & J. Grimes (Eds.), *Best practices in school psychology IV* (pp. 553–563). National Association of School Psychologists.

Fuchs, L. S. (2003). Assessing intervention responsiveness: Conceptual and technical issues. *Learning Disabilities Research & Practice*, *18*, 172–186.

Gallas, S., Marie, J. P., Leroi, A. M., & Verin, E. (2010). Sensory transcutaneous electrical stimulation improves post-stroke dysphagic patients. *Dysphagia*, *25*, 291–297.

Galletta, E. E., Conner, P., Vogel-Eyny, A., & Marangolo, P. (2016). Use of tDCS in aphasia rehabilitation: A systematic review of the behavioral interventions implemented with noninvasive brain stimulation for language recovery. *American Journal of Speech-Language Pathology*, *25*, S854–S867.

García-Casares, N., Barros-Cano, A., & García-Arnés, J. A. (2022). Melodic intonation therapy in post-stroke non-fluent aphasia and its effects on brain plasticity. *Journal of Clinical Medicine*, *11*(12), 3503.

Gartner-Schmidt, J. (2006). Voice therapy for the treatment of voice disorders. In B. J. Bailey, J. T. Johnson, & R. D. Newlands (Eds.), *Head and neck surgery: Otolaryngology* (4th ed., pp. 883–894). Lippincott Williams & Wilkins.

Gartner-Schmidt, J., Gherson, S., Hapner, E. R., Muckala, J., Roth, D., Schneider, S., & Gillespie, A. I. (2016). The development of conversation training therapy: A concept paper. *Journal of Voice*, *30*(5), 563–573.

Gauthier, K., & Genesee, F. (2011). Language development in internationally adopted children: A special case of early second language learning. *Child Development*, *82*(3), 887–901.

Geers, A. E. (2002). Factors affecting the development of speech, language, and literacy in children with early cochlear implantation. *Language, Speech, and Hearing Services in Schools*, *33*, 172–183.

Geller, E., & Foley, G. M. (2009). Expanding the "ports of entry" for speech-language pathologists: A relational and reflective model for clinical practice. *American Journal of Speech-Language Pathology*, *18*, 4–21.

Gengoux, G. W., Schwartzman, J. M., Millan, M. E., Schuck, R. K., Ruiz, A. A., Weng, Y., . . . Hardan, A. Y. (2021). Enhancing social initiations using naturalistic behavioral intervention: Outcomes from a randomized controlled trial for children with autism. *Journal of Autism and Developmental Disorders*, *51*(10), 3547–3563.

Gentry, J. R. (2000). A retrospective on invented spelling and a look forward. *The Reading Teacher*, *54*, 318–332.

Gibson, J. L., Newbury, D. F., Durkin, K., Pickles, A., Conti-Ramsden, G., & Toseeb, U. (2021). Pathways from the early language and communication environment to literacy outcomes at the end of primary school; the roles of language development and social development. *Oxford Review of Education*, *47*(2), 260–283.

Gierut, J. A. (1998). Treatment efficacy: Functional phonological disorders in children. *Journal of Speech, Language, and Hearing Research*, *41*, 85–100.

Gierut, J. A. (2001). Complexity in phonological treatment: Clinical factors. *Language, Speech, and Hearing Services in Schools*, *32*, 229–241.

Gierut, J. A. (2007). Phonological complexity and language learnability. *American Journal of Speech-Language Pathology*, *16*, 1–12.

Gierut, J. A., Elbert, M., & Dinnsen, D. A. (1987). A functional analysis of phonological knowledge and generalization learning in misarticulating children. *Journal of Speech and Hearing Research*, *30*, 462–479.

Gifford, R. H., Loiselle, L., Natale, S., Sheffield, S. W., Sunderhaus, L. W. S., Dietrich, M., & Dorman, M. F. (2018). Speech understanding in noise for adults with cochlear implants: Effects of hearing configuration, source location certainty, and head movement. *Journal of Speech, Language, and Hearing Research*, *61*(5), 1306–1321.

Gillespie, A., & Graham, S. (2014). A meta-analysis of writing interventions for students with learning disabilities. *Exceptional Children*, *80*(4), 454–473.

Gilmore, N., Ross, K., & Kiran, S. (2019). The intensive cognitive-communication rehabilitation program for young adults with acquired brain injury. *American Journal of Speech-Language Pathology*, *28*(1S), 341–358.

Giraud, A. L., Neumann, K., Bachoud-Levi, A. C., von Gudenberg, A. W., Euler, H. A., Lanfermann, H., & Preibisch, C. (2008). Severity of dysfluency correlates with basal ganglia activity in persistent developmental stuttering. *Brain and Language*, *104*(2), 190–199.

Glade, R., Bowers, L., & Baldwin, C. (2018). Incorporating informational counseling in treatment for individuals with hearing loss and their families. *Perspectives of the ASHA Special Interest Groups*, *3*(9), 13–26.

Glennen, S. (2014). A longitudinal study of language and speech in children who were internationally adopted at different ages. *Language, Speech, and Hearing Services in Schools, 45*(3), 185–203.

Glennen, S. (2015). Internationally adopted children in the early school years: Relative strengths and weaknesses in language abilities. *Language, Speech, and Hearing Services in Schools, 46*(1), 1–13.

Goebel, M. (1986). *A computer-aided fluency establishment trainer*. Annandale Fluency Clinic.

Goel, R., Hong, J., Findling, R., & Ji, N. (2018). An update on pharmacotherapy of autism spectrum disorder in children and adolescents. *International Review of Psychiatry, 30*(1), 78–95.

Godfroid, A., & Hopp, H. (2022). *The routledge handbook of second language acquisition and psycholinguistics*. Routledge.

Golding-Kushner, K. (2000). *Therapy techniques for cleft palate speech and related disorders*. Singular Publishing.

Goldin-Meadow, S., Goodrich, W., Sauer, E., & Iverson, J. (2007). Young children use their hands to tell their mothers what to say. *Developmental Science, 10*(6), 778–785.

Goldman-Eisler, F. (1968). *Psycholinguistics: Experiments in spontaneous speech*. Academic Press.

Goldstein, B. (2000). *Cultural and linguistic diversity resource guide for speech-language pathologists*. Cengage Learning.

Golom, F. D., & Schreck, J. S. (2018). The journey to interprofessional collaborative practice: Are we there yet? *Pediatric Clinics, 65*(1), 1–12.

Goodglass, H., Kaplan, E., & Barresi, B. (2001). *The assessment of aphasia and related disorders* (3rd ed.). Lippincott Williams & Wilkins.

Goodglass, H., & Wingfield, A. (1998). The changing relationship between anatomic and cognitive explanation in the neuropsychology of language. *Journal of Psycholinguistic Research, 27*, 147–165.

Goral, M., & Conner, P. S. (2013). Language disorders in multilingual and multicultural populations. *Annual Review of Applied Linguistics, 33*, 128–161.

Gordon-Brannon, M. E., & Weiss, C. E. (2007). *Clinical management of articulatory and phonological disorders* (3rd ed.). Lippincott Williams & Wilkins.

Gotham, K., Pickles, A., & Lord, C. (2012). Trajectories of autism severity in children using standardized ADOS scores. *Pediatrics, 130*, 1278–1284.

Goy, H., Fernandes, D. N., Pichora-Fuller, M. K., & van Lieshout, P. (2013). Normative voice data for younger and older adults. *Journal of Voice, 27*(5), 545–555.

Graham, M. S. (2005). Taking it to the limits: Achieving proficient esophageal speech. In P. C. Doyle & R. L. Keith (Eds.), *Contemporary considerations in the treatment and rehabilitation of head and neck cancer* (pp. 521–543). Pro-Ed.

Graham, S., & Harris, K. R. (1989). Improving learning disabled students' skills at composing essays: Self-instructional strategy training. *Exceptional Children, 56*, 201–214.

Graham, S., Liu, X., Bartlett, B., Ng, C., Harris, K. R., Aitken, A., . . . Talukdar, J. (2018). Reading for writing: A meta-analysis of the impact of reading interventions on writing. *Review of Educational Research, 88*(2), 243–284.

Graham, S., Olinghouse, N. G., & Harris, K. R. (2009). Teaching composing to students with learning disabilities: Scientifically-supported recommendations. In G. Troia (Ed.), *Writing instruction and assessment for struggling writers* (pp. 165–186). Guilford Press.

Graham, S., & Perin, D. (2007). *Writing next: Effective strategies to improve writing of adolescents in middle and high schools. A Report to Carnegie Corporation of New York*. Carnegie Corporation.

Grandin, T. (2010). *Thinking in pictures: My life with autism*. Random House.

Graves, M. F. (1986). Vocabulary learning and instruction. In E. Z. Rothkopk & L. C. Ehri (Eds.), *Review of research in education* (pp. 49–89). American Educational Research Association.

Gray, C. (1994). *Comic strip conversations*. Jenison Public Schools.

Gray, C. A. (1995). *Social stories: Improving responses of students with autism with accurate social information*. Aspen.

Gray, C. A. (1998). Social stories and comic strip conversations with students with Asperger syndrome and high-functioning autism. In E. Schopler, G. B. Mesibov, & L. J. Kunce (Eds.), *Asperger syndrome or high-functioning autism?* (pp. 167–198). Plenum.

Gray, C. A., & Garand, J. D. (1993). Social stories: Improving responses of students with autism with accurate social information. *Focus on Autistic Behavior, 8*(1), 1–10.

Green, J., Charman, T., McConachie, H., Aldred, C., Slonims, V., Howlin, P., . . . Pickles, A. (2010). Parent-mediated communication-focused treatment in children with autism (PACT): A randomised controlled trial. *Lancet, 375*(9732), 2152–2160.

Greenspan, S. (1990). How emotional development relates to learning [Video program guide]. In S. Greenspan (Ed.), *Floor time: Tuning in to each child* [Suppl.]. Scholastic.

Greenspan, S. I. (1998). Commentary: Guidance for constructing clinical practice guidelines for developmental and learning disorders: Knowledge vs. evidence-based approaches. *Journal of Developmental and Learning Disorders, 2*, 171–192.

Gregory, H. H. (1979). Controversial issues: Statement and review of the literature. In H. H. Gregory (Ed.), *Controversies about stuttering therapy* (pp. 1–62). University Park Press.

Gregory, H. H. (2003). *Stuttering therapy: Rationale and procedures*. Allyn & Bacon.

Grigos, M., Hayden, D., & Eigen, J. (2010). Perceptual and articulatory changes in speech production following PROMPT treatment. *Journal of Medical Speech Language Pathology, 18*(4), 46–53.

Grillo, E. U., Koenig, M. A., Gunter, C. D., & Kim, S. (2015). Teaching CSD graduate students to think critically, apply evidence, and write professionally. *Communication Disorders Quarterly, 36*(4), 241–251.

Groher, M., & Crary, M. (2020). *Dysphagia: Clinical management in adults and children* (3rd ed.). Mosby.

Grolig, L. (2020). Shared storybook reading and oral language development: A bioecological perspective. *Frontiers in Psychology, 11*, 1818. https://doi.org/10.3389/fpsyg.2020.01818

Grossman, R. B., Bemis, R. H., Skwerer, D. P., & Tager-Flusberg, H. (2013). Lexical and affective prosody in children with high-functioning autism. *Journal of Speech, Language, and Hearing Research, 53*(3), 778–793.

Guadagnoli, M. A., & Lee, T. D. (2004). Challenge point: A framework for conceptualizing the effects of various practice conditions in motor learning. *Journal of Motor Behavior, 36*, 212–224.

Guglielmino, G., Moraes, B. T. D., Villanova, L. C., Padovani, M., & Biase, N. G. D. (2018). Comparison of botulinum toxin and propranolol for essential and dystonic vocal tremors. *Clinics, 73*, 188.

Guitar, B. (2019). *Stuttering: An integrated approach to its nature and treatment* (3rd ed.). Lippincott Williams & Wilkins.

Guitar, B., & Marchinkoski, L. (2001). Influence of mothers' slower speech on their children's speech rate. *Journal of Speech, Language, and Hearing Research, 44*, 853–861.

Guralnick, M. J. (Ed.) (1997). *The effectiveness of early intervention.* Paul H. Brookes.

Guralnick, M. J. (2011). Why early intervention works: A systems perspective. *Infants and Young Children, 24*, 6–28.

Guralnick, M. J. (2012). Preventative interventions for preterm children: Effectiveness and developmental mechanisms. *Journal of Developmental and Behavioral Pediatrics, 33*, 352–364.

Guralnick, M. J. (2013). Developmental science and preventative interventions for children at environmental risk. *Infants and Young Children, 26*, 270–285.

Gutstein, S., & Sheely, R. K. (2002). *Relationship development intervention with children, adolescents and adults: Social and emotional development activities for Asperger syndrome, autism, PDD and NLD.* Jessica Kingsley.

Haley, K. L., Cunningham, K. T., Barry, J., & de Riesthal, M. (2019). Collaborative goals for communicative life participation in aphasia: The FOURC model. *American Journal of Speech-Language Pathology, 28*(1), 1–13.

Hall, P. K. (2000a). A letter to the parent(s) of a child with developmental apraxia of speech. Part I: Speech characteristics of the disorder. *Language, Speech, and Hearing Services in Schools, 31*, 169–172.

Hall, P. K. (2000b). A letter to the parent(s) of a child with developmental apraxia of speech. Part II: The nature and causes of DAS. *Language, Speech, and Hearing Services in Schools, 31*, 173–175.

Hall, P. K. (2000c). A letter to the parent(s) of a child with developmental apraxia of speech. Part III: Other problems often associated with the disorders. *Language, Speech, and Hearing Services in Schools, 31*, 176–178.

Hall, P. K. (2000d). A letter to the parent(s) of a child with developmental apraxia of speech. Part IV: Treatment of DAS. *Language, Speech, and Hearing Services in Schools, 31*, 179–181.

Hall, T. E., Meyer, A., & Rose, D. H. (Eds.). (2012). *Universal design for learning in the classroom: Practical applications.* Guilford Press.

Halle, J. W., Marshall, A. M., & Spradlin, J. E. (1979). Time delay: A technique to increase language use and generalization in retarded children. *Journal of Applied Behavior Analysis, 12*, 431–439.

Halliday, M. A. K. (1975). *Learning how to mean: Explorations in the development of language.* Edward Arnold.

Hallock, H., Collins, D., Lampit, A., Deol, K., Fleming, J., & Valenzuela, M. (2016). Cognitive training for post-acute traumatic brain injury: A systematic review and meta-analysis. *Frontiers in Human Neuroscience, 10*, 537.

Ham, R. (1986). *Techniques of stuttering therapy.* Prentice Hall.

Ham, R. E. (1999). *Clinical management of stuttering in older children and adults.* Pro-Ed.

Hamilton, M. B., Mont, E. V., & McLain, C. (2018). Deletion, omission, reduction: Redefining the language we use to talk about African American English. *Perspectives of the ASHA Special Interest Groups, 3*(1), 107–117.

Harley, J. (2018). The role of attention in therapy for children and adolescents who stutter: Cognitive behavioral therapy and mindfulness-based interventions. *American Journal of Speech-Language Pathology, 27*(3S), 1139–1151.

Haro-Martínez, A., Pérez-Araujo, C. M., Sanchez-Caro, J. M., Fuentes, B., & Díez-Tejedor, E. (2021). Melodic intonation therapy for post-stroke non-fluent aphasia: Systematic review and meta-analysis. *Frontiers in Neurology, 12*, 1303. https://doi.org/10.3389/fneur.2021.700115

Harris, K. R., & Graham, S. (1996). *Making the writing process work: Strategies for composition and self-regulation.* Brookline Books.

Hart, B. M., & Risley, T. R. (1974). Using preschool materials to modify the language of disadvantaged children. *Journal of Applied Behavior Analysis, 7,* 243–256.

Hart, B. M., & Rogers-Warren, A. (1978). A milieu approach to teaching language. In R. Schiefelbusch (Ed.), *Language intervention strategies* (pp. 193–235). University Park Press.

Harvey, D. Y., & Hamilton, R. (2022). Noninvasive brain stimulation to augment language therapy for post-stroke aphasia. *Handbook of Clinical Neurology, 185,* 241–250.

Hassink, J., & Wendt, O. (2010). Remediation of phonological disorders in preschool children: Evidence for the cycles approach. *EBP Briefs, 5*(2), 1–6.

Hawley, L., & Newman, J. (2010). Group interactive structured treatment (GIST): A social competence intervention for individuals with brain injury. *Brain Injury, 24*(11), 1292–1297.

Hayden, D., Eigen, J., Walker, A., & Olsen, L. (2010). PROMPT: A tactually grounded model. In L. Williams, R. McLeod, & R. McCauley (Eds.), *Interventions for speech sound disorders in children* (pp. 453–474). Paul H. Brookes.

Hayes, J., & Flower, L. (1987). On the structure of the writing process. *Topics in Language Disorders, 7,* 19–30.

Healey, E. C., Trautman, L. S., & Susca, M. (2004). Clinical applications of a multidimensional approach for the assessment and treatment of stuttering. *Contemporary Issues in Communication Science and Disorders, 31,* 40–48.

Heidlage, J. K., Cunningham, J. E., Kaiser, A. P., Trivette, C. M., Barton, E. E., Frey, J. R., & Roberts, M. Y. (2020). The effects of parent-implemented language interventions on child linguistic outcomes: A meta-analysis. *Early Childhood Research Quarterly, 50,* 6–23.

Hegarty, N., Titterington, J., McLeod, S., & Taggart, L. (2018). Intervention for children with phonological impairment: Knowledge, practices and intervention intensity in the UK. *International Journal of Language and Communication Disorders, 53*(5), 995–1006.

Hegde, M. N., & Davis, D. (2010). *Clinical methods and practicum in speech-language pathology* (5th ed.). Delmar Cengage Learning.

Helm, N. A. (1979). Management of palilalia with a pacing board. *Journal of Speech and Hearing Disorders, 44,* 350–353.

Helm-Estabrooks, N., & Albert, M. L. (2004). *Manual of aphasia and aphasia therapy.* Pro-Ed.

Helm-Estabrooks, N., & Holland, A. (1998). *Approaches to the treatment of aphasia.* Singular Publishing.

Helmick, K. (2010). Cognitive rehabilitation for military personnel with mild traumatic brain injury and chronic post-concussional disorder: Results of April 2009 consensus conference. *NeuroRehabilitation, 26*(3), 239–255.

Herder, C., Howard, C., Nye, C., & Vanryckeghem, M. (2006). Effectiveness of behavioral stuttering treatment: A systematic review and meta-analysis. *Contemporary Issues in Communication Science and Disorders, 33,* 61–73.

Highman, C., Hennessy, N., & Leitão, S. (2013). Early development in infants at risk of childhood apraxia of speech: A longitudinal investigation. *Developmental Neuropsychology, 38*(3), 197–210.

Hill, A. E., Ward, E., Heard, R., McAllister, S., McCabe, P., Penman, A., . . . Walters, J. (2021). Simulation can replace part of speech-language pathology placement time: A randomised controlled trial. *International Journal of Speech-Language Pathology, 23*(1), 92–102.

Hillis, A. E., & Newhart, M. (2008). Cognitive neuropsychological approaches to treatment of language disorders: Introduction. In R. Chapey (Ed.), *Language intervention strategies in aphasia and related neurogenic communication disorders* (pp. 595–604). Lippincott Williams & Wilkins.

Hintze, J. M., Ludlow, C. L., Bansberg, S. F., Adler, C. H., & Lott, D. G. (2017). Spasmodic dysphonia: A review. Part 1: Pathogenic factors. *Otolaryngology–Head and Neck Surgery, 157*(4), 551–557.

Hirsch, S. (2017). Combining voice, speech science and art approaches to resonant challenges in transgender voice and communication training. *Perspectives of the ASHA Special Interest Groups, 2*(10), 74–82.

Hodson, B. (2010). *Evaluating and enhancing children's phonological systems: Research and theory to practice.* Phonocomp Publishers.

Hodson, B. W. (2004). *Hodson assessment of phonological patterns* (3rd ed.). Pro-Ed.

Hodson, B. W., & Paden, E. P. (1981). Phonological processes which characterize unintelligible and intelligible speech in early childhood. *Journal of Speech and Hearing Disorders, 46,* 369–373.

Hodson, B. W., & Paden, E. P. (1983). *Targeting intelligible speech: A phonological approach to remediation.* Pro-Ed.

Hoffman, L., Ireland, M., Hall-Mills, S., & Flynn, P. (2013). Evidence-based speech-language pathology practices in schools: Findings from a national survey. *Language, Speech, and Hearing Services in Schools, 44,* 266–280.

Holland, A. (1995). *Current realities of aphasia rehabilitation: Time constraints, documentation demands, and functional outcomes* [Paper presentation]. Mid-America Rehabilitation Hospital, Overland Park, KS.

Holland, A. L. (2008). Semantic memory and language processing in aphasia and dementia. *Seminars in Speech and Language, 29,* 3–4.

Holland, A. L., Fromm, D. S., De Ruyter, F., & Stein, M. (1996). Treatment efficacy: Aphasia. *Journal of Speech and Hearing Research, 39*, 27–39.

Holland, A. L., & Nelson, R. L. (2018). *Counseling in communication disorders: A wellness perspective* (3rd ed.). Plural Publishing.

Holland, A. L., & Ramage, A. E. (2004). Learning from Roger Ross: A clinical journey. In J. F. Duchan & S. Byng (Eds.), *Challenging aphasia therapies: Broadening the discourse and extending the boundaries* (pp. 118–129). Psychology Press.

Hoover, J. J., Baca, L., Wexler-Love, E., & Saenz, L. (2008). *National implementation of response to intervention (RTI): Research summary.* National Association of State Directors of Education.

Hoover, J. J., & Patton, J. R. (2009). Role of special educators in multi-tiered instruction. *Intervention in School and Clinic, 43*, 195–202.

Hopf, S. C., Crowe, K., Verdon, S., Blake, H. L., & McLeod, S. (2021). Advancing workplace diversity through the culturally responsive teamwork framework. *American Journal of Speech-Language Pathology, 30*(5), 1949–1961.

Houle, N., Goudelias, D., Lerario, M. P., & Levi, S. V. (2022). Effect of anchor term on auditory-perceptual ratings of feminine and masculine speakers. *Journal of Speech, Language, and Hearing Research, 65*(6), 2064–2080.

Howell, J., & Dean, E. (1994). *Treating phonological disorders in children* (2nd ed.). Whurr.

Howell, P. (2007). Signs of developmental stuttering up to age eight and at 12 plus. *Clinical Psychology Review, 27*(3), 287–306.

Howell, P., & Davis, S. (2011). Predicting persistence of and recovery from stuttering by the teenage years based on information gathered at age 8 years. *Journal of Developmental and Behavioral Pediatrics, 32*(3), 196–205.

Hsieh, M. Y., Lynch, G., & Madison, C. (2018). Intervention techniques used with autism spectrum disorder by speech-language pathologists in the United States and Taiwan: A descriptive analysis of practice in clinical settings. *American Journal of Speech-Language Pathology, 27*(3), 1091–1104.

Hsu, A. S., Chater, N., & Vitányi, P. (2011). The probabilistic analysis of language acquisition: Theoretical, computational, and experimental analysis. *Cognition, 120*(3), 380–390.

Huang, S., & Kan, P. F. (2019). Working with culturally and linguistically diverse populations. In M. W. Hudson & M. DeRuiter (Eds.). *Professional issues in speech-language pathology and audiology* (pp. 485–504). Plural Publishing.

Huang, Y. T., Byrd, A. S., Asmah, R., & Domanski, S. (2023). Evaluating "meaningful differences" in learning and communication across SES backgrounds. *Annual Review of Linguistics, 9*, 589–608.

Hudgins, C. V., & Numbers, F. C. (1942). An investigation of the intelligibility of speech of the deaf. *Genetic Psychology Monographs, 25*, 289–392.

Hudley, A. H. C., Mallinson, C., Bucholtz, M., Flores, N., Holliday, N., Chun, E., & Spears, A. (2018). Linguistics and race: An interdisciplinary approach towards an LSA statement on race. *Proceedings of the Linguistic Society of America, 3*(1), 81.

Hudock, D., & Kalinowski, J. (2014). Stuttering inhibition via altered auditory feedback during scripted telephone conversations. *International Journal of Language & Communication Disorders, 49*(1), 139–147.

Hughes, C. A., & Dexter, D. D. (2011). Response to intervention: A research-based summary. *Theory into Practice, 50*(1), 4–11.

Hull, R. (2009). *Introduction to aural rehabilitation.* Plural Publishing.

Hunting Pompon, R., Burns, M., & Kendall, D. L. (2015). Counseling the caregiver: Focusing on caregivers—in addition to the client—may help improve treatment outcomes. Here's how to tailor that care. *The ASHA Leader, 20*(7), 30–32.

Hurkmans, J., Jonkers, R., Boonstra, A. M., Stewart, R. W., & Reinders-Messelink, H. A. (2012). Assessing the treatment effects in apraxia of speech: Introduction and evaluation of the Modified Diadochokinesis Test. *International Journal of Language and Communication Disorders, 47*(4), 427–436.

Hwa-Froelich, D. A., & Matsuo, H. (2019). Pragmatic language performance of children adopted internationally. *American Journal of Speech-Language Pathology, 28*(2), 501–514.

Hyodo, M., Asano, K., Nagao, A., Hirose, K., Nakahira, M., Yanagida, S., & Nishizawa, N. (2021). Botulinum toxin therapy: A series of clinical studies on patients with spasmodic dysphonia in Japan. *Toxins, 13*(12), 840.

Hyter, Y. D., & Salas-Provance, M. B. (2021). *Culturally responsive practices in speech, language, and hearing sciences.* Plural Publishing.

ICP Core Competencies, (2016). *ICP core competencies for interprofessional collaborative practice: 2016 update.* Interprofessional Education Collaborative.

Individuals with Disabilities Education Act. (2011). [IDEA is a law ensuring free appropriate public education to eligible children with disabilities.]. http://idea.ed.gov

Ingber, S., & Dromi, E. (2010). Actual versus desired family-centered practice in early intervention for children with hearing loss. *Journal of Deaf Studies and Deaf Education, 15*(1), 59–71.

Ingersoll, B., & Lalonde, K. (2010). The impact of object and gesture imitation training on language use in children with autism spectrum disorder. *Journal of Speech, Language, and Hearing Research, 53*(4), 1040–1051.

Ingham, J. C. (2003). Evidence-based treatment of stuttering: I. Definition and application. *Journal of Fluency Disorders, 28*, 197–207.

Ingham, R. J., & Bothe, A. K. (2001). Recovery from early stuttering: Additional issues within the Onslow & Packman-Yairi & Ambrose (1999) exchange. *Journal of Speech, Language, and Hearing Research, 44*, 862–867.

Interprofessional Education Collaborative Expert Panel. (2011). *Core competencies for interprofessional collaborative practice: Report of an expert panel.* Interprofessional Education Collaborative.

Jackson, C., & Schatschneider, C. (2014). Rate of language growth in children with hearing loss in an auditory-verbal early intervention program. *American Annals of the Deaf, 158*(5), 539–554.

Jackson, E., Quesal, R., & Yaruss, J. S. (2012). *What is stuttering (revisited)* [Presentation]. International Stuttering Awareness Day Online Conference. https://isad.live

Jacobs, M., Briley, P. M., Fang, X., & Ellis, C. (2021). Telepractice treatment for aphasia: Association between clinical outcomes and client satisfaction. *Telemedicine Reports, 2*(1), 118–124.

Jacobson, E. (1938). *Progressive relaxation.* University of Chicago Press.

Jakobson, R. (1968). *Child language: Aphasia and phonological universals.* Mouton.

Jakobson, R. (1964). Towards a linguistic typology of aphasic impairments. *Disorders of Language, 21*, 42.

Jakubowitz, M., & Edwards-Gaither, L. (2023). *Telepractice: A clinical guide for speech-language pathologists.* Plural Publishing.

Jick, H., & Kaye, J. A. (2012). Epidemiology and possible causes of autism. *Pharmacotherapy, 23*, 1524–1530.

Johansson, B. B. (2011). Current trends in stroke rehabilitation. A review with focus on brain plasticity. *Acta Neurologica Scandinavica, 123*(3), 147–159.

Johnson, M., Baxter, S., Blank, L., Cantrell, A., Brumfitt, S., Enderby, P., & Goyder, E. (2016). The state of the art in non-pharmacological interventions for developmental stuttering. Part 2: Qualitative evidence synthesis of views and experiences. *International Journal of Language and Communication Disorders, 51*(1), 3–17.

Johnston, E., Martin, S., McLarnon, M., & Hill, C. (2021). Pharyngoplasty for speech disorders following brain injury. *Journal of Craniofacial Surgery, 32*(2), 458–460.

Jones, J. H., Gliga, T., Bedford, R., Charman, T., & Johnson, M. K. (2013). Developmental pathways to autism: A review of prospective studies of infants at risk. *Neuroscience Bio-behavioral Review, 39*, 1–33.

Justice, L. M. (2006). Evidence-based practice, response to intervention, and the prevention of reading difficulties. *Language, Speech, and Hearing Services in Schools, 37*, 284–297.

Justice, L. M., McGinty, A. S., Piasta, S. B., Kaderavek, J. N., & Fan, X. (2010). Print-focused read-alouds in preschool classrooms: Intervention effectiveness and moderators of child outcomes. *Language, Speech, and Hearing Services in Schools, 41*(4), 504–520.

Justice, L. M., Skibbe, L. E., McGinty, A. S., Piasta, S. B., & Petrill, S. (2011). Feasibility, efficacy, and social validity of home-based storybook reading intervention for children with language impairment. *Journal of Speech, Language, and Hearing Research, 54*(2), 523–538.

Kaipa, R., & Peterson, A. M. (2016). A systematic review of treatment intensity in speech disorders. *International Journal of Speech-Language Pathology, 18*(6), 507–520.

Kaiser, A. P., & Warren, S. F. (1986). Incidental language teaching: A critical review. *Journal of Speech and Hearing Disorders, 51*, 291–299.

Kaiser, K., Villalobos, M. E., Locke, J., Iruka, I. U., Proctor, C., & Boyd, B. (2022). A culturally grounded autism parent training program with Black parents. *Autism, 26*(3), 716–726.

Kallhoff, L., & Wambaugh, J. (2021). Generalization outcomes of Sound Production Treatment (SPT) for acquired apraxia of speech: Relationship to treatment dosage. *Aphasiology, 37*(3), 1–26.

Kalk, L. G., Law, J. K., Landa, R., & Law, P. A. (2010). Onset patterns prior to 36 months in autism spectrum disorders. *Journal of Autism and Developmental Disorders, 40*, 1389–1402.

Kamhi, A., Pollock, K., & Harris, J. (1996). *Communication development and disorders in African-American children.* Paul H. Brookes.

Kamhi, A. G. (2014). Improving clinical practice for children with language and learning disorders. *Language, Speech, and Hearing Services in Schools, 45*, 92–103.

Kang, C. (2021). Progress, challenges, and future perspectives in genetic researches of stuttering. *Journal of Genetic Medicine, 18*(2), 75–82.

Kanner, L. (1943). Autistic disturbances of affective contact. *Nervous Child, 2*, 217–250.

Kasari C. (2014). Are we there yet? The state of early prediction and intervention in autism spectrum disorder. *Journal of the American Academy of Child and Adolescent Psychiatry, 53*(2), 133–134. https://doi.org/10.1016/j.jaac.2013.11.007

Kavale, K. A., Holdnack, J. A., Mostert, M. P., & Schmied, C. M. (2003, December 4–5). *The feasibility of a responsiveness to intervention approach for the identification of specific learning disability: A psychometric alternative* [Paper presentation]. National Research

Center on Learning Disabilities Responsiveness to Intervention Symposium, Kansas City, MO.

Kayser, H. (1998). *Assessment and intervention resource for Hispanic children.* Singular Publishing.

Kearney, C. A., & Rede, M. (2021). The heterogeneity of selective mutism: A primer for a more refined approach. *Frontiers in Psychology, 12,* 700745. https://doi.org/10.3389/fpsyg.2021.700745

Kearns, K. P. (1985). Response elaboration training for patient-initiated utterances. In R. H. Brookshire (Ed.), *Clinical aphasiology* (pp. 196–204). BRK Publishers.

Kenny, B., Lincoln, M., & Balandin, S. (2010). Experienced speech-language pathologists' response to ethical dilemmas: An integrated approach to ethical reasoning. *American Journal of Speech-Language Pathology, 19,* 121–134.

Kent, R. D. (1984). Stuttering as a temporal programming disorder. In R. F. Curlee & W. H. Perkins (Eds.), *Nature and treatment of stuttering: New directions* (pp. 283–301). College-Hill Press.

Kent, R. D. (2000). Research on speech motor control and its disorders: A review and prospective. *Journal of Communication Disorders, 33,* 391–427.

Kent, R. D. (2015). Nonspeech oral movements and oral motor disorders: A narrative review. *American Journal of Speech-Language Pathology, 24,* 763–789.

Kertesz, A. (1979). *Aphasia and associated disorders: Taxonomy, localization and recovery.* Grune & Stratton.

Kertesz, A., & McCabe, P. (1977). Recovery patterns and prognosis in aphasia. *Brain, 100,* 1–18.

Khan, L., & Lewis, N. (2002). *Khan-Lewis phonological analysis.* American Guidance Service.

Kichloo, A., Albosta, M., Dettloff, K., Wani, F., El-Amir, Z., Singh, J., . . . Chugh, S. (2020). Telemedicine, the current COVID-19 pandemic and the future: A narrative review and perspectives moving forward in the USA. *Family Medicine and Community Health, 8*(3), e000530.

Kielar, A., Patterson, D., & Chou, Y. H. (2022). Efficacy of repetitive transcranial magnetic stimulation in treating stroke aphasia: Systematic review and meta-analysis. *Clinical Neurophysiology, 140,* 196–227.

Kim, S., & Jo, U. (2013). Study of accent-based music speech protocol development for improving voice problems in stroke patients with mixed dysarthria. *NeuroRehabilitation, 32*(1), 185–190.

Kinsella, E. A., Smith, K., Bhanji, S., Shepley, R., Modor, A., & Bertrim, A. (2020). Mindfulness in allied health and social care professional education: A scoping review. *Disability and Rehabilitation, 42*(2), 283–295.

Kiran, S., Meier, E. L., & Johnson, J. P. (2019). Neuroplasticity in aphasia: A proposed framework of language recovery. *Journal of Speech, Language, and Hearing Research, 62*(11), 3973–3985.

Kiran, S., & Thompson, C. K. (2019). Neuroplasticity of language networks in aphasia: Advances, updates, and future challenges. *Frontiers in Neurology, 10,* 295.

Kirk, K. I., Ying, E., Miyamoto, R. T., O'Neill, T., Lento, C. L., & Fears, B. (2002). Effects of age at implantation in young children. *Annals of Otology, Rhinology, and Laryngology, 111,* 69–73.

Kjellmer, L., Fernell, E., Gillberg, C., & Norrelgen, F. (2018). Speech and language profiles in 4-to 6-year-old children with early diagnosis of autism spectrum disorder without intellectual disability. *Neuropsychiatric Disease and Treatment, 14,* 2415–2427.

Klatte, I. S., Lyons, R., Davies, K., Harding, S., Marshall, J., McKean, C., & Roulstone, S. (2020). Collaboration between parents and SLTs produces optimal outcomes for children attending speech and language therapy: Gathering the evidence. *International Journal of Language & Communication Disorders, 55*(4), 618–628.

Kleim, J. A., & Jones, T. A. (2008). Principles of experience-dependent neural plasticity: Implications for rehabilitation after brain damage. *Journal of Speech, Language, and Hearing Research, 51*(1), S225–S239.

Klein, A., & Johns, M. (2009). *Laryngeal dissection and phonosurgical atlas.* Plural Publishing.

Klima, E., & Bellugi, U. (1966). Syntactic regularities in the speech of children. In J. Lyons & R. J. Wales (Eds.), *Psycholinguistics papers* (pp. 183–203). Edinburgh University Press.

Knoors, H., & Marschark, M. (Eds.). (2018). *Evidence-based practices in deaf education.* Oxford University Press.

Knowles, T., Adams, S., Abeyesekera, A., Mancinelli, C., Gilmore, G., & Jog, M. (2018). Deep brain stimulation of the subthalamic nucleus parameter optimization for vowel acoustics and speech intelligibility in Parkinson's disease. *Journal of Speech, Language, and Hearing Research, 61*(3), 510–524.

Kohnert, K., Ebert, K. D., & Pham, G. T. (2020). *Language disorders in bilingual children and adults.* Plural Publishing.

Kolk, H. H. J. (1991). Is stuttering a symptom of adaption or of impairment? In H. F. M. Peters, W. Hulstijn, & C. W. Starkweather (Eds.), *Speech motor control and stuttering* (pp. 189–204). Elsevier Science.

Kolk, H. H. J., & Postma, A. (1997). Stuttering as a covert repair phenomenon. In R. F. Curlee & G. M. Siegel (Eds.), *Nature and treatment of stuttering* (pp. 182–203). Allyn & Bacon.

Königs, M., Beurskens, E. A., Snoep, L., Scherder, E. J., & Oosterlaan, J. (2018). Effects of timing and intensity of neurorehabilitation on functional outcome after traumatic brain injury: A systematic review and meta-analysis. *Archives of Physical Medicine and Rehabilitation, 99*(6), 1149–1159.

Korner-Bitensky, N. (2013). When does stroke rehabilitation end? *International Journal of Stroke, 8*(1), 8–10.

Krekeler, B. N., Rowe, L. M., & Connor, N. P. (2021). Dose in exercise-based dysphagia therapies: A scoping review. *Dysphagia, 36*, 1–32.

Krekeler, B. N., Vitale, K., Yee, J., Powell, R., & Rogus-Pulia, N. (2020). Adherence to dysphagia treatment recommendations: A conceptual model. *Journal of Speech, Language, Hearing Research, 63*(6), 1641–1657.

Kress, G. (2009). *Multimodality: A social semiotic approach to contemporary communication.* Routledge.

Kübler-Ross, E. (1969). *On death and dying.* Macmillan.

Kuehn, D., & Moller, K. (2000). State of the art: Speech and language issues in the cleft palate population. *Cleft Palate Craniofacial Journal, 37*, 348.

Kummer, A. W. (2008). *Cleft palate and craniofacial anomalies: Effects on speech and resonance* (2nd ed.). Delmar Cengage Learning.

Kummer, A. W. (2018). *Cleft palate and craniofacial conditions.* Jones & Bartlett Learning.

Kuo, J., & Hu, X. (2002). Counseling Asian American adults with speech, language, and swallowing disorders. *Contemporary Issues in Communication Sciences and Disorders, 29*, 35–42.

LaFrance, D. L., Weiss, M. J., Kazemi, E., Gerenser, J., & Dobres, J. (2019). Multidisciplinary teaming: Enhancing collaboration through increased understanding. *Behavior Analysis in Practice, 12*(3), 709–726.

Lam, J. H. Y., Lee, S. M. K., & Tong, X. (2021). Parents' and students' perceptions of telepractice services for speech-language therapy during the COVID-19 pandemic: Survey study. *JMIR Pediatrics and Parenting, 4*(1), e25675.

Lammers, M. J. W., van der Heijden, G. J. M. G., Pourier, V. E. C., & Grolman, W. (2014). Bilateral cochlear implantation in children: A systematic review and best evidence synthesis. *Laryngoscope, 124*(7), 1694–1699.

Landa, R. (2018). Efficacy of early interventions for infants and young children with, and at risk for, autism spectrum disorders, *International Review of Psychiatry, 30*(1), 25–39.

Langdon, C., & Blacker, D. (2010). Dysphagia in stroke: A new solution. *Stroke Research and Treatment, 2010*, 1–6. https://doi.org/10.4061/2010/570403

Langdon, H. W., & Cheng, L. R. (2002). *Collaborating with interpreters and translators.* Thinking Publications.

Lansford, K. L., Liss, J. M., Caviness, J. N., & Utianski, R. L. (2011). A cognitive-perceptual approach to conceptualizing speech intelligibility deficits and remediation practice in hypokinetic dysarthria. *Parkinson's Disease,* [150962]. https://doi.org/10.4061/2011/150962

Lanter, E., Watson, L. R., Erickson, K. A., & Freeman, D. (2012). Emergent literacy in children with autism: An exploration of developmental and contextual dynamic processes. *Language, Speech, and Hearing in Schools, 43*(3), 308–324.

LaPointe, L. L., & Katz, R. C. (2002). Neurogenic disorders of speech. In G. H. Shames & N. B. Anderson (Eds.), *Human communication disorders* (6th ed., pp. 472–509). Allyn & Bacon.

Larkman, C. S., Mellahn, K., Han, W., & Rose, M. L. (2022). Aphasia rehabilitation when speech pathologists and clients do not share the same language: A scoping review. *Aphasiology, 37*(4), 1–23.

Lass, N. J., & Pannbacker, M. (2008). The application of evidence-based practice to nonspeech oral motor treatments. *Language, Speech, and Hearing Services in Schools, 39*, 408–421.

Lavoie, M., Bier, N., & Macoir, J. (2019). Efficacy of a self-administered treatment using a smart tablet to improve functional vocabulary in post-stroke aphasia: A case-series study. *International Journal of Language & Communication Disorders, 54*(2), 249–264.

Lavoie, M., Macoir, J., & Bier, N. (2017). Effectiveness of technologies in the treatment of post-stroke anomia: A systematic review. *Journal of Communication Disorders, 65*, 43–53.

Law, J., Garrett, Z., & Nye, C. (2004). The efficacy of treatment for children with developmental speech and language delay/disorder: A meta-analysis. *Journal of Speech, Language, and Hearing Research, 47*, 924–943.

Law, J., Levickis, P., Rodríguez-Ortiz, I. R., Matić, A., Lyons, R., Messarra, C., . . . Stankova, M. (2019). Working with the parents and families of children with developmental language disorders: An international perspective. *Journal of communication disorders, 82*, 105922. https://doi.org/10.1016/j.jcomdis.2019.105922

Law, M. L., Singh, J., Mastroianni, M., & Santosh, P. (2022). Parent-mediated interventions for infants under 24 months at risk for autism spectrum disorder: A systematic review of randomized controlled trials. *Journal of Autism & Developmental Disorders, 52*(6), 2553–2574.

Leech, K. A., & Rowe, M. L. (2021). An intervention to increase conversational turns between parents and young children. *Journal of Child Language, 48*(2), 399–412.

Leach, E., Cornwall, P., Fleming, J., & Haines, T. (2010). Patient centered goal-setting in a subacute rehabilitation setting. *Disability and Rehabilitation, 32*(2), 159–172.

Leach, J. M., Scarborough, H., & Rescorla, L. (2003). Late-emerging reading disabilities. *Journal of Educational Psychology, 95*, 211–224.

Lee (2011). Size matters: Early vocabulary as a predictor of language and literacy competence. *Applied Psycholinguistics, 32*(1), 69–92.

Leinonen-Davis, E. (1988). Assessing the functional adequacy of children's phonological systems. *Clinical Linguistics and Phonetics, 2,* 257–270.

Lê, K., Coelho, C., & Fiszdon, J. (2022). Systematic review of discourse and social communication interventions in traumatic brain injury. *American Journal of Speech-Language Pathology, 31*(2), 991–1022.

Leonard, R., & Kendall, K. (2008). *Dysphagia assessment and treatment planning: A team approach* (2nd ed.). Plural Publishing.

Lew, H. L., Garvert, D. W., Pogoda, T. K., Hsu, P. T., Devine, J. M., White, D. K., . . . Goodrich, G. L. (2009). Auditory and visual impairments in patients with blast-related traumatic brain injury: Effect of dual sensory impairment on Functional Independence Measure. *Journal of Rehabilitation, Research, and Development, 46*(6), 819–826.

Lewis, A., Rudd, C. J., & Mills, B. (2018). Working with children with autism: An interprofessional simulation-based tutorial for speech pathology and occupational therapy students. *Journal of Interprofessional Care, 32*(2), 242–244.

Lewis, B. A., Freebairn, L. A., Hansen, A., Gerry Taylor, H., Iyengar, S., & Shriberg, L. D. (2004). Family pedigrees of children with suspected childhood apraxia of speech. *Journal of Communication Disorders, 37*(2), 157–175.

Liao, C. Y., Ganz, J. B., Wattanawongwan, S., Haas, A. N., Ura, S. K., Vannest, K. J., & Morin, K. L. (2022). Parent coaching in a multimodal communication intervention for children with autism. *Focus on Autism and Other Developmental Disabilities, 37*(3), 158–168.

Lim, S. R., Goldberg, D. M., & Flexer, C. (2018). Auditory-verbal graduates—25 years later: Outcome survey of the clinical effectiveness of the listening and spoken language approach for young children with hearing loss. *The Volta Review, 118*(1–2), 5–40.

Lindgren, K. A., Folstein, S. E., Tomblin, J. B., & Tager-Flusberg, H. (2009). Language and reading abilities of children with autism spectrum disorders and specific language impairment and their first-degree relatives. *Autism Research, 2*(1), 22–38.

Lloyd, C. A., & Masur, E. F. (2014). Infant behaviors influence mothers' provision of responsive and directive behaviors. *Infant Behavior and Development, 37*(3), 276–285.

Logemann, J. A. (1998). *Evaluation and treatment of swallowing disorders* (2nd ed.). Pro-Ed.

Lord, C., Petkova, E., Hus, V., Gan, W., Lu, F., Martin, D. M., . . . Risi, S. (2012). A multisite study of the clinical diagnosis of different autism spectrum disorders. *Archives of General Psychiatry, 69*(3), 306–313.

Lovaas, O. I., Koegel, R., Simmons, J. Q., & Long, S. J. (1973). Some generalization and follow-up measures on autistic children in behavior therapy. *Journal of Applied Behavior Analysis, 6*(1), 161–165.

Love, R. (2000). *Childhood motor speech disability* (2nd ed.). Allyn & Bacon.

Lowe, H., Henry, L., Müller, L. M., & Joffe, V. L. (2018). Vocabulary intervention for adolescents with language disorder: A systematic review. *International Journal of Language and Communication Disorders, 53*(2), 199–217

Lowit, A., Egan, A., & Hadjivassiliou, M. (2020). Feasibility and acceptability of Lee Silverman Voice Treatment in progressive ataxias. *The Cerebellum, 19*(5), 701–714.

Lundberg, I., Olofsson, A., & Wall, S. (1980). Reading and spelling skills in the first school years predicted from phonemic awareness skills in kindergarten. *Scandinavian Journal of Psychology, 21,* 159–173.

Luterman, D. (2006). The counseling relationship. *The ASHA Leader, 11*(4), 8–9.

Luterman, D. (2020). On teaching counseling: Getting beyond informational counseling. *American Journal of Speech-Language Pathology, 29*(2), 903–908.

Luterman, D. M. (2017). *Counseling persons with communication disorders and their families* (6th ed.). Pro-Ed.

Lynch, E., & Hanson, M. (Eds.). (2011). *Developing cross cultural competence: A guide for working with children and their families* (4th ed.). Paul H. Brookes.

Lyon, J. G. (1998). Treating real-life functionality in a couple coping with severe aphasia. In N. Helm-Estabrooks & A. Holland (Eds.), *Approaches to the treatment of aphasia* (pp. 203–239). Singular Publishing.

Maas, E., & Farinella, K. (2012). Random versus blocked practice in treatment for childhood apraxia of speech. *Journal of Speech, Language, and Hearing Research, 55*(2), 561–578.

MacArthur, C. A. (2000). New tools for writing: Assistive technology for students with writing difficulties. *Topics in Language Disorders, 20,* 85–100.

MacArthur, C. A. (2009). Reflections on research on writing and technology for struggling writers. *Learning Disabilities Research and Practice, 24,* 93–103.

MacDonald, S. (2017). Introducing the model of cognitive-communication competence: A model to guide evidence-based communication interventions after brain injury. *Brain Injury, 31*(13–14), 1760–1780.

MacDonald, S., & Wiseman-Hakes, C. (2010). Knowledge translation in ABI rehabilitation: A model for consolidating and applying the evidence for cognitive communication interventions. *Brain Injury, 24*(3), 486–508.

MacWhinney, B. (2001). The competition model: The input, the context, and the brain. In P. Robinson (Ed.), *Cognition and second language instruction* (pp. 69–90). Cambridge University Press.

MacWhinney, B. (2004). A multiple process solution to the logical problem of language acquisition. *Journal of Child Language, 31*(4), 883–914.

Madhushankara, M., Bhat, S., & Prasad, K. (2023). Design of wearable electrolarynx with automatic control. *Journal of Medical Signals and Sensors, 12*(4), 317–325.

Magee, W. L., Clark, I., Tamplin, J., & Bradt, J. (2017). Music interventions for acquired brain injury. *Cochrane Database of Systematic Reviews, 2017*(1), https://doi.org/10.1002/14651858.CD006787.pub3

Maggio, M. G., De Luca, R., Molonia, F., Porcari, B., Destro, M., Casella, C., . . . Calabro, R. S. (2019). Cognitive rehabilitation in patients with traumatic brain injury: A narrative review on the emerging use of virtual reality. *Journal of Clinical Neuroscience, 61*, 1–4.

Magill, R. A. (1998). *Motor learning: Concepts and applications.* McGraw-Hill.

Mahler, L. A., & Ramig, L. O. (2012). Intensive treatment of dysarthria secondary to stroke. *Clinical Linguistics and Phonetics, 26*(8), 681–694.

Mahoney, J., Hew, M., Vertigan, A., & Oates, J. (2022). Treatment effectiveness for vocal cord dysfunction in adults and adolescents: A systematic review. *Clinical and Experimental Allergy, 52*(3), 387–404.

Manning, W. H. (2010). *Clinical decision making in fluency disorders* (3rd ed.). Cengage.

Manolson, A. (1985). *It takes two to talk: A parent's guide to helping children communicate.* The Hanen Centre.

Marchina, S., Norton, A., & Schlaug, G. (2023). Effects of melodic intonation therapy in patients with chronic nonfluent aphasia. *Annals of the New York Academy of Sciences, 1519*(1), 173-185.

Marian, V., & Hayakawa, S. (2021). Measuring bilingualism: The quest for a "bilingualism quotient." *Applied Psycholinguistics, 42*(2), 527–548.

Marks, L. (2018). *A stitch of time: The year a brain injury changed my language and life.* Simon & Schuster.

Marshall, J., Best, W., Cocks, N., Cruice, M., Pring, T., Bulcock, G., . . . Caute, A. (2012). Gesture and naming therapy for people with severe aphasia: A group study. *Journal of Speech, Language, and Hearing Research, 55*(3), 726–738.

Marshalla, P. R. (1985). The role of reflexes in oral motor learning: Techniques for improved articulation. *Seminars in Speech and Language, 6*, 317–335.

Marsland, E., & Bowman, J. (2010). An interactive education session and follow-up support as a strategy to improve clinicians' goal-writing skills: A randomized controlled trial. *Journal of Evaluation in Clinical Practice, 16*(1), 3–13.

Martin, F. N., & Clark, J. G. (1996). *Hearing care for children.* Allyn & Bacon.

Martin, F. N., & Clark, J. G. (2019). *Introduction to audiology* (13th ed.). Pearson.

Martin, J. (2013). Quality standards for (re)habilitation. *Cochlear Implants International, 14*(S2), S34–S38.

Martin, P. I., Naeser, M. A., Ho, M., Doron, K. W., Kurland, J., Kaplan, J., . . . Pascual-Leone, A. (2009). Overt naming fMRI preand post-TMS: Two nonfluent aphasia patients, with and without improved naming post-TMS. *Brain and Language, 111*(1), 20–35.

Martins, R. H. G., do Amaral, H. A., Tavares, E. L. M., Martins, M. G., Gonçalves, T. M., & Dias, N. H. (2016). Voice disorders: Etiology and diagnosis. *Journal of Voice, 30*(6), 761.e1–761.e9.

Mathers-Schmidt, B. A. (2001). Paradoxical vocal fold motion: A tutorial on a complex disorder and the speech-language pathologist's role. *American Journal of Speech-Language Pathology, 10*, 111–125.

Mattingly, E., & Roth, C. R. (2022). Traumatic brain injury in older adults: Epidemiology, etiology, rehabilitation, and outcomes. *Perspectives of the ASHA Special Interest Groups, 7*(4), 1166-1181.

Mauszycki, S. C., Bailey, D. J., & Wambaugh, J. L. (2017). Acquired apraxia of speech: The relationship between awareness of errors in word productions and treatment outcomes. *American Journal of Speech-Language Pathology, 26*(2s), 664–673.

Mauszycki, S. C., & Wambaugh, J. (2011). Acquired apraxia of speech: A treatment overview. *The ASHA Leader, 16*(5), 16–19.

Mauszycki, S. C., & Wambaugh, J. L. (2020). Acquired apraxia of speech: Comparison of electropalatography treatment and Sound Production Treatment. *American Journal of Speech-Language Pathology, 29*(1S), 511–529.

McAuliffe, M. J., Fletcher, A. R., Kerr, S. E., O'Beirne, G. A., & Anderson, T. (2017). Effect of dysarthria type, speaking condition, and listener age on speech intelligibility. *American Journal of Speech-Language Pathology, 26*(1), 113–123.

McCabe, P., Murray, E., Thomas, D., & Evans, P. (2017). *Clinician manual for rapid syllable transition treatment (REST).* Camperdown, Australia: The University of Sydney.

McCathren, R. B., Yoder, P. J., & Warren, S. F. (1999). The relationship between prelinguistic vocalization and later expressive vocabulary in young children with developmental delay. *Journal of Speech, Language, and Hearing Research, 42*, 915–924.

McCauley, R. J., Strand, E., Lof, G. L., Schooling, T., & Frymark, T. (2009). Evidence-based systematic review: Effects of nonspeech oral motor exercises on speech. *American Journal of Speech-Language Pathology, 18*, 343–360.

McCauley, R. J., & Strand, E. A. (2008). Treatment of childhood apraxia of speech: Clinical decision making in the use of nonspeech oral motor exercises. *Seminars in Speech and Language, 29*, 284–293.

McCurtin, A., Murphy, C. A., & Roddam, H. (2019). Moving beyond traditional understandings of evidence-based practice: A total evidence and knowledge approach (TEKA) to treatment evaluation and clinical decision making in speech-language pathology. *Seminars in Speech and Language, 40*(5), 370–393.

McGinty, A. S., Breit-Smith, A., Fan, X., Justice, L. M., & Kaderavek, J. N. (2011). Does intensity matter? Preschoolers' print knowledge development with a classroom-based intervention. *Early Childhood Research Quarterly, 26*(3), 255–267.

McKenna, V. S., Zhang, B., Haines, M. B., & Kelchner, L. N. (2017). A systematic review of isometric lingual strength training programs in adults with and without dysphagia. *American Journal of Speech-Language Pathology, 26*(2), 524–539.

McLeod, S., & Baker, E. (2016). *Children's speech: An evidence-based approach to assessment and intervention.* Pearson.

McManus, B. M., Richardson, Z., Schenkman, M., Murphy, N., & Morrato, E. H. (2019). Timing and intensity of early intervention service use and outcomes among a safety-net population of children. *JAMA Network Open, 2*(1), e187529–e187529.

McNeil, M. R., Katz, W. F., Fossett, T. R. D., Garst, D. M., Szuminsky, N. J., Carter, G., & Lim, K. Y. (2010). Effects of online augmented kinematic and perceptual feedback on treatment of speech movements in Apraxia of Speech. *Folia Phoniatrica et Logopaedica, 63*(3), 127–133.

McNeil, M. R., Robin, D. A., & Schmidt, R. A. (1997). Apraxia of speech: Definition, differentiation, and treatment. In M. R. McNeil (Ed.), *Clinical management of sensorimotor speech disorders* (pp. 311–344). Thieme.

McReynolds, L., & Bennett, S. (1972). Distinctive feature generalization in articulation training. *Journal of Speech and Hearing Disorders, 37*, 462–470.

Medina, A. M., & Mead, J. S. (2021). An exploration of mindfulness in speech-language pathology. *Communication Disorders Quarterly, 42*(4), 257–265.

Medina, A. M., Pareja, D., Berlanga, E., Crawford, C., & Tormo, A. (2023). Concepts of family support in stuttering: A multicultural perspective. *Language, Speech, and Hearing Services in Schools, 8*(2), 343–357.

Mehegan, C. C., & Dreifuss, F. E. (1972). Hyperlexia: Exceptional reading ability in brain damaged children. *Neurology, 22*, 1105–1111.

Melnick, K. S., Conture, E. G., & Ohde, R. N. (2003). Phonological priming in picture naming in young children who stutter. *Journal of Speech, Language, and Hearing Research, 46*, 1428–1443.

Mendoza Ramos, V., Paulyn, C., Van den Steen, L., Hernandez-Diaz Huici, M. E., De Bodt, M., & Van Nuffelen, G. (2021). Effect of boost articulation therapy (BArT) on intelligibility in adults with dysarthria. *International Journal of Language & Communication Disorders, 56*(2), 271–282.

Mesibov, G. B., & Shea, V. (2010). The TEACCH program in the era of evidence-based practice. *Journal of Autism and Developmental Disorders, 40*(5), 570–579.

Meulenbroek, P., Ness, B., Lemoncello, R., Byom, L., MacDonald, S., O'Neil-Pirozzi, T. M., & Moore Sohlberg, M. (2019). Social communication following traumatic brain injury part 2: Identifying effective treatment ingredients. *International Journal of Speech-Language Pathology, 21*(2), 128–142.

Meulenbroek, P., O'Neil-Pirozzi, T. M., Sohlberg, M. M., Lemoncello, R., Byom, L., Ness, B., . . . Phillips, B. (2022). Tutorial: The speech-language pathologist's role in return to work for adults with traumatic brain injury. *American Journal of Speech-Language Pathology, 31*(1), 188–202.

Meyer, T. K., Spiekerman, C., Kaye, R., Blitzer, A., Kamizi, R. S., Jiang, L., & Weaver, E. M. (2021). Association of laryngeal botulinum neurotoxin injection with work productivity for patients with spasmodic dysphonia. *JAMA Otolaryngology–Head & Neck Surgery, 147*(9), 804–810.

Milisen, R. (1954a). A rationale for articulation disorders. *Journal of Speech and Hearing Disorders, 4*, 5–17.

Milisen, R. (1954b). A rationale for articulation disorders. *Journal of Speech and Hearing Disorders, Monograph Supplement, 4*, 6–17.

Miller, A. J. (2008). Neuroscience of swallowing: Strategies for rehabilitation. *Perspectives on Swallowing and Swallowing Disorders, 17*, 121–127.

Mitchum, C. C., & Berndt, R. S. (2008). Testing the interplay of structure and meaning in aphasic sentence production. *Aphasiology, 22*, 853–865.

Montanari, E. G., Abel, R., Graßer, B., & Tschudinovski, L. (2018). Do bilinguals create two different sets of vocabulary for two domains? *Linguistic Approaches to Bilingualism, 8*(4), 502–522.

Moore, C. A., & Ruark, J. L. (1996). Does speech emerge from earlier appearing motor behaviors? *Journal of Speech and Hearing Research, 39*, 1034–1047.

Morello, A. N. D. C., Beber, B. C., Fagundes, V. C., Cielo, C. A., & Rieder, C. R. (2020). Dysphonia and dysarthria in people with Parkinson's disease after subthalamic nucleus deep brain stimulation: Effect of frequency modulation. *Journal of Voice, 34*(3), 477–484.

Morgan, A. T., Murray, E., & Liegeois, F. J. (2018). Interventions for childhood apraxia of speech. *Cochrane Database of Systematic Reviews*, (5), https://doi.org/10.1002/14651858.CD006278.pub3

Morris, R. J., Gorham-Rowan, M. M., & Scholz, K. (2018). Assessing and teaching critical thinking in communication science and disorders. *Teaching and Learning in Communication Sciences and Disorders, 2*(1), 4.

Mowrer, D. E. (1988). *Methods of modifying speech behaviors* (2nd ed.). Waveland Press.

Mozeiko, J., Abolafia, V., Garneau, A., & Coelho, C. (2020). Intensive sound production treatment for severe, chronic apraxia of speech. *Aphasiology, 34*(9), 1164–1181.

Mozeiko, J., Myers, E. B., & Coelho, C. A. (2018). Treatment response to a double administration of constraint-induced language therapy in chronic aphasia. *Journal of Speech, Language, and Hearing Research, 61*(7), 1664–1690.

Mulhern, T., Lydon, S., Healy, O., Mollaghan, G., Ramey, D., & Leoni, M. (2017). A systematic review and evaluation of procedures for the induction of speech among persons with developmental disabilities. *Developmental Neurorehabilitation, 20*(4), 207–227.

Muñoz-Vigueras, N., Prados-Román, E., Valenza, M. C., Granados-Santiago, M., Cabrera-Martos, I., Rodríguez-Torres, J., & Torres-Sánchez, I. (2021). Speech and language therapy treatment on hypokinetic dysarthria in Parkinson disease: Systematic review and meta-analysis. *Clinical Rehabilitation, 35*(5), 639–655.

Muris, P., & Ollendick, T. H. (2021). Current challenges in the diagnosis and management of selective mutism in children. *Psychology Research and Behavior Management, 14*, 159–167.

Murphy, K. A., Justice, L. M., O'Connell, A. A., Pentimonti, J. M., & Kanderavek, J. K. (2016). Understanding risk for reading difficulties in children with language impairment. *Journal of Speech, Language, and Hearing Research, 59*(6), 1436–1447.

Murray, C. S., Woodruff, A. L., & Vaughn, S. (2010). First-grade student retention within a 3-tier reading framework. *Reading and Writing Quarterly, 26*, 26–50.

Murray, E., McCabe, P., & Ballard, K. J. (2015). A randomized controlled trial for children with childhood apraxia of speech comparing rapid syllable transition treatment and the Nuffield dyspraxia programme (3rd ed.). *Journal of Speech, Language, and Hearing Research, 58*, 669–686.

Murray, L., & Clark, H. (2006). *Neurogenic disorders of language.* Delmar Cengage Learning.

Murry, T., Carrau, R. L., & Chan, K. (2020). *Clinical management of swallowing disorders.* Plural Publishing.

Myers, B., & Bell, T. (2020). Adapting vocal function exercises for voice masculinization. *Perspectives of the ASHA Special Interest Groups, 5*(4), 861–866.

Myers, F., Bakker, K., St. Louis, K., & Raphael, L. (2012). Disfluencies in cluttered speech. *Journal of Fluency Disorders, 37*, 9–19.

Nagdee, N., Sebothoma, B., Madahana, M., Khoza-Shangase, K., & Moroe, N. (2022). Simulations as a mode of clinical training in healthcare professions: A scoping review to guide planning in speech-language pathology and audiology during the COVID-19 pandemic and beyond. *South African Journal of Communication Disorders, 69*(2), 905.

Nagshabandi, B. S., Zinnershine, L., & Shune, S. E. (2023). A review of factors contributing to adults' adherence to dysphagia dietary recommendations through an ecological lens. *American Journal of Speech-Language Pathology, 32*(1), 341–357.

Nation, K. (2005). Picture naming and developmental reading disorders. *Journal of Research in Reading, 28*, 28–38.

National Autism Center. (2009). *Evidence-based practice and autism in the schools: A guide to providing appropriate intervention to students with autism spectrum disorders.*

National Autism Center. (2015). *Findings and conclusions: National standards project, phase 2.*

National Center for Education Statistics. (2019). https://nces.ed.gov/programs/digest/d21/tables/dt21_204.20.asp

National Institute of Neurological Disorders and Stroke. (2010). *Deep brain stimulation for movement disorders information page.* http://www.ninds.nih.gov/Disorders/All-Disorders/Deep-Brain-StimulationMovement-Disorders-Information-Page

Nelson, K. (1973). Structure and strategy in learning to talk. *Monographs of the Society for Research in Child Development, 38*(1-2, Serial No 149), 136. https://doi.org/10.2307/1165788

Nelson, N. W. (2014). Classroom-based writing assessment. In C. A. Stone, E. R. Silliman, B. J. Heren, & G. P. Wallach (Eds.), *Handbook of language and literacy: Development and disorders* (2nd ed., pp. 524–544). Guilford Press.

Newson, J. (1979). The growth of shared understanding between infant and care-giver. In M. Bullowa (Ed.), *Before speech* (pp. 207–243). Cambridge University Press.

Nickerson, R. S. (1998). Confirmation bias: A ubiquitous phenomenon in many guises. *Review of General Psychology, 2*, 175–220.

Nikjeh, D. A. (2019). Ethical decision making: Coding and compliance dilemmas for speech-language pathologists. *Perspectives of the ASHA Special Interest Groups, 4*(6), 1289–1297.

Ninio, A., & Bruner, J. (1978). The achievement and antecedents of labeling. *Journal of Child Language, 5*, 1–14.

Niparko, J. K. (2009). *Cochlear implants: Principles and practices* (2nd ed.). Lippincott Williams & Wilkins.

Nippold, M. A. (2017). Reading comprehension deficits in adolescents: Addressing underlying language abilities. *Language, Speech, and Hearing Services in Schools, 48*(2), 125–131.

Nippold, M. (1998). *Later language development: The school age and adolescent years* (2nd ed.). Pro-Ed.

Nippold, M. A., Hesketh, L. J., Duthie, J. K., & Mansfield, T. C. (2005). Conversational versus expository discourse: A study of syntactic development in children, adolescents and adults. *American Journal of Speech-Language Pathology, 10*, 169–179.

Nippold, M. A., Leonard, L. B., & Kail, R. (1984). Syntactic and conceptual factors in children's understanding of metaphors. *Journal of Speech and Hearing Research, 27*, 197–205.

Nittrouer, S. (1993). The emergence of mature gestural patterns is not uniform: Evidence from an acoustic study. *Journal of Speech and Hearing Research, 36*, 959–972.

Nober, E. H. (1967). Articulation of the deaf. *Exceptional Child, 33*, 611–621.

Noblitt, B., Alfonso, K. P., Adkins, M., & Bush, M. L. (2018). Barriers to rehabilitation care in pediatric cochlear implant recipients. *Otology & Neurotology, 39*(5), e307.

Nolan, I. T., Morrison, S. D., Arowojolu, O., Crowe, C. S., Massie, J. P., Adler, R. K., . . . Francis, D. O. (2019). The role of voice therapy and phonosurgery in transgender vocal feminization. *Journal of Craniofacial Surgery, 30*(5), 1368–1375.

Nouwens, F., Dippel, D. W., de Jong-Hagelstein, M., Visch-Brink, E. G., Koudstaal, P. J., & de Lau, L. M (2013). Rotterdam-Aphasia Therapy Study (RATS)3: The efficacy of intensive cognitive-linguistic therapy in the acute stage of aphasia; design of a randomised controlled trial. *Trials, 14*(1), 24.

Odom, S. L. (2019). Peer-based interventions for children and youth with autism spectrum disorder: History and effects. *School Psychology Review, 48*(2), 170–176.

Odom, S. L., Boyd, B. A., Hall, L. J., & Hume, K. A. (2010). Evaluation of comprehensive treatment models for individuals with autism spectrum disorders. *Journal of Autism and Developmental Disorders, 40*, 425–437.

Ogle, D. (1986). K-W-L: A teaching model that develops active reading of expository text. *The Reading Teacher, 39*, 564–571.

Ohlsson, A. C., Dotevall, H., Gustavsson, I., Hofling, K., Wahle, U., & Österlind, C. (2020). Voice therapy outcome—A randomized clinical trial comparing individual voice therapy, therapy in group, and controls without therapy. *Journal of Voice, 34*(2), 303.e17–303.e26.

Oller, D. (1980). The emergence of the sounds of speech in infancy. In G. Yeni-Komshian, J. Cavanaugh, & C. Ferguson (Eds.), *Child phonology. Volume 1: Production* (pp. 93–112). Academic Press.

Oller, D. K. (1975). Simplification as the goal of phonological processes in child speech. *Language Learning, 24*, 299–303.

Oller, D. K., & Kelly, C. A. (1974). Phonological substitution processes of a hard-of-hearing child. *Journal of Speech and Hearing Disorders, 39*, 65–74.

O'Neil-Pirozzi, T. M. (2011). Evidence supports metacognitive strategy instruction for particular executive functions in young to middle-aged adults with chronic traumatic brain injury. *Evidence-Based Communication Assessment and Intervention, 5*, 85–88.

Onslow, M., & Andrews, C. (1994). A control/experimental trial of an operant treatment for early stuttering. *Journal of Speech and Hearing Research, 37*, 1244–1260.

Onslow, M., & Packman, A. (1999a). The Lidcombe program of early stuttering intervention. In N. B. Ratner & E. C. Healy (Eds.), *Stuttering research and practice: Bridging the gap* (pp. 193–210). Lawrence Erlbaum.

Onslow, M., & Packman, A. (1999b). Treatment recovery and spontaneous recovery from early stuttering: The need for consistent methods in collecting and interpreting data. *Journal of Speech, Language, and Hearing Research, 42*, 398–401.

Orosco, M. J., & Klingnen, J. (2010). One school's implementation of RTI with English language learners. *Journal of Learning Disabilities, 43*, 269–288.

Owens, R. E. (2011). *Language development: An introduction* (8th ed.). Allyn & Bacon.

Packman, A. (2012). Theory and therapy in stuttering: A complex relationship. *Journal of Fluency Disorders, 37*(4), 225–233.

Packman, A., Onslow, M., Webber, M., Harrison, E., Arnott, S., Bridgman, K., . . . Lloyd, W. (2014). *The Lidcombe Program Treatment Guide*. Lidcombe Program Trainers Consortium. https://www.lidcombeprogram.org/helpful-resources/helpful-downloads/

Pamplona, M. C., Ysunza, A., & Ramirez, P. (2004). Naturalistic intervention in cleft palate children. *International Journal of Pediatric Otorhinolaryngology, 68*, 75–81.

Panebianco, M., Marchese-Ragona, R., Masiero, S., & Restivo, D. A. (2020). Dysphagia in neurological diseases: A literature review. *Neurological Sciences, 41*, 3067–3073.

Park, J. S., & Hwang, N. K. (2021). Chin tuck against resistance exercise for dysphagia rehabilitation: A systematic review. *Journal of Oral Rehabilitation, 48*(8), 968–977.

Park, M. N., Moulton, E. E., & Laugeson, E. A. (2022). Parent-assisted social skills training for children with autism spectrum disorder: PEERS for preschoolers. *Focus on Autism and Other Developmental Disabilities*, *38*(2), 80–89.

Patterson, F., Fleming, J., & Doig, E., (2016). Group based delivery of interventions in traumatic brain injury rehabilitation: A scoping review. *Disability and Rehabilitation*, *38*(20), 1961–1986.

Paul, D. R., Blosser, J., & Jakubowitz, M. D. (2006). Principles and challenges for forming successful literacy partnerships. *Topics in Language Disorders*, *26*, 5–22.

Paul, R. (2007). *Language disorders from infancy to adolescence: Assessment and intervention.* Mosby.

Paul, R. (2017). What works for treating language disorders in children. *Journal of the American Academy of Child and Adolescent Psychiatry*, *56*(10), S127.

Paul, R., Augustyn, A., Klin, A., & Volkmar, F. R. (2005). Perception and production of prosody by speakers with autism spectrum disorders. *Journal of Autism and Developmental Disorders*, *35*(2), 205–220.

Paul, R., Norbury, C., & Gosse, C. (2018). *Language disorders from infancy through adolescence: Listening, speaking, reading, writing, and communicating* (5th ed.). Elsevier.

Paul, R., & Roth, F. P. (2011). Characterizing and predicting outcomes of communication delays in infants and toddlers: Implications for clinical practice. *Language, Speech, and Hearing Services in Schools*, *42*(3), 331–340.

Payten, C. L., Chiapello, G., Weir, K. A., & Madill, C. J. (2022). Frameworks, terminology and definitions used for the classification of voice disorders: A scoping review. *Journal of Voice*, *36*(2), https://doi.org/10.1016/j.jvoice.2022.02.009

Peach, R. K. (2013). The cognitive basis for sentence planning difficulties in discourse after traumatic brain injury. *American Journal of Speech-Language Pathology*, *22*(2), S285–S297.

Pedersen, M., & McGlashan, J. (2012). Surgical versus non-surgical interventions for vocal cord nodules. *Cochrane Database of Systematic Reviews*, *2012*(6). https://doi.org/10.1002/14651858.CD001934.pub2

Pedersen, P., Draguns, J., Lonner, W., & Trimble, J. (2002). *Counseling across cultures.* Sage.

Pedersen, P. M., Vintner, K., & Olsen, T. S. (2004). Aphasia after stroke: Type, severity, and prognosis. *Cerebrovascular Diseases*, *17*, 35–43.

Pelatti, C. Y., Justice, L. M., Pentimonti, J. M., & Schmitt, M. B. (2013). Fostering children's emergent literacy development: The role of family practices. In C. A. Stone, E. R. Silliman, B. J. Ehren, & G. P. Wallach (Eds.), *Handbook of language and literacy: Developmental disorders* (pp. 190–203). Guilford Press.

Pellicano, E. (2012). Do autistic symptoms persist across time? Evidence of substantial change in symptomatology over a 3-year period in cognitively able children with autism. *American Journal on Intellectual and Developmental Disabilities*, *117*(2), 156–166.

Pellicano, E. (2013). Testing the predictive power of cognitive atypicalities in autistic children: Evidence from a 3-year follow-up study. *Pediatrics*, *130*, 1278–1284.

Pellowski, M. W., & Conture, E. G. (2002). Characteristics of speech disfluency and stuttering behaviors in 3- and 4-year-old children. *Journal of Speech, Language, and Hearing Research*, *45*, 20–34.

Peng, Z. E., Hess, C., Saffran, J. R., Edwards, J. R., & Litovsky, R. Y. (2019). Assessing fine-grained speech discrimination in young children with bilateral cochlear implants. *Otology and Neurotology*, *40*(3), e191–e197.

Pentimonti, J. M., Zucker, T. A., Justice, L. M., & Kaderavek, J. N. (2010). Informational text use in preschool classroom read-alouds. *The Reading Teacher*, *63*(8), 656–665.

Peterson-Falzone, S., Trost-Cardamone, J., Karnell, M., & Hardin-Jones, M. (2006). *The clinician's guide to treating cleft palate speech.* Mosby Elsevier.

Peterson-Falzone, S. J., Hardin-Jones, M. S., & Karnell, M. (2001). *Cleft palate speech.* Mosby.

Peterson-Falzone, S. J., Trost-Cardamone, J., Karnell, M. P., & Hardin-Jones, M. A. (2016). *The clinician's guide to treating cleft palate speech-e-book.* Elsevier Health Sciences.

Pfeiffer, D. L., Pavelko, S. L., Hahs-Vaughn, D. L., & Dudding, C. C. (2019). A national survey of speech-language pathologists' engagement in interprofessional collaborative practice in schools: Identifying predictive factors and barriers to implementation. *Language, Speech, and Hearing Services in Schools*, *50*(4), 639–655.

Pfost, M., Blatter, K., Artelt, C., Stanat, P., & Schneider, W. (2019). Effects of training phonological awareness on children's reading skills. *Journal of Applied Developmental Psychology*, *65*, 101067. https://doi.org/10.1016/j.appdev.2019.101067

Phillips, B. M., Tabulda, G., Ingrole, S. A., Burris, P. W., Sedgwick, T. K., & Chen, S. (2016). Literate language intervention with high-need prekindergarten children: A randomized trial. *Journal of Speech, Language, and Hearing Research*, *59*(6), 1409–1420.

Piaget, J. (1951). *Plays, dreams and imitation in childhood.* Heinemann.

Piaget, J. (1954). *Origins of intelligence.* Basic Books.

Piaget, J. (1973). *The child and reality: Problems of genetic psychology* (A. Rosin, Trans). Grossman.

Picou, E., & Tharpe, A. M. (2015). Standardized patients: Potential to improve student training in aural rehabilitation. *Perspectives on Public Health Issues Related to Hearing and Balance, 16*(1), 4–14.

Pierce, J. E., Menahemi-Falkov, M., O'Halloran, R., Togher, L., & Rose, M. L. (2019). Constraint and multimodal approaches to therapy for chronic aphasia: A systematic review and meta-analysis. *Neuropsychological Rehabilitation, 29*(7), 1005–1041.

Pinker, S. (1989). *Learnability and cognition: The acquisition of argument structure.* MIT Press.

Pinker, S. (1996). *Language learnability and language development.* Harvard University Press.

Pionek Stone, B., Kratochwill, T. R., Sladezcek, I., & Serlin, R. (2002). Treatment of selective mutism: A best-evidence synthesis. *School Psychology Quarterly, 17*(2), 168–190.

Plotkin, S., Gerber, J. S., & Offit, P. A. (2009). Vaccines and autism: A tale of shifting hypotheses. *Clinical and Infectious Diseases, 48,* 456–461.

Plowman, E. K., Hentz, B., & Ellis, C. (2011). Poststroke aphasia prognosis: A review of patient-related and stroke-related factors. *Journal of Evaluation in Clinical Practice, 18*(3), 689–694.

Poole, E. (1934). Genetic development of articulation of consonant sounds in speech. *Elementary English Review, 11,* 159–161.

Postma, A. (2000). Detection of errors during speech production: A review of speech monitoring models. *Cognition, 77*(2), 97–132.

Prater, R. J., Swift, R. W., Deem, J. F., & Miller, L. (1999). *Manual of voice therapy* (2nd ed.). Pro-Ed.

Prather, E., Hedrick, D., & Kern, C. (1975). Articulation development in children aged two to four years. *Journal of Speech and Hearing Disorders, 40,* 179–191.

Preston, D. R., Bayley, R., & Escalante, C. (2022). *Variation and second language acquisition* (Vol. 28). John Benjamins Publishing.

Prins, D., & Ingham, R. J. (2009). Evidence-based treatment and stuttering: Historical perspective. *Journal of Speech, Language, and Hearing Research, 52*(1), 254–263.

Prizant, B. M. (1983). Language acquisition and communicative behavior in autism toward an understanding of the whole of it. *Journal of Speech and Hearing Disorders, 48*(3), 296–307.

Prizant, B. M., & Duchan, J. F. (1981). The functions of immediate echolalia in autistic children. *Journal of Speech and Hearing Disorders, 46*(3), 241–249.

Prizant, B. M., Wetherby, A. M., Rubin, E., & Laurent, A. C. (2003). The SCERTS Model: A transactional, family-centered approach to enhancing communication and socioemotional abilities of children with autism spectrum disorder. *Infants & Young Children, 16*(4), 296–316.

Procter, T., & Joshi, A. (2022). Cultural competency in voice evaluation: Considerations of normative standards for sociolinguistically diverse voices. *Journal of Voice, 36*(6), 793–801.

Pulvermuller, F., Hauk, O., Zohsel, K., Neininger, B., & Mohr, B. (2005). Therapy-related reorganization of language in both hemispheres of patients with chronic aphasia. *NeuroImage, 28,* 481–489.

Pulvermuller, F., Kujala, T., Shtyrov, Y., Simola, J., Tiitinen, H., Alku, P., . . . Näätänen, R. (2001). Memory traces for words as revealed by the mismatch negativity. *NeuroImage, 14,* 607–616.

Pu, T., Huang, M., Kong, X., Wang, M., Chen, X., Feng, X., . . . Xu, F. (2021). Lee Silverman voice treatment to improve speech in Parkinson's disease: A systemic review and meta-analysis. *Parkinson's Disease, 2021,* 3366870.

Quach, W., & Tsai, P. T. (2017). Preparing future SLPs for the clinical world of cultural-linguistic diversity. *Perspectives of the ASHA Special Interest Groups, 2*(14), 82–102.

Qualls, C. D. (2012). Neurogenic disorders of speech, language, cognition-communication, and swallowing. In D. E. Battle (Ed.), *Communication disorders in multicultural and international populations* (4th ed., pp. 148–163). Mosby.

Quinn, S., & Kidd, E. (2019). Symbolic play promotes non-verbal communicative exchange in infant–caregiver dyads. *British Journal of Developmental Psychology, 37*(1), 33–50.

Radomski, M. V., Anheluk, M., Bartzen, M. P., & Zola, J. (2016). Effectiveness of interventions to address cognitive impairments and improve occupational performance after traumatic brain injury: A systematic review. *American Journal of Occupational Therapy, 70*(3), 1–9.

Radziewicz, C., & Antonellis, C. S. (2008). Children with hearing loss: Considerations and implications. In D. K. Bernstein & E. Tiegerman-Farber (Eds.), *Language and communication disorders in children* (pp. 370–402). Allyn & Bacon.

Ralabate, P. K. (2011). Universal design for learning: Meeting the needs of all students. *The ASHA Leader, 16*(10), 14–17.

Rameau, A. (2020). Pilot study for a novel and personalized voice restoration device for patients with laryngectomy. *Head & Neck, 42*(5), 839–845.

Ramig, L. O. (1998). Speech and voice disorders in Parkinson disease and their treatment. In L. Chernery (Ed.), *Topics in geriatric rehabilitation* (pp. 28–43). Aspen.

Ramig, L. O., Pawlas, A., & Countryman, S. (1995). *The Lee Silverman Voice Treatment.* National Center for Voice and Speech.

Ramig, L. O., & Verdolini, K. (1998). Treatment efficacy: Voice disorders. *Journal of Speech, Language, and Hearing Research, 41*, 101–116.

Rapin, I., & Dunn, M. (1997). Language disorders in children with autism. *Seminars in Pediatric Neurology, 4*(2), 86–92.

Ratner, N. (1995). Treating the stuttering child with concomitant grammatical or phonological disorders. *Language, Speech, and Hearing Services in Schools, 26*, 180–186.

Ratner, N., & Bruner, J. (1978). Games, social exchange and the acquisition of language. *Journal of Child Language, 5*, 391–402.

Raymer, A. M., Kendall, D., Maher, L., Martin, N., Murray, L., Rose, M., . . . Gonzalez Rothi, L. J. (2008). Translational research in aphasia: From neuroscience to neurorehabilitation. *Journal of Speech, Language, and Hearing Research, 51*, 259–275.

Raymer, A. M., & Rothi, L. J. G. (2017). Principles of aphasia rehabilitation. In A.M. Raymer & L. J. G. Rothi (Eds.), *The Oxford handbook of aphasia and language disorders*, (pp. 307–326). Oxford University Press.

Reichow, B. (2011). Overview of meta-analyses on early intensive behavioral intervention for young children with autism spectrum disorders. *Journal of Autism and Developmental Disorders, 42*(4), 512–520.

Repetto, C., Paolillo, M. P., Tuena, C., Bellinzona, F., & Riva, G. (2021). Innovative technology-based interventions in aphasia rehabilitation: A systematic review. *Aphasiology, 35*(12), 1623–1646.

Řepová, B., Zabrodsky, M., Plzak, J., Kalfert, D., Matousek, J., & Betka, J. (2021). Text-to-speech synthesis as an alternative communication means after total laryngectomy. *Biomedical papers of the Medical Faculty of the University Palacky, Olomouc, Czechoslovakia, 165*(2), 192–197.

Richard, G. J. (2013). Language processing versus auditory processing. In D. Geffner & D. Ross-Swain (Eds.), *Auditory processing disorders: Assessment, management, and treatment* (pp. 283–299). Plural Publishing.

Riegler, L., Wade, S. L., Narad, M., & Sarver, L. (2017). POWER-A telehealth rehabilitation program for veterans: Feasibility and preliminary findings. *Perspectives of the ASHA Special Interest Groups, 2*(18), 3–14.

Rinaldi, S., Caselli, M. C., Cofelice, V., D'Amico, S., De Cagno, A. G., Della Corte, G., . . . Zoccolotti, P. (2021). Efficacy of the treatment of developmental language disorder: A systematic review. *Brain Sciences, 11*(3), 407.

Rizzo, K., Mong, L., Helser, M., Howard, N., Katz, I., & Scarborough, D. (2016). Effects of bolus size on swallow safety: A systematic review of external evidence. *EBP Briefs, 11*(3), 1–12.

Robbins, A. M. (2017). 12 guiding premises of pediatric cochlear implant habilitation. *World Journal of Otorhinolaryngology-Head and Neck Surgery, 3*(4), 235.

Robey, R. R. (1998). A meta-analysis of clinical outcomes in the treatment of aphasia. *Journal of Speech, Language, and Hearing Research, 41*, 172–187.

Robey, R. R. (2004). Levels of evidence. *The ASHA Leader, 9*(7), 5.

Robinson, T. L., Jr. (2012). Cultural diversity and fluency disorders. In D. E. Battle (Ed.), *Communication disorders in multicultural and international populations* (4th ed., pp. 164–173). Mosby.

Roelofs, R. L., Wingbermühle, E., Egger, J. I. M., & Kessels, R. P. C. (2017). Social cognitive interventions in neuropsychiatric patients: A meta-analysis. *Brain Impairment, 18*(1), 138–173.

Rogers, C. R. (1951). *Client-centered therapy*. Houghton Mifflin.

Rogers, S. J. (2009). What are infant siblings teaching us about autism in infancy? *Autism Research, 2*(3), 125–137.

Rogers, S. J., Hall, T., Osaki, D., Reaven, J., & Herbison, J. (2000). The Denver Model: A comprehensive integrated educational approach to young children with autism and their families. In J. S. Handleman & S. L. Harris (Eds.), *Preschool education programs for children with autism* (pp. 95–133). Pro-Ed.

Rohlfing, K. J. (2019). Learning language from the use of gestures. In J. S. Horst & J. von Koss Torkildsen (Eds.), *International handbook of language acquisition* (pp. 213–233). Routledge/Taylor & Francis Group.

Rohrer, D., & Pashler, H. (2010). Recent research on human learning challenges conventional instructional strategies. *Educational Researcher, 39*(5), 406–412.

Rollin, W. (2000). *Counseling individuals with communication disorders: Psychodynamic and family aspects*. Butterworth-Heinemann.

Rollins, P. R., De Froy, A., Campbell, M., & Hoffman, R. T. (2021). Mutual gaze: An active ingredient for social development in toddlers with ASD: A randomized control trial. *Journal of Autism and Developmental Disorders, 51*(6), 1921–1938.

Rose, D. H., & Meyer, A. (2000). Universal design for individual differences. *Educational Leadership, 58*, 39–43.

Rose, M., Mok, Z., & Sekine, K. (2017, March–April). Communicative effectiveness of pantomime gesture in people with aphasia. *International Journal of Language and Communication Disorders, 52*, 227–237.

Rose, M. L. (2013). Releasing the constraints on aphasia therapy: The positive impact of gesture and multimodality treatments. *American Journal of Speech-Language Pathology, 22*(2), S227–S239.

Roseberry-McKibbin, C. (2007). *Language disorders in children: A multicultural and case perspective.* Allyn & Bacon.

Roseberry-McKibbin, C. (2008). *Multicultural students with special language needs* (3rd ed.). Academic Communication Associates.

Rosenbek, J. C., & LaPointe, L. L. (1985). Treating apraxia of speech. In D. Johns (Ed.), *Clinical management of neurogenic communicative disorders* (pp. 97–152). Little, Brown.

Rossetti, L. M. (2001). *Communication intervention: Birth to three.* Delmar Cengage Learning.

Roth, F. P. (1999). Communicative intervention for children with psychiatric and communication disorders. *Child and Adolescent Psychiatric Clinics of North America, 8*(1), 137–152.

Roth, F. P., & Baden, B. (2001). Investing in emergent literacy intervention: A key role for speech-language pathologists. *Seminars in Speech and Language, 22,* 163–174.

Roth, F. P., Dougherty, D. P., Paul, D. R., & Adamczyk, D. (2010). *RTI in action: Oral language activities for K–2 classrooms.* American Speech Language-Hearing Association.

Roth, F. P., & Troia, G. A. (2006). Collaborative efforts to promote emergent literacy and efficient word recognition skills. *Topics in Language Disorders, 26,* 24–41.

Roth, F. P., & Troia, G. A. (2009). Applications of responsiveness to intervention and the speech language pathologist in elementary school settings. *Seminars in Speech and Language, 30,* 75–89.

Roth, F. P., Troia, G. A., Worthington, C. K., & Dow, K. A. (2002). Promoting the awareness of sounds in speech: An initial report of an early intervention for children with speech and language impairments. *Applied Psycholinguistics, 23,* 535–565.

Roth, F. P., Troia, G. A., Worthington, C. K., & Handy, D. (2006). Promoting awareness of sounds in speech (PASS): The effects of intervention and stimulus characteristics on the blending performance of preschool children with communication impairments. *Learning Disability Quarterly, 29,* 67–88.

Roth, F. P., Worthington, C. K., & Troia, G. A. (2009, November 19). *PASS: A phonological awareness interventional program for at-risk preschool children* [Seminar presentation]. Presented at the ASHA Annual Convention, New Orleans, LA.

Roth, F. P., Worthington, C. K., & Troia, G. A. (2012). *Promoting Awareness of Speech Sounds (PASS): A phonological awareness intervention program.* Attainment.

Roy, N., Merrill, R. M., Gray, S. D., & Smith, E. M. (2005). Voice disorders in the general population: Prevalence, risk factors, and occupational impact. *Laryngoscope, 115*(11), 1988–1995.

Ruark, J. L., & Moore, C. A. (1997). Coordination of lip muscle activity by 2-year-old children during speech and nonspeech tasks. *Journal of Speech and Hearing Research, 40,* 1373–1385.

Ruff, S., Bocklet, T., Nöth, E., Müller, J., Hoster, E., & Schuster, M. (2017). Speech production quality of cochlear implant users with respect to duration and onset of hearing loss. *ORL, 79,* 282–294.

Rumbach, A. F., Aiken, P. J., & Novakovic, D. (2022). Treatment outcome measures for spasmodic dysphonia: A systematic review. *Journal of Voice, 14*(12), 844.

Russell, J. A., Ciucci, M. R., Connor, N. P., & Schallert, T. (2010). Targeted exercise therapy for voice and swallow in person with Parkinson's disease. *Brain Research, 1341,* 3–11.

Russo, M. J., Prodan, V., Nerina Meda, N., Carcavallo, L., Muracioli, A., Sabe, L., . . . Olmos, L. (2017). High-technology augmentative communication for adults with post-stroke aphasia: A systematic review. *Expert Review of Medical Devices, 14*(5), 355–370.

Rvachew, S. (2005). Stimulability and treatment success. *Topics in Language Disorders, 25,* 207–219.

Rvachew, S., Nowak, M., & Cloutier, G. (2004). Effect of phonemic perception training on the speech production and phonological awareness skills of children with expressive phonological delay. *American Journal of Speech-Language Pathology, 13,* 250–263.

Rvachew, S., Rafaat, S., & Martin, M. (1999). Stimulability, speech perception skills, and the treatment of phonological disorders. *American Journal of Speech Language Pathology, 8,* 33–43.

Ryan, B. P. (1974). *Programmed therapy of stuttering in children and adults.* Charles C. Thomas.

Ryan, N. M., Vertigan, A. E., Bone, S., & Gibson, P. G. (2010). Cough reflux sensitivity improves with speech language pathology management of refractory chronic cough. *Cough, 6*(5), 1–8.

Ryan, W. B. F., Alnouri, G., & Sataloff, R. T. (2022). Neurectomy and myomectomy for treatment of spasmodic dysphonia. *Journal of Voice, 36,* https://doi.org/10.1016/j.jvoice.2021.07.026

Rydell, P., & Prizant, B. (1995). Assessment and intervention strategies for children who use echolalia. In K. Quill (Ed.), *Teaching children with autism: Methods to increase communication and socialization* (pp. 105–129). Delmar.

Saletta, M. (2018). Reading disabilities in adolescents and adults. *Language, Speech, and Hearing Services in Schools, 49*(4), 787–797.

Salinger, T. (2001). Assessing the literacy of young children: The case for multiple forms of evidence. In S. B. Neuman & D. K. Dickinson (Eds.), *Handbook of early literacy research* (pp. 390–418). Guilford Press.

Saltuklaroglu, T. (2012). Assessment and treatment of stuttering using altered auditory feedback. In S. J. Jaksic & M. Onslow (Eds.), *The science and practice of stuttering treatment: A symposium* (pp. 29–42). John Wiley & Sons.

Sanuki, T. (2022). Spasmodic dysphonia: An overview of clinical features and treatment options. *Auris Nasus Larynx, 50*(1), 17–22.

Sapienza, C., & Ruddy, B. H. (2021). *Voice disorders* (4th ed.). Plural Publishing.

Sapir, S., Ramig, L., & Fox, C. (2013). Voice, speech, and swallowing disorders. In S. Factor & F. Weiner (Eds.), *Parkinson disease: Diagnosis and clinical management* (pp. 77–97). Demos.

Sarant, J. Z., Harris, D. C., Galvin, K. L., Bennet, L. A., Canagasabey, M., & Busby, P. A. (2018). Social development in children with early cochlear implants: Normative comparisons and predictive factors, including bilateral implantation. *Ear and Hearing, 39*(4), 770–782.

Sarno, M. T., & Levita, E. (1971). Natural course of recovery in severe aphasia. *Archives of Physical Medicine and Rehabilitation, 52*, 175–178.

Sarno, M. T., Silverman, M., & Sands, E. (1970). Speech therapy and language recovery in severe aphasia. *Journal of Speech and Hearing Research, 13*, 607–623.

Sauer, A. K., Stanton, J., Hans, S., & Grabrucker, A. (2021). Autism spectrum disorders: Etiology and pathology. In A. M. Grabrucker (Ed.), *Autism spectrum disorders* (pp. 1–15). Exon Publications.

Sawyer, J., & Yairi, E. (2010). Characteristics of disfluency clusters over time in preschool children who stutter. *Journal of Speech, Language, and Hearing Research, 53*(5), 1191–1205.

Scaler Scott, K., Gurtizen, E., Giacumbo, K., & Kisenwether, J. (2022). A perceptual study of communication effectiveness in cluttering. *Perspectives of the ASHA Special Interest Groups, 7*(5), 1347–1356.

Scarborough, H. (1989). Index of productive syntax. *Applied Psycholinguistics, 11*, 1–22

Scarborough, H., & Dobrich, W. (1990). Development of children with early language delay. *Journal of Speech and Hearing Research, 33*, 70–83.

Scarborough, H. S. (1998). Early identification of children at risk for reading disabilities. In B. K. Shapiro, P. J. Accardo, & A. J. Capute (Eds.), *Specific reading disabilities: A view of the spectrum* (pp. 75–119). York Press.

Scarpa, A., Williams White, S. & Attwood, T. (Eds.) (2013). *CBT for children and adolescents with high functioning autism spectrum disorders*. The Guilford Press.

Schafer, E. C., Amlani, A. M., Seibold, A., and Shattuck, P. L. (2007). A meta-analytic comparison of binaural benefits between bilateral cochlear implants and bimodal stimulation. *Journal of American Academy of Audiology, 18*(9), 760–776.

Schlesinger, I. (1971). Production of utterances and language acquisition. In D. Slobin (Ed.), *The ontogenesis of grammar* (pp. 63–101). Academic Press.

Schmitt, M. B., Justice, L. M., & Logan, J. A. (2017). Intensity of language treatment: Contribution to children's language outcomes. *International Journal of Language and Communication Disorders, 52*(2), 155–167.

Schmitt, M. B., Tambyraja, S., & Siddiqui, S. (2022). Peer effects in language therapy for preschoolers with developmental language disorder: A pilot study. *American Journal of Speech-Language Pathology, 13*(4), 1854–1867.

Schneider, S. L. (2019). Update: Behavioral management of unilateral vocal fold paralysis and paresis. *Perspectives of the ASHA Special Interest Groups, 4*(3), 474–482.

Schopler, E., & Reichler, R. J. (1971). Parents as cotherapists in the treatment of psychotic children. *Journal of Autism and Childhood Schizophrenia, 1*, 87–102.

Schuck, R. K., Tagavi, D. M., Baiden, K. M., Dwyer, P., Williams, Z. J., Osuna, A., . . . Vernon, T. W. (2021). Neurodiversity and autism intervention: reconciling perspectives through a naturalistic developmental behavioral intervention framework. *Journal of Autism and Developmental Disorders, 52*(10), 4625–4645.

Schuell, H., Jenkins, J. H., & Jimenez-Pabon, E. (1964). *Aphasia in adults: Diagnosis, prognosis and treatment.* Hober-Harper.

Schumaker, J., Deshler, D., Alley, G., Warner, M., Clark, F., & Nolan, S. (1982). Error monitoring: A learning strategy for improving adolescent performance. In W. Cruickshank & J. Lerner (Eds.), *Best of ACLD* (pp. 179–183). Syracuse University Press.

Schuster, M., Lohscheller, J., Kummer, P., Hoppe, U., Eysholdt, U., & Rosanowski, F. (2003). Quality of life in laryngectomees after prosthetic voice restoration. *Folia Phoniatrica et Logopaedica, 55*, 211–219.

Schwartz, S. A. (2020). Frequent billing misconceptions and potential related dilemmas faced by speech-language pathologists. *Perspectives of the ASHA Special Interest Groups, 5*(1), 97–101.

Schwarz, M., Ward, E. C., Ross, J., & Semciw, A. (2018). Impact of thermo-tactile stimulation on the speed and efficiency of swallowing: A systematic review. *International Journal of Language and Communication Disorders, 53*(4), 675–688.

Schweigert, W. A. (1986). The comprehension of familiar and less familiar idioms. *Journal of Psychological Research, 15*, 33–45.

Scott, L. A. (2018). Teaching and improving clinical counseling skills. *Seminars in Hearing, 39*(1), 1–2.

Seikel, J. A., Drumright, D. G., & King, D. W. (2015). *Anatomy and physiology for speech, language, and hearing.* Nelson Education.

Self, T. L., Hale, L. S., & Crumrine, D. (2010). Pharmacotherapy and children with autism spectrum disorder: A tutorial for speech-language pathologists. *Language, Speech, and Hearing in Schools, 41*(3), 367–375.

Shakespeare, T. (2006). The social model of disability. *The Disability Studies Reader, 2,* 197–204.

Shames, G. H. (2000). *Counseling the communicatively disabled and their families: A manual for clinicians.* Allyn & Bacon.

Shames, G. H., & Florance, C. L. (1980). *Stutter-free speech: A goal for therapy.* Charles E. Merrill.

Sharp, H. M., & Bryant, K. M. (2003). Ethical issues in dysphagia: When patients refuse assessment or treatment. *Seminars in Speech and Language, 24,* 285–299.

Sharp, W. G., Berry, R. C., McCracken, C., Nuhu, N. N., Marvel, E., Saulnier, C. A., . . . Jaquess, D. L. (2013). Feeding problems and nutrient intake in children with autism spectrum disorders: A meta-analysis and comprehensive review of the literature. *Journal of Autism and Developmental Disorders, 43,* 2159–2173.

Sheehan, J. G. (1958). Conflict theory of stuttering. In J. Eisenson (Ed.), *Stuttering: A symposium* (pp. 121–166). Harper and Row.

Sheehan, J. G. (1968). Stuttering as a self-role conflict. In H. H. Gregory (Ed.), *Learning theory and stuttering therapy* (pp. 72–83). Northwestern University Press.

Sheehan, J. G. (1970). *Stuttering: Research and therapy.* Harper & Row.

Shine, R. E. (1980). Direct management of the beginning stutterer. *Seminars in Speech, Language, and Hearing, 1,* 339–350.

Shipley, K. G., & Roseberry-McKibbin, C. (2006). *Interviewing and counseling in communicative disorders: Principles and procedures* (3rd ed.). Pro-Ed.

Shriberg, L., Aram, D., & Kwiatkowski, J. (1997a). Developmental apraxia of speech: I. Descriptive and theoretical perspectives. *Journal of Speech, Language, and Hearing Research, 40,* 273–285.

Shriberg, L., Aram, D., & Kwiatkowski, J. (1997b). Developmental apraxia of speech: II. Toward a diagnostic marker. *Journal of Speech, Language, and Hearing Research, 40,* 286–312.

Shriberg, L., Aram, D., & Kwiatkowski, J. (1997c). Developmental apraxia of speech: III. A subtype marked by inappropriate stress. *Journal of Speech, Language, and Hearing Research, 40,* 313–337.

Shriberg, L. D., & Kwiatkowski, J. (1980). *Natural process analysis.* Wiley.

Shriberg, L. D., Strand, E. A., Fourakis, M., Jakielski, K. J., Hall, S. D., Karlsson, H. B., . . . Wilson, D. L. (2017). A diagnostic marker to discriminate childhood apraxia of speech from speech delay: I. Development and description of the Pause Marker. *Journal of Speech, Language, and Hearing Research, 60*(4), S1096–S1117.

Shumway, S., & Wetherby, A. (2009). Communicative acts by children with ASD in the second year of life. *Journal of Speech, Language, and Hearing Research, 52,* 1139–1156.

Simmons-Mackie, N. (2001). Social approaches to aphasia intervention. In R. Chapey (Ed.), *Language intervention strategies in aphasia and related neurogenic communication disorders* (pp. 246–268). Lippincott Williams & Wilkins.

Simmons-Mackie, N. (2008). Social approaches to aphasia intervention. In R. Chapey (Ed.), *Language intervention strategies in aphasia and related neurogenic communication disorders* (pp. 290–317). Lippincott Williams & Wilkins.

Simmons-Mackie, N., Raymer, A., & Cherney, L. R. (2016). Communication partner training in aphasia: An updated systematic review. *Archives of Physical Medicine & Rehabilitation, 97*(12), 2202–2221.e8.

Siposova, B., & Carpenter, M. (2019). A new look at joint attention and common knowledge. *Cognition, 189,* 260–274.

Sisskin, V. (2018). Avoidance Reduction Therapy for stuttering (ARTs®). In B. J. Amster & E. R. Klein (Eds.), *More than fluency: The social, emotional, and cognitive dimensions of stuttering* (pp. 157–186). Plural Publishing.

Skelly, M. (1979). *Amer-Ind gestural code based on universal American Indian hand talk.* Elsevier Science.

Skinner, B. F. (1953). *Science and human behavior.* Macmillan.

Skinner, B. F. (1957). *Verbal behavior.* Appleton-Century-Crofts.

Slavin, D., & Fabus, R. (2018). A case study using a multimodal approach to melodic intonation therapy. *American Journal of Speech-Language Pathology, 27*(4), 1352–1362.

Smart, E., Nalder, E., Trentham, B., & King, G. (2022). Negotiating expectations for therapy between mothers and service providers: A narrative analysis. *Disability and Rehabilitation, 44,* 1–11. https://doi.org/10.1080/09638288.2022.2117861

Smit, A. B., Hand, L., Freilinger, J., Bernthal, J., & Bird, A. (1990). The Iowa Articulation Norms Project and its Nebraska replication. *Journal of Speech and Hearing Disorders, 55,* 779–798.

Smith, A. (1999). Stuttering: A unified approach to a mulitfactorial, dynamic disorder. In N. B. Ratner & E. C. Healey (Eds.), *Stuttering research and practice: Bridging the gap* (pp. 27–44). Erlbaum.

Smith, A., & Kelly, E. (1997). Stuttering: A dynamic, multifactorial model. In R. F. Curlee & G. M. Siegel

(Eds.), *Nature and treatment of stuttering: New directions* (pp. 204–217). Allyn & Bacon.

Smith, A., Sadagopan, N., Walsh, B., & Weber-Fox, C. (2010). Increasing phonological complexity reveals heightened instability in inter-articulatory coordination in adults who stutter. *Journal of Fluency Disorders, 35*, 1–18.

Smythe, I., & Everatt, J. (2002). Dyslexia and the multicultural child: Policy into practice. *Topics in Language Disorders, 22*, 71–80.

Solomon, N. P., Makashay, M. J., Helou, L. B., & Clark, H. M. (2017). Neurogenic orofacial weakness and speech in adults with dysarthria. *American Journal of Speech-Language Pathology, 26*(3), 951–960.

Souza Mumy, A. P. G. (2023). Culturally responsive guidelines for serving families of bilingual children who stutter. *Perspectives of the ASHA Special Interest Groups, 8*(1), 164–175.

Sparks, R. W. (2001). Melodic intonation therapy. In R. Chapey (Ed.), *Language intervention strategies in aphasia and related communication disorders* (pp. 703–717). Lippincott Williams & Wilkins.

Sparks, R. W., Helm, N., & Albert, M. (1974). Aphasia rehabilitation resulting from melodic intonation therapy. *Cortex, 10*, 303.

Sparks, R. W., & Holland, A. L. (1976). Method: Melodic intonation therapy for aphasia. *Journal of Speech and Hearing Disorders, 41*, 287–297.

Speece, D. L., & Hines, S. J. (2008). Identifying children who require different instruction in a response to instruction framework. *Perspectives on Language Learning and Education, 15*, 34–40.

Spekman, N. J., & Roth, F. P. (1984). Intervention strategies for learning disabled children with oral communication disorders. *Learning Disability Quarterly, 7*, 7–18.

Spencer, C., Davison, K. E., Boucher, A. R., & Zuk, J. (2022). Speech perception variability in childhood apraxia of speech: Implications for assessment and intervention. *Language, Speech, and Hearing Services in Schools, 53*(4), 969–984.

Spencer, K. A., Yorkston, K. M., & Duffy, J. R. (2003). Behavioral management of respiratory/phonatory dysfunction from dysarthria: A flowchart for guidance in clinical decision making. *Journal of Medical Speech Language Pathology, 11*(2), xxxix–lxi.

Stachler, R. J., Francis, D. O., Schwartz, S. R., Damask, C. C., Digoy, G. P., Krouse, H. J., . . . Smith, L. J. (2018). Clinical practice guideline: Hoarseness (dysphonia)(update). *Otolaryngology–Head and Neck Surgery, 158*(1 Suppl.), S1–S42.

Stahl, B., Mohr, B., Büscher, V., Dreyer, F. R., Lucchese, G., & Pulvermüller, F. (2018). Efficacy of intensive aphasia therapy in patients with chronic stroke: A randomised controlled trial. *Journal of Neurology, Neurosurgery, and Psychiatry, 89*(6), 586–592.

Stanovich, K. E. (1986). Matthew effects in reading: Some consequences of individual differences in the acquisition of literacy. *Reading Research Quarterly, 21*, 360–406.

Stanovich, K. E. (2000). *Progress in understanding reading: Scientific foundations and new frontiers.* Guilford Press.

Stark, R. (1980). Stages of speech development in the first year of life. In G. Yeni-Komshian, J. Cavanaugh, & C. Ferguson (Eds.), *Child phonology. Volume 1: Production* (pp. 73–92). Academic Press.

Starkweather, C. W. (1985). The development of fluency in normal children. In H. H. Gregory (Ed.), *Stuttering therapy: Prevention and intervention with children* (pp. 67–100). Speech Foundation of America.

Starkweather, C. W. (1987). *Fluency and stuttering.* Prentice Hall.

Starkweather, C. W., & Gottwald, S. R. (2000). The demands and capacities model II: Clinical implications. *Journal of Fluency Disorders, 15*, 143–157.

Stead, A., Vinson, M., Michael, P., Henry, S., Fryer, M., Fitzgerald, C., & Dow, F. (2023). Simulating an end-of-life care conference using standardized patients: Examining students' professional communication. *Perspectives of the ASHA Special Interest Groups, 8*(1), 189–203.

Steel, J., Elbourn, E., & Togher, L. (2021). Narrative discourse intervention after traumatic brain injury: A systematic review of the literature. *Topics in Language Disorders 41*(1), 47–72.

Steele, R. (2009). *On aphasia pharmacotherapy.* Speech Pathology.com. http://www.speechpathology.com/articles/on-aphasia-pharmacotherapy-1187

Stein, N. L., & Glenn, C. G. (1979). An analysis of story comprehension in elementary school children. In R. O. Freedle (Ed.), *New directions in discourse processing* (Vol. 2, pp. 53–120). Ablex.

Steinbrenner, J. R., Hume, K., Odom, S. L., & Morin, K. L. (2020). *Evidence-based practices for children, youth, and young adults with autism spectrum disorder.* The University of North Carolina at Chapel Hill; Frank Porter Graham Child Development Institute; National Clearinghouse on Autism Evidence and Practice Review Team.

Stemple, J. C., Glaze, L. E., & Klaben, B. G. (2000). *Clinical voice pathology: Theory and management.* Delmar Cengage Learning.

Stevens, K., & Hanson, H. (2013). Articulatory-acoustic relations as the basis of distinctive contrasts. In W. J. Hardcastle, J. Laver, & F. E. Gibbon (Eds). *The handbook of phonetic sciences* (pp. 424–444). Blackwell.

Stinchfield-Hawk, S., & Young, E. (1938). *Children with delayed and defective speech: Motor-kinesthetic factors and their training.* Stanford University Press.

Stoel-Gammon, C., Stone-Goldman, J., & Glaspey, A. (2002). Pattern-based approaches to phonological therapy. *Seminars in Speech and Language, 23*, 3–13.

Stone, C. A., Silliman, E. R., Ehren, B. J., & Wallach, G. P. (Eds.). (2014). *Handbook of language and literacy: Development and disorders.* Guilford Press.

Stone, J. R., & Olswang, L. B. (1989). The hidden challenge in counseling. *ASHA, 31*, 27–31.

Storch, S. A., & Whitehurst, G. J. (2002). Oral language and code-related precursors to reading: Evidence from a longitudinal structural model. *Developmental Psychology, 38*(6), 934.

Storkel, H. L. (2018). The complexity approach to phonological treatment: How to select treatment targets. *Language, Speech, and Hearing Services in Schools, 49*(3), 463–481.

Storkel, H. L. (2022). Minimal, maximal, or multiple: Which contrastive intervention approach to use with children with speech sound disorders? *Language, Speech, and Hearing Services in Schools, 53*(3), 632–645.

Strain, P. S., & Hoyson, M. (2000). The need for longitudinal, intensive social skill intervention LEAP follow-up outcomes for children with autism. *Topics in Early Childhood Special Education, 20*(2), 116–122.

Strand, E. A. (2020). Dynamic temporal and tactile cueing: A treatment strategy for childhood apraxia of speech. *American Journal of Speech-Language Pathology, 29*(1), 30–48.

Strangman, N. (2003). Strategy instruction goes digital: Two teachers' perspectives on digital texts with embedded learning supports. *Reading Online, 6*, 9.

Strode, R., & Chamberlain, C. (2006). *The source for childhood apraxia of speech.* LinguiSystems.

Stuart, A., Kalinowski, J., Rastatter, M. P., Saltuklaroglu, T., & Dayalu, V. (2004). Investigations of the impact of altered auditory feedback in-the-ear devices on the speech of people who stutter: Initial fitting and 4-month follow-up. *International Journal of Language and Communication Disorders, 39*, 93–113.

Sue, D. W., & Sue, D. (2012). *Counseling the culturally diverse: Theory and practice* (6th ed.). John Wiley & Sons.

Sugden, E., Baker, E., Munro, N., Williams, A. L., & Trivette, C. M. (2018). Service delivery and intervention intensity for phonology-based speech sound disorders. *International Journal of Language and Communication Disorders, 53*(4), 718–734.

Sugden, E., Lloyd, S., Lam, J., & Cleland, J. (2019). Systematic review of ultrasound visual biofeedback in intervention for speech sound disorders. *International Journal of Language & Communication Disorders, 54*(5), 705–728.

Sullivan, H. (1953). *The interpersonal theory of psychiatry.* Norton.

Sutherland, R., Trembath, D., & Roberts, J. (2018). Telehealth and autism: A systematic search and review of the literature. *International Journal of Speech-Language Pathology, 20*(3), 324–336.

Svirsky, M. A., Teoh, S., & Neuburger, H. (2004). Development of language and speech perception in congenitally, profoundly deaf children as a function of age at cochlear implantation. *Audiology and Neuro-otology, 9*, 224–233.

Swaminathan, D., & Farquharson, K. (2018). Using response to intervention for speech sound disorders: Exploring practice characteristics and geographical differences. *Perspectives of the ASHA Special Interest Groups, 3*(16), 53–66.

Taboas, A., Doepke, K., & Zimmerman, C. (2023). Preferences for identity-first versus person-first language in a U.S. sample of autism stakeholders. *Autism, 27*(2), 565–570.

Tager-Flusberg, H., Paul, R., & Lord, C. (2005). Language and communication in autism. *Handbook of Autism and Pervasive Developmental Disorders, 1*, 335–364.

Tager-Flusberg, H., Rogers, S., Cooper, J., Landa, R., Lord, C., Paul, R., . . . Yoder, P. (2009). Defining spoken language benchmarks and selecting measures of expressive language development for young children with autism spectrum disorders. *Journal of Speech, Language, and Hearing Research, 52*(3), 643–652.

Tanaka, Y., Albert, M. L., Fujita, K., Nonaka, C., & Yokoyama, E. (2006). Treating perseveration improves naming in aphasia. *Brain and Language, 99*, 57–58.

Tanielian, T. L., & Jaycox, L. (Eds.). (2008). *Invisible wounds of war: Psychological and cognitive injuries, their consequences, and services to assist recovery* (Vol. 1). Rand Corporation.

Tanner, D. C. (2003). *The psychology of neurogenic communication disorders: A primer for health care professionals.* Allyn & Bacon.

Tanner, D. C. (2008). *The family guide to surviving stroke and communication disorders* (2nd ed.). Jones & Bartlett.

Tate, R., Kennedy, M., Ponsford, J., Douglas, J., Velikonja, D., Bayley, M., & Stergiou-Kita, M. (2014). INCOG Recommendations for management of cognition following traumatic brain injury, Part III: Executive function and self-awareness. *Journal of Head Trauma Rehabilitation, 29*(4), 338–352.

Teasell, R., Cullen, N., Marshall, S., MacKenzie, H., Bayley, M., Bateman, A., . . . Flores-Sandoval, C. (2018). *ERABI: Evidence-based review of moderate to severe acquired brain injury.* https://erabi.ca

Teasell, R. W. (2018). *Evidence-based review of stroke rehabilitation* (19th ed.). http://www.ebrsr.com/

Teixeira, L. C., & Behlau, M. (2015). Comparison between vocal function exercises and voice amplification. *Journal of Voice, 29*(6), 718–726.

Te Kaat-van den Os, D. J. A., Jongmans, M. J., Volman, C., & Lauteslager, P. E. M. (2017). Parent-implemented language interventions for children with a developmental delay: A systematic review. *Journal of Policy and Practice in Intellectual Disabilities, 14*(2), 129–137.

Templin, M. C. (1957). *Certain language skills in children.* University of Minnesota Press.

Terrell, P., & Watson, M. (2018) Laying a firm foundation: Embedding evidence-based emergent literacy practices into early intervention and preschool environments. *Language, Speech, and Hearing Services in Schools, 49*(2), 148–164.

Tetnowski, J. A., Scott, K. S., & Rutland, B. F. (2021). Fluency and fluency disorders. In J. S. Damico, N. Müller, & M. J. Ball (Eds.) *The handbook of language and speech disorders,* (2nd ed., pp. 414–444). Wiley Blackwell.

Tezcaner, Z. Ç., Gökmen, M. F., Yıldırım, S., & Dursun, G. (2019). Clinical features of psychogenic voice disorder and the efficiency of voice therapy and psychological evaluation. *Journal of Voice, 33*(2), 250–254.

Thelen, E., & Smith, L. B. (1994). *A dynamic systems approach to the development of cognition and action.* MIT Press.

Thiyagalingam, S., Kulinski, A. E., Thorsteinsdottir, B., Shindelar, K. L., & Takahashi, P. Y. (2021). Dysphagia in older adults. *Mayo Clinic Proceedings, 96*(2), 488–497.

Thomas, D. C., McCabe, P., & Ballard, K. J. (2018). Combined clinician-parent delivery of rapid syllable transition (ReST) treatment for childhood apraxia of speech. *International Journal of Speech-Language Pathology, 20*(7), 683–698.

Thomas, R. E., Alves, J., Vaska Mlis, M. M., & Magalhaes, R. (2017). Therapy and rehabilitation of mild traumatic brain injury/concussion: A systematic review. *Restorative Neurology and Neuroscience, 35*(6), 643–666.

Thompson, C. K., Shapiro, L. P., Kiran, S., & Sobecks, J. (2003). The role of syntactic complexity in treatment of sentence deficits in agrammatic aphasia: The complexity account of treatment efficacy (CATE). *Journal of Speech, Language, and Hearing Research, 46,* 591–608.

Throneburg, R. N., & Yairi, E. (2001). Durational, proportionate, and absolute frequency characteristics of disfluencies: A longitudinal study regarding persistence and recovery. *Journal of Speech, Language, and Hearing Research, 44,* 38–52.

Thurber, J. (1945). *The Thurber carnival.* Samuel French.

Tichenor, S. E., Constantino, C., & Yaruss, J. S. (2022). A point of view about fluency. *Journal of Speech, Language, and Hearing Research, 65*(2), 645–652.

Tiede, G., & Walton, K. M. (2019). Meta-analysis of naturalistic developmental behavioral interventions for young children with autism spectrum disorder. *Autism, 23*(8), 2080–2095.

Tjaden, K., & Wilding, G. (2011). Effects of speaking task on intelligibility in Parkinson's disease. *Clinical Linguistics & Phonetics, 25*(2), 155–168.

Tobey, E. A., Geers, A. E., Brenner, C., Altuna, D., & Gabbert, G. (2003). Factors associated with development of speech production skills in children implanted by age five. *Ear and Hearing, 24,* 36S–45S.

Togher, L., Wiseman-Hakes, C., Douglas, J., Stergiou-Kita, M., Ponsford, J., Teasell, R., . . . Turkstra, L. S. (2014). INCOG recommendations for management of cognition following traumatic brain injury, Part IV: Cognitive communication. *Journal of Head Trauma Rehabilitation, 29*(4), 353–368.

Tomaino, C. M. (2012). Effective music therapy techniques in the treatment of nonfluent aphasia. *Annals of the New York Academy of Sciences, 1252*(1), 312–317.

Tomasello. M. (2003). The key is social cognition. In D. Gentner & S. Goldin-Meadow (Eds.), *Language in mind: Advances in the study of language and thought* (pp. 47–57). Boston Review.

Torgesen, J. K., & Davis, C. (1996). Individual difference variables that predict response to training in phonological awareness. *Journal of Experimental Child Psychology, 63,* 1–21.

Torgesen, J. K., Wagner, R. K., & Rashotte, C. A. (1994). Longitudinal studies of phonological processing and reading. *Journal of Learning Disabilities, 27,* 276–286.

Torppa, R., & Huotilainen, M. (2019). Why and how music can be used to rehabilitate and develop speech and language skills in hearing-impaired children. *Hearing Research, 380,* 108–122.

Torres, J., Drebing, D., & Hamilton, R. (2013). TMS and tDCS in post-stroke aphasia: Integrating novel treatment approaches with mechanisms of plasticity. *Restorative Neurology and Neurosciences, 31*(4), 501–515.

Travis, L. E. (1931). *Speech pathology.* Appleton-Century.

Tyler, A. A. (2005). Planning and monitoring intervention programs. In A. G. Kamhi & K. E. Pollock (Eds.), *Phonological disorders in children: Clinical decision making in assessment and intervention* (pp. 123–137). Paul H. Brookes.

U.S. Bureau of the Census. (2015). *Census Bureau reports at least 350 languages spoken in the U.S. homes.* https://www.census.gov/newsroom/archives/2015-pr/cb15-185.html

U.S. Bureau of the Census. (2019). *Language use in the United States: 2019.* https://www.census.gov/library/publications/2022/acs/acs-50.html

U.S. Bureau of the Census. (2021). *What languages do we speak in the United States? ACS B16001.* https://www.census.gov/library/stories/2022/12/languages-we-speak-in-united-states.html

U.S. Department of Education. (2009). *Data and statistics.* https://www2.ed.gov/rschstat/landing.jhtml?src=image

U.S. Department of State. (2021). *Adoption statistics.* https://travel.state.gov/content/travel/en/Intercountry-Adoption/adopt_ref/adoption-statistics-esri.html?wcmmode=disabled

Usler, E. (2022). Communicative fluency and the experience of stuttering: A viewpoint. *Journal of Speech, Language, and Hearing Research, 65*(10), 3827–3834.

Üstün-Yavuz, M. S., Warmington, M., Gerlach, H., & St. Louis, K. O. (2021). Cultural difference in attitudes towards stuttering among British, Arab and Chinese students: Considering home and host cultures. *International Journal of Language & Communication Disorders, 56*(3), 609–619.

Vaiouli, P., & Andreou, G. (2018). Communication and language development of young children with autism: A review of research in music. *Communication Disorders Quarterly, 39*(2), 323–329.

Valian, V. (1992). Categories of first syntax: B*e, be+ing,* and nothingness. In J. M. Meisel (Ed.), *The acquisition of verb placement: Functional categories and V2 phenomena in language development* (pp. 401–422). Kluwer.

Välimaa, T., Kunnari, S., Laukkanen-Nevala, P., Lonka, E., & National Clinical Research Team. (2018). Early vocabulary development in children with bilateral cochlear implants. *International Journal of Language and Communication Disorders, 53*(1), 3–15.

Van der Kleij, F. M., Feskens, R. C., & Eggen, T. J. (2015). Effects of feedback in a computer-based learning environment on students' learning outcomes: A meta-analysis. *Review of Educational Research, 85*(4), 475–511.

Vanderploeg, R. D., Belanger, H. G., & Curtiss, G. (2009). Mild traumatic brain injury and posttraumatic stress disorder and their associations with health symptoms. *Archives of Physical Medicine and Rehabilitation, 90*(7), 1084–1093.

van de Wetering-van Dongen, V. A., Kalf, J. G., van der Wees, P. J., Bloem, B. R., & Nijkrake, M. J. (2020). The effects of respiratory training in Parkinson's disease: A systematic review. *Journal of Parkinson's Disease, 10*(4), 1315–1333.

Van Gelder, T. (2015). Using argument mapping to improve critical thinking skills. In M. Davies & R. Barnett (Eds.), *The Palgrave handbook of critical thinking in higher education* (pp. 183–192). Palgrave Macmillan.

Van Heugten, C. M., Dekker, J., Deelman, B. G., Stehmann-Saris, J. C., & Kinebanian, A. (2000). Rehabilitation of stroke patients with apraxia: The role of additional cognitive and motor impairments. *Disability and Rehabilitation, 22,* 547–554.

Van Riper, C. (1973). *The treatment of stuttering.* Prentice Hall.

Van Riper, C. (1978). *Speech correction: Principles and methods* (6th ed.). Prentice Hall.

Van Riper, C. (1982). *The nature of stuttering* (2nd ed.). Prentice Hall.

Van Sickle, A. (2016). Evidence-based intervention for individuals with acquired apraxia of speech. *EBP Briefs, 11*(2), 1–9.

Van Stan, J. H., Mehta, D. D., Petit, R. J., Sternad, D., Muise, J., Burns, J. A., & Hillman, R. E. (2017). Integration of motor learning principles into real-time ambulatory voice biofeedback and example implementation via a clinical case study with vocal fold nodules. *American Journal of Speech-Language Pathology, 26*(1), 1–10.

Van Stan, J. H., Roy, N., Awan, S., Stemple, J., & Hillman, R. E. (2015). A taxonomy of voice therapy. *American Journal of Speech-Language Pathology, 24*(2), 101–125.

Vasic, N., & Wijnen, F. (2005). Stuttering as a monitoring deficit. In R. J. Hartsuiker, R. Bastiaanse, A. Postma, & F. Wijnen (Eds.), *Phonological encoding and monitoring in normal and pathological speech* (p. 226). Psychology Press.

Velikonja, D., Tate, R., Ponsford, J., McIntyre, A., Janzen, J., & Bayley, M. (2014). INCOG recommendations for management of cognition following traumatic brain injury, Part V: Memory. *Journal of Head Trauma Rehabilitation, 29*(4), 369–386.

Verdolini Abbott, K. (2008). *Lessac-Madsen resonant voice therapy: Clinician manual.* Plural Publishing.

Vicente, M., Calandruccio, L., Miller, M. K., Browning, J. M., Oleson, J., & Leibold, L. J. (2019). Language proficiency and dominance considerations when working with Spanish–English bilingual adults. *American Journal of Audiology, 28*(3), 724–729.

Victorino, K. R., & Hinkle, M. S. (2018). The development of a self-efficacy measurement tool for counseling in speech-language pathology. *American Journal of Speech-Language Pathology, 28*(1), 108–120.

Vygotsky, L. S. (1962). *Thought and language.* MIT Press.

Vygotsky, L. S. (1978). Interaction between learning and development. In L. S. Vygotsky (Ed.), *Mind in society* (pp. 79–91). Harvard University Press.

Wagner, R. K., & Torgesen, J. K. (1987). The nature of phonological processing and its causal role in the acquisition of reading skills. *Psychological Bulletin, 101,* 192–212.

Wagner, R. K., Torgesen, J. K., & Rashotte, C. A. (1994). Development of reading-related phonological processing abilities: New evidence of bidirectional causality from a latent variable longitudinal study. *Developmental Psychology, 30*, 73–87.

Wall, M., & Myers, F. (1995). *Clinical management of childhood stuttering*. Pro-Ed.

Wallace, S. E., Farquharson, K., Berdik, M., Foote, L. T., Manspeaker, S. A., & Hankemeier, D. A. (2022). Speech-language pathologists' perspectives of interprofessional collaboration. *Journal of Interprofessional Care, 36*(6), 801–809.

Walker, D., Sepulveda, S. J., Hoff, E., Rowe, M. L., Schwartz, I. S., Dale, P. S., . . . Bigelow, K. M. (2020). Language intervention research in early childhood care and education: A systematic survey of the literature. *Early Childhood Research Quarterly, 50*(Part 1), 68–85.

Walsh, B., Usler, E., Bostian, A., Mohan, R., Gerwin, K. L., Brown, B., . . . Smith, A. (2018). What are predictors for persistence in childhood stuttering? *Seminars in Speech and Language, 39*(4), 299–312.

Walton, C., Conway, E., Blackshaw, H., & Carding, P. (2017). Unilateral vocal fold paralysis: A systematic review of speech-language pathology management. *Journal of Voice, 31*(4), 509–e7.

Wambaugh, J. L. (2021). An expanding apraxia of speech (AOS) treatment evidence base: An update of recent developments. *Aphasiology, 35*(4), 442–461.

Wambaugh, J. L., Duffy, J. R., McNeil, M. R., Robin, D. A., & Rogers, M. A. (2006). Treatment guidelines for acquired apraxia of speech: Treatment descriptions and recommendations. *Journal of Medical Speech Language Pathology, 14*, xxxv–lxvii.

Wambaugh, J. L., Kallhoff, L., & Nessler, C. (2021). Sound production treatment for acquired apraxia of speech: An examination of dosage in relation to probe performance. *American Journal of Speech-Language Pathology, 30*(1S), 425–440.

Wambuagh, J. L., & Martinez, A. L. (2000). Effects of modified response elaboration training with apraxic and aphasic speakers. *Aphasiology, 14*(5–6), 603–617.

Wambaugh, J. L., Nessler, C., & Wright, S. (2013). Modified response elaboration training: Application to procedural discourse. *American Journal of Speech Language Pathology, 22*, S409–S425.

Wambaugh, J. L., Nessler, C., Wright, S., Mauszycki, S. C., DeLong, C., Berggren, K., & Bailey, D. J. (2017). Effects of blocked and random practice schedule on outcomes of sound production treatment for acquired apraxia of speech: Results of a group investigation. *Journal of Speech, Language, and Hearing Research, 60*(6s), 1739–1751.

Wambaugh, J. L., Wright, S., Boss, E., Mauszycki, S. C., DeLong, C., Hula, W., & Doyle, P. J. (2018). Effects of treatment intensity on outcomes in acquired apraxia of speech. *American Journal of Speech-Language Pathology, 27*(1s), 306–322.

Wambaugh, J. L., Wright, S., Nessler, C., Mauszycki, S. C., Bunker, L., Boss, E., . . . Doyle, P. J. (2020). Further study of the effects of treatment intensity on outcomes of sound production treatment for acquired apraxia of speech: Does dose frequency matter? *American Journal of Speech-Language Pathology, 29*(1), 263–285.

Wampold, B. E. (2015). How important are the common factors in psychotherapy? An update. *World Psychiatry, 14*(3), 270–277.

Wan, C., Wu, L., Wu, H., Wang, S., & Wan, M. (2012). Assessment of a method for the automatic on/off control of an electrolarynx via lip deformation. *Journal of Voice, 26*(5), 674e21–30.

Wang, G., Ge, L., Zheng, Q., Huang, P., & Xiang, J. (2020). Constraint-induced aphasia therapy for patients with aphasia: A systematic review. *International Journal of Nursing Sciences, 7*(3), 349–358.

Wang, J., Pines, J., Joanisse, M., & Booth, J. R. (2021). Reciprocal relations between reading skill and the neural basis of phonological awareness in 7-to 9-year-old children. *NeuroImage, 236*, 118083.

Ward, D., & Scott, K. (Eds.). (2011). *Cluttering: A handbook of research, intervention, and education*. Psychology Press.

Ward, R., Leitão, S., & Strauss, G. (2014). An evaluation of the effectiveness of PROMPT therapy in improving speech production accuracy in six children with cerebral palsy. *International Journal of Speech Language Pathology, 16*(4) 355–371.

Ward, R., Reynolds, J. E., Pieterse, B., Elliott, C., Boyd, R., & Miller, L. (2020). Utilisation of coaching practices in early interventions in children at risk of developmental disability/delay: A systematic review. *Disability and Rehabilitation, 42*(20), 2846–2867.

Warren, S. F., Fey, M. E., & Yoder, P. J. (2007). Differential treatment intensity research: A missing link to creating optimally effective communication interventions. *Special Issue: Language and Communication, 13*, 70–77.

Warren, Z., McPheeters, M. L., Sathe, N., Foss-Feig, J. H., Glasser, M. A., & Vander-Weele, J. (2011). A systematic review of early intervention for ASD. *Pediatrics, 127*, 1303–1311.

Washington, J., & Craig, H. (1994). Dialect forms during discourse of poor, urban African-American preschoolers. *Journal of Speech and Hearing Research, 37*, 816–823.

Wasik, B. A., & Iannone-Campbell, C. (2012). Developing vocabulary through purposeful, strategic conversations. *The Reading Teacher, 66*(4), 321–332.

Watkins, K. E., Smith, S. M., Davis, S., & Howell, P. (2008). Structural and functional abnormalities of the motor system in developmental stuttering. *Brain, 131*, 50–59.

Watt, N., Wetherby, A., & Shumway, S. (2006). Prelinguistic predictors of language outcome at 3 years of age. *Journal of Speech, Language, and Hearing Research, 49*, 1224–1237.

Webster, R., Schumacher, S., & Lubker, B. (1970). Changes in stuttering frequency as a function of various intervals of DAF. *Journal of Abnormal Psychology, 75*, 45–49.

Weidner, K., & Lowman, J. (2020). Telepractice for adult speech-language pathology services: A systematic review. *Perspectives of the ASHA Special Interest Groups, 5*(1), 326–338.

Weiner, F. F. (1981). Treatment of phonological disability using the method of meaningful minimal contrast: Two case studies. *Journal of Speech and Hearing Disorders, 46*, 97–100.

Weir-Mayta, P., Green, S., Abbott, S., & Urbina, D. (2020). Incorporating IPE and simulation experiences into graduate speech-language pathology training. *Cogent Medicine, 7*(1), 1847415.

Weismer, S. E., Kaushanskaya, M., Larson, C., Mathée, J., & Bolt, D. (2018). Executive function skills in school-age children with autism spectrum disorder: Association with language abilities. *Journal of Speech, Language, and Hearing Research, 61*(11), 2641–2658.

Wertz, R. T., Collins, M. J., Weiss, D. G., Kurtzke, J. F., Friden, T., Brookshire, R. H., . . . Resurreccion, E. (1981). Veteran's Administration cooperative study on aphasia: A comparison of individual and group treatment. *Journal of Speech and Hearing Research, 24*, 580–594.

Wertz, R. T., LaPointe, L. L., & Rosenbek, J. C. (1991). *Apraxia of speech in adults: The disorder and its management.* Singular Publishing.

Wertz, R. T., Weiss, D. G., Aten, J. L., Brookshire, R. H., Garcia-Bunuel, L., Holland, A. L., . . . Goodman, R. (1986). Comparison of clinic, home, and deferred language treatment for aphasia: A Veteran's Administration cooperative study. *Archives of Neurology, 43*, 653–658.

Westby, C. (2019). A Multidimensional Approach to Stuttering. *Word of Mouth, 30*(4), 7–10

Westby, C. E. (2012). Assessing and remediating text comprehension problems. In A. G. Kamhi & H. W. Catts (Eds.), *Language and reading disabilities* (3rd ed., pp. 154–223). Pearson.

Westerveld, M. F., & Paynter, J. (2021). Introduction to the forum: Literacy in autism—Across the spectrum. *Language, Speech, and Hearing Services in Schools, 52*(1), 149–152.

Westerveld, M. F., Paynter, J., Trembath, D., Webster, A. A., Hodge, A. M., & Roberts, J. (2017). The emergent literacy skills of preschool children with autism spectrum disorder. *Journal of Autism and Developmental Disorders, 47*(2), 424–438.

Weston, A., & Bain, B. (2003, November 20). *Current vs. evidence-based practice in phonological intervention: A dilemma* [Poster session presentation]. Annual Convention of the American Speech-Language Hearing Association, Chicago, IL.

Wetherby, A., Cain, D., Yonclas, D., & Walker, V. (1988). Analysis of intentional communication of normal children from the prelinguistic to the multi-word stage. *Journal of Speech and Hearing Research, 31*, 240–252.

Wetherby, A. M., & Prizant, B. M. (2000). *Autism spectrum disorders: A transactional developmental perspective.* Paul H. Brookes.

Whitehurst, G. J., Arnold, D. S., Epstein, J. N., & Angell, A. L. (1994). A picture book reading intervention in day care and home for children from low-income families. *Developmental Psychology, 30*(5), 679–689.

Whitehurst, G. J., & Lonigan, C. J. (1998). Child development and emergent literacy. *Child Development, 69*, 848–872.

Whyte, J., Ponsford, J., Watanabe, T., & Hart, T. (2010). Traumatic brain injury. In W. R. Frontera, J. D. Delisa, B. M. Gans, N. A. Walsh, & L. Robinson (Eds.), *Delisa's physical medicine and rehabilitation: Principles and practice* (5th ed., pp. 575–623). Wolters Kluwer, Lippincott Williams & Wilkins.

Wilcox, M. J., & Woods, J. (2011). Participation as a basis for developing early intervention outcomes. *Language, Speech, and Hearing Services in Schools, 42*(3), 365–378.

Will, M. N., Currans, K., Smith, J., Weber, S., Duncan, A., Burton, J., . . . Anixt, J. (2018). Evidenced-based interventions for children with autism spectrum disorder. *Current Problems in Pediatric and Adolescent Health Care, 48*(10), 234–249.

Williams, A. L. (2002). Epilogue: Perspectives in the assessment of children's speech. *American Journal of Speech-Language Pathology, 11*, 259–263.

Williams, A. L., McLeod, S., & McCauley, R. J. (Eds.). (2010). *Interventions for speech sound disorders in children.* Paul H. Brookes.

Williams, R., & Wolfram, W. (1977). *Social dialects: Differences vs. disorders.* American Speech-Language-Hearing Association.

Wilson, S. M., & Schneck, S. M. (2020). Neuroplasticity in post-stroke aphasia: A systematic review and meta-analysis of functional imaging studies of reorganization of language processing. *Neurobiology of Language, 2*(1), 22–82.

Wingate, M. E. (1964). Recovery from stuttering. *Journal of Speech and Hearing Disorders, 29*, 312–321.

Wingate, M. E. (1976). *Stuttering: Theory and treatment.* Irvington.

Wiseman-Hakes, C., Ryu, H., Lightfoot, D., Kukreja, G., Colantonio, A., & Matheson, F. I. (2020). Examining the efficacy of communication partner training for improving communication interactions and outcomes for individuals with traumatic brain injury:

A systematic review. *Archives of Rehabilitation Research and Clinical Translation, 2*(1), 100036.

Wittke, K., & Spaulding, T. J. (2018). Which preschool children with specific language impairment receive language intervention? *Language, Speech, and Hearing Services in Schools, 49,* 59–71.

Witwer, A. N., & Lecavalier, L. (2008). Examining the validity of autism spectrum disorder subtypes. *Journal of Autism Developmental Disorders, 38,* 1611–1624.

Wolf, M. (1984). Naming, reading, and the dyslexias: A longitudinal overview. *Annals of Dyslexia, 34,* 87–136.

Wolf, M. (1991). Naming speed and reading: The contribution of the cognitive neurosciences. *Reading Research Quarterly, 26,* 123–141.

Wolstencroft, J., Robinson, L., Srinivasan, R., Kerry, E., Mandy, W., & Skuse, D. (2018). A systematic review of group social skills interventions, and meta-analysis of outcomes, for children with high functioning ASD. *Journal of Autism and Developmental Disorders, 48*(7), 2293–2307.

Wong, B. Y. L. (2000). Writing strategies instruction for expository essay writing for adolescents with and without learning disabilities. *Topics in Language Disorders, 20,* 29–44.

Woods, J. J., & Brown, J. A. (2011). Family capacity building and child outcomes to support social development in young children with ASD. *Topics in Language Disorders, 31,* 235–246.

World Health Organization. (2001). *ICF: International classification of functioning, disability, and health report.* http://www.who.int/classifications/icf/en/

World Professional Association for Transgender Health. (2016). [International organization devoted to evidence-based care, advocacy, and research in transgender health.]. https://www.wpath.org

Worrall, L., Sherratt, S., Rogers, P., Howe, T., Hersh, D., Ferguson, A., & Davidson, B. (2011). What people with aphasia want: Their goals according to the ICF. *Aphasiology, 25*(3), 309–322.

Woynaroski, T., Yoder, P. J., Fey, M. E., & Warren, S. F. (2014). A transactional model of spoken vocabulary variation in toddlers with intellectual disabilities. *Journal of Speech, Language, and Hearing Research, 57*(5), 1754–1763. https://doi.org/10.1044/2014_JSLHR-L-13-0252

Wren, Y., Harding, S., Goldbart, J., & Roulstone, S. (2018). A systematic review and classification of interventions for speech-sound disorder in preschool children. *International Journal of Language & Communication Disorders, 53*(3), 446–467.

Yairi, E., & Ambrose, N. G. (1999). Early childhood stuttering I: Persistency and recovery rates. *Journal of Speech, Language, and Hearing Research, 42,* 1097–1112.

Yairi, E., & Ambrose, N. G. (2001). Longitudinal studies of childhood stuttering: Evaluation of critiques. *Journal of Speech, Language, and Hearing Research, 44,* 867–872.

Yairi, E., & Ambrose, N. (2013). Epidemiology of stuttering: 21st century advances. *Journal of Fluency Disorders, 38,* 66–87.

Yairi, E., & Seery, C. (2021). *Stuttering: Foundations and clinical applications* (3rd ed.). Plural Publishing.

Yalom, I. (1980). *Existential psychotherapy.* Basic Books.

Yamaji, C., & Maeshima, S. (2021). Spontaneous recovery and intervention in aphasia. In D. C. Jianu & D. F. Mureşanu (Eds.), *Aphasia compendium* (pp. 81–89). Intech Open.

Yang, S. N. (2017). Current evidence for post stroke aphasia treatment. *Brain Neurorehabilitation, 10*(2), e15.

Yaruss, J. S. (1998). Describing the consequences of disorders: Stuttering and the International Classification of Impairments, Disabilities, and Handicaps. *Journal of Speech, Language, and Hearing Research, 49,* 249–257.

Yaruss, S. (2010). Assessing quality of life in stuttering treatment outcomes research. *Journal of Fluency Disorders, 35,* 190–202.

Yavas, M., & Lamprecht, R. (1988). Processes and intelligibility in disordered phonology. *Clinical Linguistics and Phonetics, 2,* 329–345.

Yawn, R. J., O'Connell, B. P., Dwyer, R. T., Sunderhaus, L. W., Reynolds, S., Haynes, D. S., & Gifford, R. H. (2018). Bilateral cochlear implantation versus bimodal hearing in patients with functional residual hearing: A within-subjects comparison of audiologic performance and quality of life. *Otology and Neurotology, 39*(4), 422–427.

Yilmaz-Na, E., & Sönmez, E. (2023). Having qualified arguments: Promoting Pre-service teachers' critical thinking through deliberate computer-assisted argument mapping practices. *Thinking Skills and Creativity, 47,* 101216. https://doi.org/10.1016/j.tsc.2022.101216

Yirmiya, N., & Charman, T. (2010). The prodome of autism: Early behavioral and biological signs, regression, periand post-natal development and genetics. *Journal of Child Psychology and Psychiatry, 51*(4), 432–458.

Yiu, E. M. L., Lo, M. C., & Barrett, E. A. (2017). A systematic review of resonant voice therapy. *International Journal of Speech-Language Pathology, 19*(1), 17–29.

Ylvisaker, M., Szekeres, S. F., & Feeney, T. J. (2008). Communication disorders associated with traumatic brain injury. In R. Chapey (Ed.), *Language intervention strategies in adult aphasia* (5th ed., pp. 879–962). Lippincott, Williams, & Wilkins.

Ylvisaker, M., Turkstra, L., Coelho, C., Yorkston, K., Kennedy, M., Sohlberg, M., & Avery, J. (2007).

Behavioural interventions for children and adults with behaviour disorders after TBI: A systematic review of the evidence. *Brain Injury, 21*(8), 769–805.

Yoder, P., Fey, M. E., & Warren, S. F. (2012). Studying the impact of intensity is important but complicated. *International Journal of Speech-Language Pathology, 14*(5), 410–413.

Yopp, R. H., & Yopp, H. K. (2012). Young childrens' limited and narrow exposure to informational text. *The Reading Teacher, 65*(7), 480–490.

Yorkston, K. M. (1996). Treatment efficacy: Dysarthria. *Journal of Speech and Hearing Research, 39*, S46–S57.

Yorkston, K. M., Beukelman, D. R., & Bell, K. R. (1988). *Clinical management of dysarthric speakers.* Little, Brown.

Yorkston, K. M., Miller, R. M., & Strand, E. A. (2013). *Management of speech and swallowing in degenerative diseases* (3rd ed.). Pro-Ed.

Youmans, G., Holland, A., Muñoz, M., & Bourgeois, M. (2005). Script training and automaticity in two individuals with aphasia. *Aphasiology, 19*(3–5), 435–450.

Youmans, G., Youmans, S. R., & Hancock, A. B. (2011). Script training treatment for adults with apraxia of speech. *American Journal of Speech-Language Pathology, 20*(1), 23–37.

Yuan, S. N. V., & Ip, H. H. S. (2018). Using virtual reality to train emotional and social skills in children with autism spectrum disorder. *London Journal of Primary Care, 10*(4), 110–112.

Yu, C., Shane, H., Schlosser, R. W., O'Brien, A., Allen, A., Abramson, J., & Flynn, S. (2018). An exploratory study of speech-language pathologists using the Echo Show™ to deliver visual supports. *Advances in Neurodevelopmental Disorders, 2*(3), 286–292.

Zakszeski, B. N., & DuPaul, G. J. (2017). Reinforce, shape, expose, and fade: A review of treatments for selective mutism (2005–2015). *School Mental Health, 9*(1), 1–15.

Zebrowski, P. M. (1994). Stuttering. In J. B. Tomblin, H. L. Morris, & D. C. Spriestersbach (Eds.), *Diagnosis in speech-language pathology* (pp. 215–245). Singular Publishing.

Zebrowski, P. M. (1997). Assisting young children who stutter and their families: Defining the role of the speech-language pathologist. *American Journal of Speech-Language Pathology, 6*(2), 19–28.

Zemlin, W. R. (1998). *Speech and hearing science.* Allyn & Bacon.

Zero to Three. (2012). *National Center for Infants, Toddlers, and Families.* http://www.zerotothree.org

Zhang, J., Yu, J., Bao, Y., Xie, Q., Xu, Y., Zhang, J., & Wang, P. (2017). Constraint-induced aphasia therapy in post-stroke aphasia rehabilitation: A systematic review and meta-analysis of randomized controlled trials. *PLoS ONE, 12*(8), e0183349.

Zheng, C., Lynch, L., & Taylor, N. (2016). Effect of computer therapy in aphasia: A systematic review. *Aphasiology, 30*(2–3), 211–244.

Index

B

Babbling, **163**
Baselines, pretreatment, 6
Basic Interpersonal Communication Skills (BICS), 375
Behavior modification, 17–22
Behavioral model of learning, 16
Behavioral objectives, 10, 12, **14**
BICS (Basic Interpersonal Communication Skills), 375
Bilingual, defined, 367
Biofeedback mechanism, 264
Branching, 10
Broader ASD phenotype (BAP), 200
Broca's aphasia, **227, 242**
Broca's area, 235, 276
Brown's 14 grammatical morphemes, **134–135**
Bucco-facial VAT, **237**
Bulbar palsy, **262**

C

Cajun English, 367
CALPS (Cognitive-Academic Language Proficiency Skills), 375
CAP (central auditory processing), 120
CAPD (central auditory processing disorder), 120
Carryover/generalization, 11, 110, 118
CBLEs (computer-based learning experiences), 395
CCSS (Common Core State Standards), 161–164
Central auditory processing (CAP), 120
Central auditory processing disorder (CAPD), 120
Central nervous system, 120, 276
Cerebellar disorders, **262**
Cerebrovascular accident (CVA), 42, 223
Chant talk, 328
Chewing, 328
Childhood apraxia of speech (CAS), 104–109. *See also* Apraxia of speech (AOS)
  example profile, **107**
  sample activities, 107-109
  speech production characteristics for, 104
  therapy approaches for, 105, 106, 144, 167
  working with children with,
Children who stutter (CWS), 296, 298, 302. *See also* Stuttering
Chorea, **262**
CILT (constraint-induced language therapy), 233–234
CLD. *See* Cultural and linguistic diversity
Cleft palates, 93–95,
  example profile, 95–98
  sample activities, 96–97
  speech sound errors in children with, 95
  timeline for child with, 93–94
Cleft palates working with children with, 93–95
Client-specific strategy, 8–9

Clinical reports, 45
  formats, 46–54
  philosophy, 45
  proofreading tips for, 54–55
  technical writing style for, 45–46
Clinical skills, of SLPs, 5
Clinician-client relationship, 26–27
Clinicians. *See* Speech-language pathologists (SLPs)
Closed head injury (CHI), 251
Cluster reduction, 76, 88, 112
Cochlear implants (CIs), 100
Code of Ethics (ASHA), 4, 367
Code-switching, 367, 384
Coding, websites for, 395–397
Cognitive biases, knowledge of, 388
Cognitive communication impairments, 251
Cognitive development, stages of, 121
Cognitive-Academic Language Proficiency Skills (CALPS), 375
Collaboration, 33–35
Collaborative models, 33–34
  consultative, 34
  self-contained, 34
  team teaching, 34
Common Core State Standards (CCSS), 161–164
Communicative intentions, **126, 127**
  expressed at single-word level, **127**
  preverbal, **126**
Compare-contrast essay structure, 188–189
Compensatory approaches,
Comprehension, 113, 114, **131, 137, 155**, 220
Computer-based learning experiences (CBLEs), 395
Computer-driven therapy, 166
Condition statements, for behavioral objectives, 13
Conduction aphasia, **225**
Conductive (peripheral) hearing loss, 98
Confidential voice technique, 329
Consequences, 17
Consonant-injection method, 344–345
Consonants
  age of acquisition of English, **79**
  frequency of occurrence in English, **91**
Constraint-induced language therapy (CILT), 233–234
Constructivism, 16–17
Contact ulcers, 324
Conversation initiation, 255–256
Conversion dysphonias, 325
Cooing, **125**
Core vocabulary phonological therapy, 75
Correspondence, professional, 58
Cortex, **225**, 260, 291
Cough suppression techniques, 329
Counseling, 353–354
  checklist, **362**
  client and family emotional reactions, 357